Multiple Sclerosis from Both Sides of the Desk

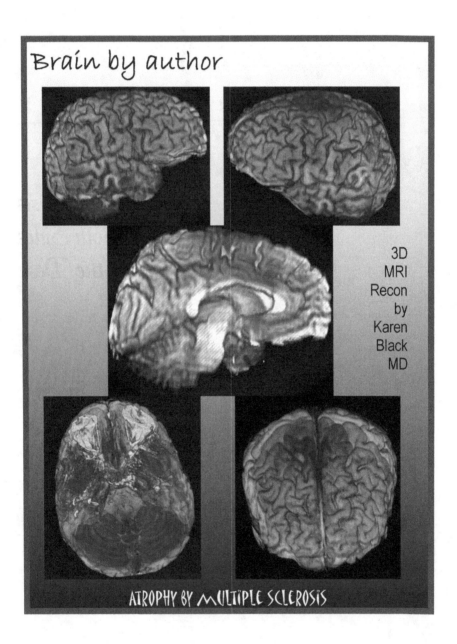

Brain by author

3D
MRI
Recon
by
Karen
Black
MD

ATROPHY BY MULTIPLE SCLEROSIS

Multiple Sclerosis from Both Sides of the Desk

Two Views of MS through One Set of Eyes

VINCENT F. MACALUSO, MD

⊙iUniverse®

MULTIPLE SCLEROSIS FROM BOTH SIDES OF THE DESK
TWO VIEWS OF MS THROUGH ONE SET OF EYES

The information, ideas, and suggestions in this book are not intended as a substitute for professional medical advice. Before following any suggestions contained in this book, you should consult your personal physician. Neither the author nor the publisher shall be liable or responsible for any loss or damage allegedly arising as a consequence of your use or application of any information or suggestions in this book.

iUniverse books may be ordered through booksellers or by contacting:

iUniverse
1663 Liberty Drive
Bloomington, IN 47403
www.iuniverse.com
1-800-Authors (1-800-288-4677)

Because of the dynamic nature of the Internet, any web addresses or links contained in this book may have changed since publication and may no longer be valid. The views expressed in this work are solely those of the author and do not necessarily reflect the views of the publisher, and the publisher hereby disclaims any responsibility for them.

Any people depicted in stock imagery provided by Thinkstock are models, and such images are being used for illustrative purposes only. Certain stock imagery © Thinkstock.

ISBN: 978-1-4917-5745-1 (sc)
ISBN: 978-1-4917-5746-8 (hc)
ISBN: 978-1-4917-5747-5 (e)

Library of Congress Control Number: 2015900137

Print information available on the last page.

iUniverse rev. date: 7/08/2015

To my son, Vincent, for helping me to become a better man.

To my daughter, Abigail, for appreciating the
remarks I make under my breath.

And to my wife, Lauren, for being the singularity
of goodness that holds my world together.

Your time is limited, so don't waste it
living someone else's life.

Don't be trapped by dogma, which is
living with the results of other
people's thinking.

Don't let the noise of others'
opinions drown out your own inner
voice.

And most important,
have the courage to follow your
heart and intuition.

They somehow already know what
you truly want to become.

Everything else is secondary.

Steve Jobs
Stanford Commencement Address
2005

Contents

EPILOGUE

Table of Figures

List of Tables

Foreword

From 1981 to 1994, I split my time practicing adult outpatient psychiatry at Georgetown and serving as associate dean for students at the med school. The latter had me overseeing the academic and psychological well-being of the med students.

Products of a rigorous admissions process, the med students were collectively bright, enthusiastic, hardworking, and generous. Individually, they were a wondrous bazaar of personalities, talents, and interests. Academic or disciplinary problems were rare. Problems, if they arose, were generally of a personal or emotional nature. They were a delight to work with.

In the course of time, one young man appeared on the scene, Vincent Macaluso, articulate and witty (no surprise when I found out he was a New Yorker, a graduate of Regis, the scholarship Jesuit prep school), interested in almost everything but specifically in editing the school newspaper. Over time, we became friends. When his diagnosis of multiple sclerosis came, he shared it, and subsequently we shared his adventures navigating the rocks and shoals of the clinical years and neurology residency. He introduced me to Lauren, and they invited me to be the priest at their wedding. The years rolled by. I've marveled at his courage, patience, and perseverance, and I've rejoiced in his progress, personal (great kids!) and professional.

And here is his book, Vince sharing himself in his many roles: physician, scholar, patient, husband, father, friend, comedian, teacher, healer.

A careful reader might note that although Vince lists religion as one of the major influences in his life, his text has no explicit mention of God or church. But the book is one man's story of love received and love shared: parental love, years of patient study utilizing the brain and talents God gave him, meeting challenges and overcoming obstacles, keeping a happy, joyful spirit, and building a generous, competent, compassionate care for others. Jesuit education aims to educate "men and women for others"—students who develop the gifts God gives them and who, in gratitude, spend them generously in the service of others. Love and gratitude are shown not just in words but in actions: Vince's life and Vince's book show them both.

Our Italian friends would term this book an *abbondanza*, a grand feast of scientific knowledge and practical wisdom, a buffet cavalcade of experiences and emotions. Fasten your seat belt: sample, savor, chew, learn, laugh, enjoy, and give thanks.

Jon J. O'Brien, SJ, DO
Georgetown University
Washington, DC 20057

Preface

I have had MS since 1987 but was diagnosed in 1991 between my first and second years of medical school. As I went through med school and residency and became a husband and father, MS always played a part in my life. I knew I wanted to write a book about MS, but I didn't know if I had anything new to contribute to the many books available on the subject. While I had my personal experiences and had thoroughly learned about the disease during my medical training and practice, I still didn't know how to put it all together. If I undertook the project of writing a book about MS, I wanted it to have a unique purpose. There are some tremendous medical texts out there handling what many doctors believe to be the main troubles affecting those of us with MS. I respect and laud them for their thorough work. Likewise, there are some excellent stories about how individuals have dealt with the challenges that MS has presented to them. I cheer all people who are proactive in dealing with the significant challenges that life offers. I wanted my literary contribution in the MS world to be a synthesis of my medical and MS lives. Fortunately, I had some experiences that helped me to define my task.

In 2007, I was asked to speak at the national sales meeting for Biogen Idec—the company that makes the drug that I currently use to treat my multiple sclerosis. I made an impression at the meeting not only with the words I said but also in the way I said them. For the most part, people think that we physicians are boring people. So do I. When we get up in front of a group of people and start talking, we can forget that our audiences have not spent the majority of their lives developing intimate relationships with textbooks. Much of a doctor's life is a solitary one. Our lives are spent learning from books, cadavers, slides, a few teachers, each other, and eventually from patients. We are, quite often, socially challenged.

I sat through thousands of hours of medical lectures where an *expert* doctor would take an interesting topic and then surreptitiously suck the life out of both the topic and the students. The lecturer would do this by using a combination of a monotone voice, an unintelligible accent, confusing slides, and absolutely no sign of any organizational scheme that we could use to remember the material. On a number of occasions, I seriously thought about stabbing myself in the eye with a pencil so I could have some sort of meaningful, sensate experience before I died from boredom. It was then that I swore to myself that if I ever got the chance to teach anybody about anything, I would make sure that I would

1. remain a cognizant, feeling human;
2. simplify any and all concepts to the simplest level; and
3. maintain the audience's interest.

Because of this promise and my love of good stand-up comedy, I always infuse my shows with plenty of humor, pictures, data, movies, some sarcasm, and plenty of eye contact. My shows are educational, funny, and inspirational. This, I feel, is the essence of teaching.

At the sales meeting, the woman running the program asked how I would like to be introduced. I told her that I would like to show a rap video that my family and I had made. (Okay. I made my family make a rap video. It was the end of a long weekend where we had been trapped indoors because of bad weather. Tensions were running high. My wife and I were considering whether or not we still really needed *both* of the kids. So I set up the video camera and hung up a sheet as a backdrop, and we each took turns singing the words to a rap that I had made up about multiple sclerosis. After I shot all the footage, I set the whole thing to a beat and edited it on my Mac.) It was a nice thirty-second piece that I hoped would get the crowd going. After the video was played, I had the audio guys blast "Back in Black" by AC/DC. Everyone was on their feet cheering. I jogged from the back of the room and leapt onto the stage. I felt like a rock star. I did some stand-up, and then I told everyone what it's like being a doctor who also had MS. I killed![1] The following week, requests started pouring in for me to give talks at locations all over the country about MS—both from a medical point of view and from a patient's point of view. Soon after the show, my schedule was full. I had forty-five gigs booked in thirty-five different cities. I was on tour.

The thing about being on tour is that it takes a lot of time and energy. Given the fact that I was a husband, a father of two, a doctor and had a major neurological disease, I was already pushing the limits. Now I had committed to a thirty-five-city tour, and I realized that I had a lot on my plate. Family has always been my top priority (followed closely by nachos and watching my favorite stand-up comedians), so I wanted to make sure that I did not spend any more time away from home than necessary. I managed to schedule all my presentations to be Friday night/Saturday morning combinations so that I could say good-bye to the wife and kids on Friday morning, leave my home Friday at midday, do the shows, and be on my way back home within twenty-two to twenty-eight hours after having left so I could kiss the kids good night on Saturday and my wife and I could settle in for our weekly game of canasta.[2]

During the tour, I had the chance to meet many people. The doctors I met across the country were great. They were mostly neurologists who were interested in trying to find out how they could improve their MS patients' care. One thing I learned was that while many of the physicians in certain regions of the country wanted to use a certain therapy for their patients with MS, their decision-making process was sometimes influenced by what the local insurance monopoly dictated. Some doctors I met wanted to give therapy Q, but the insurance company put requirements that the patient be tried on drugs X, Y, and Z first before they would approve drug Q, even though there was no scientific data backing up this policy. In another location, the insurance company said that the doctor's office could administer a medication but the doctor had to buy the drug from the insurance company's pharmacy. The thing was that the insurance company's pharmacy had jacked up the price so much that the doctor would wind up losing money on the project after filing for reimbursement from the insurance company. It was disturbing.

I also met some physicians who didn't really enjoy the time they spent with their MS patients. Some said that MS patients took too much time in their schedule. Others complained that their MSers would bring in a stack of papers that had all sorts of misinformation downloaded from the Internet. They said that they couldn't understand what we MSers meant when we said, "It feels like my whole back is on fire all the time" or "I slept for sixteen hours yesterday, and I still don't have enough energy to get off the couch." Who can blame them? In medical school and residency, we learn about things that can be measured, touched, heard, seen, and smelled. These, for the most part, are tangible things. The intangible things, like sensations that are outside of the norm (called paresthesias), are hard to teach and impossible to learn if the student doesn't accept the fact that some things don't follow the logic of medical reasoning. Comprehension of something that isn't tangible and trying to fit it into the dogma of medical knowledge is an art. As in any art, there are some people who can create it, there are some who can appreciate it, and there are some who just don't get it. From my experiences working with colleagues in medicine, I've seen two groups of doctors who can understand what it feels like to have MS. The first is the group of doctors who have multiple sclerosis and feel comfortable sharing this side of their lives with their patients. We have an inside line on what the disease feels like and what issues need to be dealt with. Then there's a collection of doctors who have been blessed with a combination of open-mindedness, intelligence, and caring. Even though they don't have the disease, these special people can appreciate the feelings that we MSers have as observers and use their medical and social talents to help us out.

Then, of course, there are doctors who just don't get us. Sometimes they look at us as roadblocks on their otherwise concrete medical highway. For these otherwise fine physicians, I would like to offer this. The clinical care of MS patients is challenging both intellectually and emotionally. To serve these patients well, we need to recognize and accept something:

> *What we know about how an MSer feels is greatly*
> *outweighed by what we do not know.*

If this is not your cup of tea, that's cool. Have coffee instead, and leave MS for the docs who thrive on it.

Aside from the medical aspect of the tour, the people that I met and the places that I visited were amazing. Many people (patients, caregivers, doctors, hotel employees, taxi drivers) had interesting questions, ideas, and stories. During my shows, I have a question-and-answer session at the end. I leave note cards on the attendees' tables before the show. I tell them that if they have a question during the show, they can either raise their hand or, if they do not feel comfortable speaking in front of other people, write it down on the note card. After the show was over, I would collect the cards and answer their questions as best I could. At the same time, I would listen to the patients and caregivers who offered their own experiences in dealing with MS issues in their lives. The questions were always interesting. I always made sure to let everyone know that all questions are great. People would sometimes say, "But I don't want to sound stupid." I would tell them that the thing to remember is that there is no such thing as a stupid question. Then I would add that there actually is one stupid question:

> *The only stupid question is the one that goes unasked.*

The greatness of a question comes not only from the question itself but also from how much thinking the question can engender. If you ask a question that no one has asked before, you've found a key to a whole new world of discovery. By asking a question, a person is stimulating others to think. And even if a question might sound simple to one person, there are ten other people who are glad that someone asked it.

It was also enlightening to fly into and out of so many different cities. Some were big (Chicago and Atlanta). Some were small (Lincoln, Nebraska, and Camp Hill, Pennsylvania). Some audiences were louder (Brooklyn, New York) than others (Waltham, Massachusetts). But one thing was a constant. The MSers I met around the country, no matter how different they looked or moved or sounded, shared a common denominator. They were not going to let multiple sclerosis stop them from doing what they wanted to do. And the supporting cast around us MSers (husbands, wives, parents, kids, cousins, neighbors, pets) are a stalwart group who put up with tremendous challenges and should be lauded right along with the folks who have been affected by our *challenging* disease.

By the end of the tour, I felt that I had started to see more clearly what the purpose of my contribution to literary medical science was. My calling was to speak from both sides of the MS world. I have arranged most of this book as a series of "chapter-couplets." The first half of each couplet teaches about a topic from a medical science point of view ("... from a Neurological Point of View"). The content is factual, and valid medical references are cited. The second half of each couplet is written as prose and reflects my experiences, both as an MSer and as a physician ("... from the Other Side of the Desk"). Through this dualistic presentation of the world of MS in my life, I hope to help patients, caregivers, nurses, doctors, and whoever else is interested understand that they cannot understand what the world is like in the mind of another individual. Hopefully, if this concept is appreciated, it will help to fortify the gains that have been made to slow down our disease and then help to launch a unified onslaught of creative ideas that initiates the termination sequence of the medical condition called multiple sclerosis.

VFM

---

[1] In medical school, they advised us not to use this phrase on a regular basis.

[2] Sometimes, if the kids went to bed early, we would play canasta two or three times.

Acknowledgments

In terms of the people who helped me to get this far in life, I want to thank:

My Family
Mom and Dad, Liz, Jenny, Amy, Aunt Ann, Grandma and Grandpa, Uncle Joe, the Sbrollinis, Tom and all the Cartys, Matt and all the Gilmores, Fr. Jon J. O'Brien SJ DO, my godfather Joe and his family and last, but far from least, Carla, Joey, and Sarina Dinardo.

My Friends
Scott and Susan Ehrler, Emil and Vivica Albanese, Paul and Gina Vambutas, Rich and Johnny Lynch, the Lynches, Dr. Steve Machnicki, Rebecca Sparrow, Dr.and Mrs. Peter and Deb Harvey, Ray Paprocky, Kathleen Pierce and the other great ABMs, Fred and Cory, Dr. Santo Terranova, Victor Schwartz, the Muccinis, the Josephs, Mr. and Mrs. Peter and Carmen Colletta, Mrs. Ann Marie Petrucci and Ms. Irene Constantino, all my friends from Dougalston, Mr. Ted Tierney, Fr. Emilio, and my executive assistants, Mercedes Cuascut, Ayja Cuascut, and Donna Fabbricante.

My Teachers
Mrs. Arcidiocono, Mr. Amara, Mrs. McKenzie, Mr. Young, Mme. Zezulin, Mr. Blatchford, Mr. Vose, Mr. Driscoll, Mr. Weimann, Mr. Sabatelli, Fr. Schwizter, Mr. Dimichele, Dr. Vaiganos, Mr. Walsh, Mr. and Mrs. Hannon, Mr. Barrett, Fr. Callahan, Fr. Kelly, Fr. DiGiacomo, Dr. Herbert J. Manz, Dr. Wesley Norman, Drs. John and Nancy Richert, Dr. Carlo Tornatore, Dr. Stan Cohan, Dr. Robert Laureno, Dr. Mike Sirdofsky, Dr. Marshall Balish, Shari from radiology and Graham from housekeeping at the Washington DC VA, Dr. Mitch Wallin, Dr. Roy Goodman, Dr. Mitch Freedman, Dr. Rick Munschauer, Dr. Steve Kulick, Dr. Frank Loh, Dr. Steve Schwartzberg, Dr. Tim Vartanian, Dr. Al Sandrock, Dr. David Langer, Dr. Michael Schulder, Dr. David Chalif, Dr. Avi Setton, Dr. Karen Black (along with Frank Scalia and Daniel Adams), and my most important medical teachers, my patients.

First

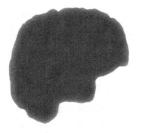

*Each friend represents a
world in us, a world possibly
not born until they arrive,
and it is only by this meeting
that a new world is born.*
—Anais Nin, author
1903–1977

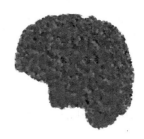

MY HOUSE IS YOUR HOUSE

Welcome. This is my life. My life consists of my family and friends, being a doctor, comedy, multiple sclerosis, teaching, religion, computing, woodworking, writing, jogging, nookie, thinning hair, the Yankees, reading Spenser novels, and thinking about God.

These are all things that are parts of my life. They're things that came into my life, and I treasure all of them because they're what make my life unique. This is Vincent Macaluso's life. I do not live with any of them. They live with me.

It's my house. It is up to me to keep the things that I have control of in balance. I value my family beyond all else in this world. My wife is the axis of my existence. We are blessed with two beautiful children. The four of us work through life together. We are a close family, in a cozy house. This allows us to create a tremendous home.

I love laughing. I love it when I laugh so hard it hurts and I can't catch my breath. Sometimes I get lucky and I laugh so hard that I can't catch my breath, and I start to black out, and I fall down. Then, when I'm lying on the floor, I start to think about how funny it must have looked when I keeled over. For me, that's a win-win-win situation.

I like watching *The Colbert Report* because it makes me think about the things going on in the world around me. Dr. Colbert's character brings up the absurdity of a situation or creates absurdity when there is none just to be a nudge. He goes fast, and you have to look and read and listen and think all at the same time. Stephen Colbert is smart. He challenges us. He has hair that does not move.

On the topic of hair, mine started an exodus several years ago. I didn't worry about it because I realized that I was getting older and it was a natural part of life. But as it grew thinner, I saw some pictures of myself and thought I would look better with hair—at least for a few more years. I started medication to keep my hair, and it had been working pretty well to slow down the loss. Unfortunately, the numbers continue to dwindle despite the medication. The countless many are becoming the cherished few. Well, I did what I could, but if this is my lot, so be it. I know I could get hair transplants done, but my two children are approaching the launch pad for college, and I think the money would be better spent maximizing what's inside their heads instead of maximizing what's on top of mine. I think of the hair loss situation the same way I think about Joe Torre and the Yankees. They had a good time together, but once they no longer benefitted from being together, they parted ways.

Multiple sclerosis entered my life over twenty-seven years ago. At first I didn't know what was happening. It was like some unwanted houseguest had arrived. My life was going on as usual, but suddenly I started to have strange feelings. Tingling here, decreased sensation there. I had trouble concentrating. Learning wasn't as easy as it had always been. This flighty guest came and went with neither rhyme nor reason. At first, I didn't know its name, but after diagnosis, I found out what it really was—an unruly guest. Sometimes with unruly guests, guidelines have to be set down. I had to find out what MS was all about. I had to find out what I could do to keep it in control. I also had to realize that some things I did not have control over. I decided to forget about that part so I could focus on the things that I could control in dealing with this *morbus non grata*. It was a big house I was running. Just because I found a chink in the foundation, I was not going to let the rest of what I had built get torn down.

I found a nice neurologist who specialized in MS.

I learned as much as I could about MS.

I got on a therapy to slow down MS.

I let my neurologist know if something new came up so we could decide what intervention we should make—if any.

I kept my eyes and ears open for new therapies that were coming.

I did not fight MS.

I saw what the situation was, and I did what I could to continue to make my home beautiful.

I asked for help.

I had good people around me who helped me when I asked for help.

I had people around me who helped even when I did not ask for it.

Or know that I needed it.

I was lucky that I had been able to lay such a good foundation for my home so that it was rock solid and ready to withstand storms when they hit.

While MS initially appeared daunting and unwelcomed when it showed up at my door, it turned out to be a crucial guest in my life. It helped me realize that while it is *my* life, it is still just that.

Life.

In life, there are no certainties.

There are joys.

There are marriages.

There are children.

There are diseases.

There are good people.

There are deaths.

There are challenges.

There are jobs.

There are careers.

There are disappointments.

There are successes.

There is laughter.

There are houses.

There is your house.

There is my house.

This book is written from both sides of the desk. The first half of most topics is written by me, Vincent Macaluso, MD, from a neurological point of view. In these sections, I'm writing to teach about the factual things in MS—what the disease is, how to treat it, and so on. The second half of most topics is written by me, Vincent Macaluso, a guy with a wife, two kids, a mortgage, a lawn mower that might or might not turn over after several pulls, and a burning desire to make people laugh. It is in these sections that I get creative. Everything written here is experiential. I write about how it feels to have MS, to take medications, to get a neurological examination, to receive life-changing news. The most important chapter, "The MS ICE," is where doctor and patient meet, put their thoughts together, and try to make a contribution to the worlds of patients, doctors, and anyone who wants to learn about MS.

All right. I'm gonna go exercise for a while, then make some nachos and watch some stand-up comedy and think about poetry and "fire and ice" and the nature of God, and maybe I'll have a beer.

The door to my world is open.

I hope you enjoy it.

Second

WHAT MS IS FROM A NEUROLOGICAL POINT OF VIEW

What we've got here is failure to communicate.
—Captain, Road Prison 36, *Cool Hand Luke*

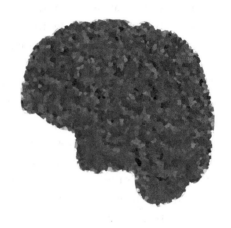

W e will begin our journey in the central nervous system (CNS), which is made of the brain and spinal cord (see figure 1). Of the two, the star is the brain. In fact, it's so special it's sequestered in its own private room—the skull. The fact that the brain is kept separate from the rest of the body makes it even more mysterious. Before CT and MRI imaging came along, the only way to see what it looked like was to cut open its protective case and take a look around. When seen up close, such as during surgery, it doesn't appear to be doing much. The surface glistens and pulses

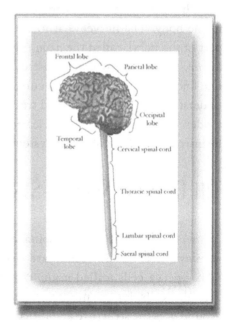

Figure 1. The CNS.
The CNS is composed of the brain and the spinal cord.

slightly with each heartbeat. At first glance, it appears to be similar to other organs, like the liver or kidneys. Upon closer inspection, however, its surface appears convoluted, like a walnut. How come it doesn't appear uniform like the other organs?

Unlike other organs, the brain does not do a fixed number of tasks, repeatedly, for the entire life of a person. It's the organ that has a new job each and every day. It has to be expandable but cannot grow any bigger. It does this by having its many different computer processors, called *neurons*, make new connections based upon the tasks that they're given. It upgrades continuously. Our brains are made of about one hundred billion neurons. They're organized into different functions, placed in different locations, set in a thin, gelatinous matrix, and then stuffed into an irregularly shaped carrying case. This is what gives it a walnut-like appearance.

Extending from the base of the brain is its partner, the spinal cord. It too has some nerves that have special functions, but its major function is to act as a conduit. It's the main highway carrying information from the brain to the body and from the body to the brain. Multiple sclerosis (MS) is a disease that affects the nerves that are in the brain and spinal cord.

The central nervous system (CNS) is what controls almost all the actions in the body. The nerves that make up the CNS send signals out along a part of the nerve called the *axon*. The axon has insulation around it called *myelin*. In MS, the myelin is destroyed by the body's immune system. No one knows exactly why this occurs, but starting in the 1970s, methods for understanding, diagnosing, and treating this disease have made enormous strides. In this chapter, you will learn more about the CNS and you will also be introduced to the immune system and multiple sclerosis.

THE CENTRAL NERVOUS SYSTEM

As mentioned, the brain and spinal cord make up what is called the *central nervous system* (CNS).[3] There are two main cell types that make up the CNS—nerve cells (called *neurons*) and supporting cells (called *glial cells*). The glial cells, for the most part, make the skeleton that the nerves grow around. It is the structure and function of the nerve cells, however, that are the focus of the story. Figure 2 shows what a nerve looks like when you look at it very closely.

In total, there are about one hundred billion cells (nerve and glial cells

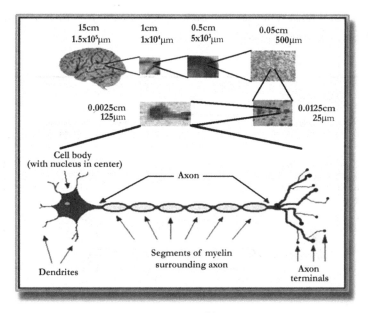

Figure 2. Diagram of the neuron.

combined) in your CNS.[4] Those one hundred billion cells are arranged into many different regions that have many different functions. Most of those different regions make multiple connections to other functional areas of the CNS via pathways (also called *tracts, fasciculi,* or *projections*). For example, some of the pathways go from your eyes to another part of your brain that tells you that you see your best friend coming. Other tracts go from the part of your brain that saw the shape of your best friend to another part of your brain that stored the memory that your best friend still owes you ten dollars. Other pathways contain the nerves that go from your brain all the way down to your hand that lets you put your hand out as you approach your friend. There are other pathways that go to the language center in another part of your brain to say something to your friend. And then there is yet another part of your brain that makes the final decision as to whether you say "Hi. How are you?" and shake your friend's hand or say, "Hey, you owe me ten bucks, and I want my money," and you put your hand out, palm side up, waiting for the ten dollars.

While learning all the different functional areas and discreet pathways that the one hundred billion nerves in your brain and spinal cord make, there is one easy thing to remember. All nerves essentially work the same way. The nerves are set up very much like the computer in your home.[5] Let's say your computer has a fancy picture on it, and you want to send it to someone over the Internet (see figure 3).

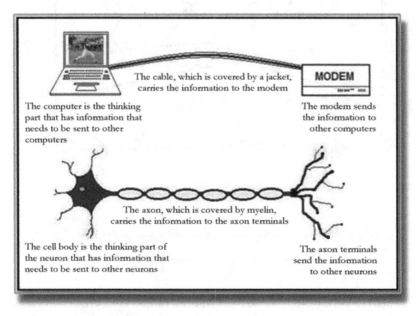

The cable, which is covered by a jacket, carries the information to the modem

MODEM

The computer is the thinking part that has information that needs to be sent to other computers

The modem sends the information to other computers

The axon, which is covered by myelin, carries the information to the axon terminals

The cell body is the thinking part of the neuron that has information that needs to be sent to other neurons

The axon terminals send the information to other neurons

Figure 3. A nerve is like a computer with an external modem.

The computer sends the bits of the digital file along a cable to your modem. Your modem then modulates the picture into bits of information that can be sent over the Internet to your friend's modem (see figure 4). Your friend's modem then demodulates the information into data that her computer can interpret and display as a picture. Each neuron in our brain plays all of these parts. A neuron is 1) a computer, 2) a cable, and 3) a modem. For our purposes, the Internet will be the space between the axon terminal of the first nerve and the dendrites on the cell body of the next nerve. This space is called the *synapse*. The body's "Internet" transmits information from the axon terminal of one nerve to the dendrites on the cell body of the next by using neurotransmitters.[6]

In our analogy, the computer is the thinking part of the nerve, which is called the *cell body*. The dendrites on the cell body are the receivers of information—the "demodulating" half of your modem. The cell body is the central processing unit of the nerve. It integrates the input from the dendrites and then sends its message, through a cable called the *axon*, to the nerve terminal, which then acts like the "modulating" part described above.

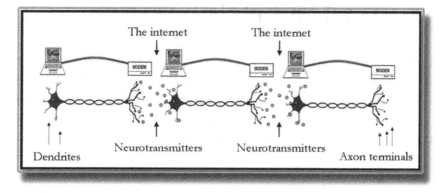

Figure 4. Neurotransmitters are like the Internet.

In multiple sclerosis, the important part of the nerve is the cable coming off the cell body, which is called the *axon*. Like the insulation that surrounds the cable coming off your computer, there is an insulation that surrounds the axon. This insulation is called *myelin*. Myelin is the thing that is under attack in MS. Hold that thought. We'll get back to it after we talk about the immune system.

THE IMMUNE SYSTEM

The other crucial element to know about in MS is the immune system. This is the system in your body that fights off the bugs that try to invade your body. If you cut your finger or someone sneezes on you, bugs (like viruses and bacteria) try to get inside you and take over. The thing that prevents the bug from taking over your body is the immune system.

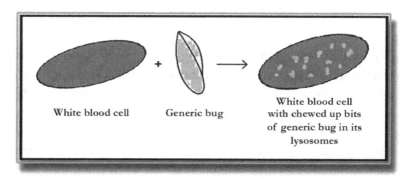

Figure 5. Artist's rendition of how the immune system works.

NOW, LET'S PUT THESE TWO IDEAS TOGETHER

In multiple sclerosis, the body's immune system, for unknown reasons, turns on itself. Instead of just fighting off bugs and other invaders, it starts to attack the myelin that surrounds the axons in the CNS (see figure 6). This is called *demyelination*. When an axon is demyelinated, it can no longer carry the information from the cell body to the axon terminal of the nerve. If the message cannot be transmitted, then whatever function the nerve was in charge of doing (like telling a muscle to contract or helping a person pay attention when reading about neurobiology) cannot be executed! This can cause a lot of trouble for a person with MS (as well as for the people around the person with MS).[7]

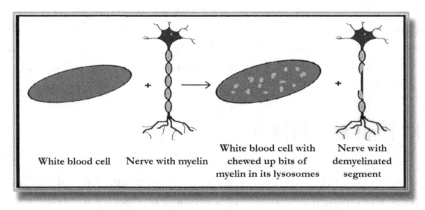

| White blood cell | Nerve with myelin | White blood cell with chewed up bits of myelin in its lysosomes | Nerve with demyelinated segment |

Figure 6. Artist's rendition of what happens when the immune system starts to attack the myelin around the axon of a nerve.

No one knows exactly why a person's immune system decides to turn on itself. There are many ideas about why this happens. It could be that a person is exposed to something in the environment, such as a virus or some other foreign substance, which looks like myelin on a molecular level. Normally, when the immune system sees a virus, it makes antibodies based upon the molecular structure of the virus. By doing this, if and when the antibody sees the same molecular structure again, it will be ready to immediately launch an attack and prevent a full-blown infection.[8] Possibly, in MS, if an invading virus has a molecular structure similar to the molecular structure of myelin, the antibodies that were made for the virus could then start to attack the myelin.

Table 1. Autoimmune diseases and the tissues that they affect.

Disease	Tissue under attack
Multiple sclerosis	Myelin surrounding nerve axons in central nervous system
Insulin dependent diabetes mellitus	Insulin producing (beta) cells in the pancreas
Systemic lupus erythematosus	Various tissues in the body
Sjøgren's disease	Moisture producing glands (like salivary and lacrimal glands)
Sarcoidosis	Various tissues in the body
Rheumatoid arthritis	Synovial membrane that covers joints
Guillain-Barré syndrome	Myelin surrounding nerve axons of peripheral nervous system
Vasculitis	The walls of blood vessels

There is good evidence that our genetic makeup plays a role in having our immune system start attacking tissues within our own body.[9,10] Most MS experts believe that the cause of MS is almost certain to be multifactorial (a combination of genes and something in the environment). In their paper, *Genetics of Multiple Sclerosis: Swimming in an Ocean of Data*, Sergio E. Baranzini and Dorothee Nickles put together the results of the largest genome-wide association study for MS, as of 2011.[11] Their synthesis confirmed the association of twenty-three genes with MS and reported about twenty-one other suspect genes. They also report on the data implicating the *CYP27B1* gene variant as a heritable factor that prevents proper conversion of vitamin D from its inactive 25-hydroxyvitamin D form to its active 1,25 dihydroxyvitamin D form.[12] The paper goes on to describe other statistically valid and reliable data, including the "brother and sister" relationship of MS with other autoimmune diseases like Crohn's disease, diabetes mellitus type I, asthma, psoriasis, celiac disease, rheumatoid arthritis, and Grave's disease. The number of newly discovered genes and gene variants associated with MS increases on a regular basis. At an MS consortium meeting in 2014, it was announced that the number of genes associated with MS was up to 159.

Other potential causes of MS will be discussed again in the chapter dedicated to the immune system.

Conclusion

So there you have the essence of MS. After a nerve is demyelinated, it cannot transmit the message from the cell body, along the axon, to the axon terminal and allow for neurotransmitter release to communicate with the next cell.[13] If it affects a visual pathway, a person might have trouble with vision. If it affects a coordination tract, movements can become clumsy. If it affects a behavior fasciculus, initiative can be impaired or lost.[14] We don't know the exact causes of MS, but we have many clues. The next chapter will discuss more of the specifics about how the immune system causes demyelination. Then, in subsequent chapters, we will discuss how to slow this whole process down.

---

[3] The nerves that come off the spinal cord are part of the peripheral nervous system (PNS). We won't be dealing with them in this book because MS only occurs in the CNS. The PNS version of MS is called Guillain-Barré syndrome (GBS). Feel free to learn more about it on the Internet. The National Institute of Neurological Disorders and Stroke has a great website for it. The address is: http://www.ninds.nih.gov/disorders/gbs/gbs.htm.

[4] *The Scientific American Book of the Brain* (New York: Scientific American, 1999), 3.

[5] For our purposes, we will only talk about computers that are hardwired to the Internet. As of right now, wireless neuronal networks are not available. This is good because the rate plans would be ridiculously expensive. I have basic cable, and I can't understand why my home TV, phone, and Internet bill is over three hundred dollars a month while the bill for my cell phone (which lets me watch TV, talk, and surf) costs eighty-nine dollars per month!

[6] Neurotransmitters are chemicals that neurons release from their axon terminals to communicate with other nerves. Some common neurotransmitters include acetylcholine, epinephrine, norepinephrine, serotonin, glutamate, GABA, and dopamine. Please see the MS ICE chapter for more information about neurotransmitters and receptors.

[7] Don't worry. Keep reading. There is a lot of good stuff coming.

[8] This is the concept behind vaccinations.

[9] J. Link, I. Kockum, A. R. Lorentzen, B. A. Lie, E. G. Celius, H. Westerlind, M. Schaffer et al., Department of Clinical Neuroscience, Karolinska Institutet, Stockholm, Sweden, "Importance of Human Leukocyte Antigen (HLA) Class I and II Alleles on the Risk of Multiple Sclerosis," *PLoS One* 7, no. 5 (2012): e36779. Epub 2012 May 7.

[10] S. E. Baranzini and D. Nickles, Department of Neurology, University of California, San Francisco, California, USA, sebaran@cgl.ucsf.edu, "Genetics of multiple sclerosis: swimming in an ocean of data," *Current Opinion in Neurology* 25, no. 3 (June 2012): 239–45.

[11] S. Sawcer, G. Hellenthal, M. Pirinen et al., "Genetic risk and a primary role for cell-mediated immune mechanisms in multiple sclerosis," *Nature* 476 (2011): 214–219.

[12] S. V. Ramagopalan, D. A. Dyment, M. Z. Cader et al., "Rare variants in the CYP27B1 gene are associated with multiple sclerosis," *Annals of Neurology* 70 (2011): 881–886.

[13] I will not discuss the exact way that the nerve impulse is carried down the axon in this chapter. The scientific term for the process is called *saltatory conduction*. There is a brief description of the process in The MS ICE chapter. You can find a more complete description of what saltatory conduction is all about at http://faculty.washington.edu/chulder/salt.html. There is a more in-depth description of how the neuron works, which starts at http://www.khanacademy.org/video/anatomy-of-a-neuron?playlist=Biology.

[14] Pathway=tract=fasciculus=bundle. One of the hardest things I had to deal with when learning neuroscience as an undergraduate, and then again as a medical student, was that everyone used different terminology for the same thing. I was too scared to ask a question because I was afraid that I would look like an idiot. I know now that if I have a question, at least 30 percent of the other people probably have the same question going through their heads as well.

Third

What MS Is from the Other Side of the Desk

I wrote the following piece in 1998, after graduating from my neurology residency. My wife and I had moved to our home in New York with our new baby daughter, Abigail. I had had MS for eleven years and had been on beta-interferon 1a, intramuscular for almost three years. The purpose of the following story is to help introduce a central concept of this book. A very large percentage of people with MS have behavior changes that are disabling in ways different from physical changes. Behavior and cognition are very much guided by the front part of the brain, called the frontal lobes. If a person with intact frontal lobes sees a chore that needs to be done, like folding the clothes or cleaning the bathroom, they have initiative to get up and start doing it. People with intact frontal lobes can also pay attention and complete a task. People with intact frontal lobes have good emotional control and don't say socially inappropriate things. The main character in the following story has MS and has trouble with all of these things. The cause of the trouble, as will be discussed in The MS ICE chapter, comes not from focal MS lesions (such as the white spots that can sometimes be seen on MRI) but rather from the elevated pressure within the brain itself that causes a generalized, reversible dysfunction of certain pathways that govern initiative, concentration, and emotional control.

A DAY AND A NIGHT IN AN MS LIFE

The heat was melting Joseph's will to live as he sat in his office, sweating. Over the phone, he could hear Steph walking up the stairs on the way to their bedroom. He had just come back from the hospital after seeing some consultations when he realized he had forgotten his …

"Cell phone. Yep. It's here on your nightstand."

"Thank God," he muttered into the receiver. "At least I didn't lose it." He looked at his watch—10:50 a.m. "Would you be able to bring it to me here at the office?" he asked as sweat ran down the side of his face into his ear.

"I just finished feeding Gabby and put her down for a nap. I wanted to get some exercise, and then I have to go food shopping."

That's not an answer, Joseph thought to himself. *Why can't she just tell me what time she can come?*

"So you wouldn't be able to leave until when?" he reworded, impatiently.

"Well, I also have to get a gift for your sister for her birthday …" she continued. The sweat in his ear made it sound like they were talking via ham radio.

"Soooo, when do you think you would be able to leave by?" he said, thinking that it really wasn't a hard question to answer.

After another pause, she answered. "Probably around two."

"So you wouldn't get down here until about three," he said as he calculated her potential trip: forty miles each way, baby in car, at least twenty-five dollars for gas and tolls, total driving time of about two hours. He realized that it wasn't worthwhile for her to bring the phone to him. After a few more seconds of thinking, he realized that he was a fool for even considering it as an option.

There was silence on the line.

"I guess it doesn't make sense for you to bring the phone all the way down here," he said.

"Probably not," she replied. He started to wonder why Steph bothered to put up with him. He felt like an idiot. He had been forgetting more things than one would expect of a doctor, or any adult for that matter. Heck, he had seen videos of high-functioning golden retrievers that forgot fewer things than he did.

"Do you ever make a list of the things that you need to do each morning before you leave?" Steph asked. "You know. So you don't have trouble like this so often?"

"Sure I make lists," he said. "Go up to my desk in the attic. All my lists are up there. Except, of course, for the few that I remember to take with me."

"Where do you keep the lists that you remember to take with you?"

"The living room," Joe replied.

"And why do you keep them there?" she continued, sounding like a mother asking her child why he left his mittens at school.

"Because I have to put them down so I can take my vitamins, find my computer bag, put on my coat, and do whatever else I have to do before I leave for work."

"So why don't you pick the lists up after you put them down?" she asked, not understanding Joseph's thinking.

"Because I forget that I put them down," he explained, with the tone of an impatient ten-year-old.

"Why don't you put each list in your pocket after you make it?"

"I can't do that. It would just get scrunched up."

"Can't you put it in your wallet?" she asked, sounding logical.

Joseph looked down at the lump hanging off the side of his thigh in his pants pocket.

"I could," he answered. "But it would just get lost in there with all of the lottery tickets, receipts, laundry tickets, reminder notes I wrote to myself to clean out my wallet, and coupons for one free, medium-sized drink with purchase of one medium burger on or before some date that passed long ago."

There was no response.

The silence on the phone line was filled with Joseph's internal voice asking when he had become so disorganized. He hadn't always been this way. When he was a child in grammar school, he always kept his important papers in his plan book. He used to work at his desk every night. The homework books were stacked on the left side of the desk. As he started and completed each subject, he would take the book, do the work, and then stack the book on the right side of the desk. In high school, he used a portable file-folder system for papers and continued to use the desk-book-stack system. In college, things started out okay. During freshman year, he used notebooks for each subject. He worked at resource centers more. He did well. Everything was neat and clean and tidy.

Sophomore year started okay, but then he got a girlfriend. It was his first *real* girlfriend—a girlfriend who helped him realize that there was a tremendous number of other things to be learned aside from what was taught in a classroom. His parents told him that he was in love and that he should be careful. Others told him that he should pull back from the socializing and hit the books more. The most disturbing thing, however, was something he had noticed about himself that others could not see. He noticed that *he* had changed. For the first time in his life, he didn't care whether he was ready for classes or assignments or exams. His GPA started dropping. He had to drop some classes (which he had to make up the following summer). He started acting childishly.

Some of his social deeds, in retrospect, were also completely inappropriate for a college student (as well as for most kindergarteners). Eventually, the relationship with his girlfriend went south, and after getting over the devastation, he tried to buckle down. He graduated college, but the learning was no longer as easy as it had been. The academic challenges in medical school, residency, and as a young physician were like trying to climb a scholastic Mount Everest every day. Something had happened during sophomore year in college that changed who Joseph was.

"Friggin' Ivy League," Joseph muttered to himself.

Steph's voice came over the phone. "The living room is a mess," she commented. He could hear her walking back down the stairs.

"Yeah. The baby's toys are all over the place," he answered as the phone slipped from between his shoulder and ear. He wiped the sweat off the receiver and put it to his other sweaty ear.

"True," she continued, "but there are copies of *The New Yorker* lying everywhere, and I know Gabby doesn't read them."

"Maybe not cover to cover," he contested. "But I have heard her laughing at some of Woody Allen's pieces."

"If she likes them so much, why are all the covers ripped off?" she pressed.

"I don't know. Maybe she's frustrated that he hasn't written anything in a while." He heard no response from his wife. Normally, he'd get a chuckle; today, nothing.

"It's for an arts project Gabby will have to do one day," he tried to explain. "My mom always used to save things for me to use in school if I ever needed them. I figure I better start doing the same for Gabby so she'll have the best-looking dioramas in the school."

"I'm just so sick of this mess," Steph continued. The desperation in her voice was rising like the oppressive sun was outside.

"I'll clean them up when I get home," he said, trying to put some happiness back in her voice.

"And your tool bag?"

"I told Gabby that if she left my power drill out again, then she was going to have to put the swing set together herself!"

The silence grew louder.

"Sorry," he apologized. "I was leaving them out because I still have to change the knobs on the cabinets that you asked me to put on two weeks ago."

"Do you need the power saw for that?"

"No, but when I was getting the hardware for the cabinets, I realized that I could get started on the project to refinish my mom's old stereo cabinet, and I had to cut some pieces of wood to size ..."

"And so that's why there are piles of lumber in the dining room."

"You're in my thoughts," he said, trying to convey the idea that their love was so deep, words were no longer necessary for communication. The lack of response told him that she was thinking (telekinetically telling him) that she would have been better off getting a dog than getting married.

"We have to clean up before my parents get here this weekend," she added. "Should I put them outside?"

No, they can sleep in the guestroom like they normally do, Joseph thought to himself.

Hahahahaha!

Great line! Quick—use it, one part of Joseph's brain thought.

"No ..."

Wait! Stop! Don't say it! the other side of his brain started to shout.

"... they ..."

The room is rough tonight, the voice continued.

"... can ..."

You're zero for three, his conscience pleaded. *Cut your losses! Stop!*

"... be put away in the basement when I get home," he answered. "Yeah. You don't want lumber out in humid weather like this. It might warp." *Holy cheese and crackers. It was hard to keep myself from saying that line,* Joseph thought as he came back out of his head.

"I'll see you when I get home tonight. Okay?" he added.

"Sure," she answered. Her voice was tired.

"Love ya," Joseph said.

"Love you too ..." Steph's voice trailed off. He held the receiver to his ear until he heard her hang up. He felt physically and emotionally drained, and it wasn't even noon yet. He went over to the air register by the window to see if the air-conditioner was going. He could feel cool air coming out, but he still felt uncomfortably warm. Outside the window in the street, he could see the heat building. The sun was approaching its zenith. Electric company workers were digging up some power lines. Their shirts were soaked with sweat. He looked down at some bushes and noticed two bees hovering around some lilacs right in front of his window. That's all they were doing. Hovering. Not zipping around, bouncing from flower to flower. Just hanging in midair, hovering. They were probably complaining to each other about the heat.

> *"Hey, Morey. Can you believe this heat?"*
> *"Ach! Irv, it's not the heat! It's the humidity!" Morey replied.*
> *"But the heat ain't no taste of honey neither!" Irv complained.*
> *"Ahh. The queen's meshugeneh. Let's go down to the boardwalk and get a coupla egg creams."*

At least they don't have to go to the hospital, he thought to himself. Plus, they didn't have to wear suits. They were wearing yellow-and-black, sleeveless jumpsuits.

"At least your uniforms breathe," Joseph muttered to himself. He looked at his charcoal suit. "Me. I'm wearing a greenhouse." He closed the blinds and turned from the window. His jacket was stuck to his shirt, with sweat making it feel like he was wearing a basket of wet laundry. The jacket carried his collapsible neuro hammer, a pack of patient cards, a PDA, a candy bar, a wad of tissues, a checkbook, and a bunch of handouts to give to the residents at the hospital. The weight of his jacket pulled his necktie up against his throat. It felt like he was being choked by an unmotivated strangler.

Taking off his jacket, he loosened his tie, sat back down, and looked around the office. Diplomas and licenses hung on the wall in front of him. He had never liked seeing doctors' offices decorated with framed pieces of academic validation. He thought it was pompous. The practice asked for them before he started. When he arrived for his first day, they had framed and posted the documents on a wall in his office. He guessed they needed to make the place look professional. When he looked at them, he felt conflicted. Obviously, at one point, his thinking had been better than it was now. Despite being a neurologist, he still couldn't figure out what had gone on in his brain that had caused the change. He had been diagnosed with multiple sclerosis, after having the onset of double vision between his first and second years of medical school. Ever since, he felt run down all the time. He could still move and talk normally, but his thoughts seemed all over the place. He couldn't keep track of his cell phone, his medical bag, and many other important things. At least he hadn't forgotten his anniversary, he thought. He glanced at the calendar.

Nope. Not yet.

The thing he was most concerned about, however, was forgetting to do something for his patients. That was one of the reasons he spent so much time with them. He was not going to let his disorganized mind put them in jeopardy. He spoke with them and listened to their stories during residency. By spending the extra time, he was able to make sure he had covered all the bases. At the same time, it was then that he discovered that listening is sometimes the best medication. Unfortunately, now that he was in practice, he had to see a lot more patients. This left little room for the listening. As more demands were being put on him, Joseph's life was becoming a woeful existence. He loved taking care of people but hated the way he was being forced to do it.

He sat for several more minutes. After the sweat had dried on his face, he gathered up his bag, jacket, and patient list and went out to reception. Jess, his sardonic nurse, was sitting at her desk.

"Hey," Jess started. "Any news about your phone?"

"I called Steph. She says that she found my phone on the nightstand."

"Well, at least it's not lost," she said encouragingly.

"True," he said, trying to smile.

"Here are some new friends for you to see," Jess said as she placed a piece of paper on the counter. *Sonofamotherfather,* Joseph thought. More consults. He looked at each name on the list. He didn't think about the person or the diagnosis. He thought about having to slog through traffic, watching the heat shimmy off the hood of his car. He thought about how much time he was going to have to spend suffocating in warm, stagnant hospital rooms. He thought about the slaglike air cutting off the oxygen supply to whatever life remained in his soul. His thoughts drained any desire to do anything. He looked at Jess. *First, she pulls me in close with sympathy, and then she stabs me in the back with a three-by-five-inch index card.* He felt betrayed.

"I don't know if I have the energy," he replied.

As he continued to stare at the list, the image he saw doubled as his eyes started to cross.

"What's the matter with your eyes?" she asked.

"I don't know. I just feel so wiped out," he replied.

Jess stared at the young physician. "You look like you've been hit by a truck," she said. "You should go home and get some rest."

Joseph looked at Jess. "What?" he asked. "I can't go home. I've got to see the new patients."

"Have you seen what you look like?" she asked as she took the list out of his hand. "I'll get someone to cover the consults."

Joseph stepped back from the desk. He had felt exhausted, but now he felt terrible. Jess had seen something that Joe couldn't see. He trusted that she knew what she was doing.

"Okay," he muttered as he turned to go.

"But before you go," Jess continued, "stop by radiology to see Gerry. She wants you to do your monkey-man impression for her."

"Monkey-man?" Joseph asked.

"You know. The thing where you skip around and then you fall to the ground."

"Oh yeah," he answered. "How did she find out about that?"

"I told her," she said. "It's funny. Go do it, and I'll see you tomorrow," she added. She waved Joe off and started to dial a number on her phone. He nodded and started walking toward radiology. As he walked, he realized he should stop by the restroom before leaving for home.

The bathroom was one of the few respites that Joseph had at work. The cool marble tile on the floors and walls acted as a sink for the heat that was stored in his warm clothes. It was clean, and unlike his bathroom at home, there were no leaks that he had to deal with. Plus, there was no cell phone reception in the bathroom. It was his temporary isolation tank. He hung up his jacket, and after standing in the cool room for about thirty seconds, he felt a bit of his initiative return. He stopped at the sink to wash his hands. He kept them under the cool stream of water for a minute. The mirror over the vanity reflected some of what he felt. The image was heavy—eyelids hanging, shoulders drooped. He had a tired face. He splashed some water on his face and then wiped it away from his eyes with his fingers. While the cool water on his face dripped into the sink, he looked into the mirror. Now he looked soggy and tired, but at least he felt a bit better. After his hand found a towel, he dried himself off and walked toward radiology.

"There he is!" screeched Gerry when she saw him walking toward her desk. "Do the monkey-man thing for me! No, wait! Let me get Lisa." He could feel her excited, happy energy inflate his thick and heavy world as she went over to the file cabinet and started pulling on Lisa's arm.

"Lisa, come heeeeah!" she pleaded. "Ya gotta see this!"

"See what?" Lisa asked, with minimal inflection in her voice.

"This! This!" Gerry looked at Joseph. "Gahead! Gahead! Do it!" she said in her dense New Yorker accent. He looked at Lisa. Lisa, who rarely smiled and often looked unhappy, had a good sense of humor. That was one of the things he liked about her. He had been one of the few doctors who could get her to smile on a regular basis.

"It's not that big of a deal," he said.

Lisa shrugged. "Just do it so Gerry will shut up," she said.

"Okay," he said. Joseph looked to make sure there were no patients around. When it was clear, he started doing a walk-skip, chimp-like gait back and forth in front of them. Gerry started to turn purple from holding in laughter. He then stopped, looked at them, and collapsed to the floor. Gerry let out a "Wraaaaagh!" followed by a series of silent head dips and body rocking. She was purple by the time she started to breathe again.

"Whasso funny 'bout dat?" Lisa asked.

"I don't know," he replied as he got up. "I just like doing it because I like to see her laugh."

Gerry took in another deep breath so she could continue laughing. As Joseph and Lisa continued to watch her, they both started feeling a little better. After another ten seconds, Gerry slowed her laughing. She pointed at Joseph.

"You're monkey-man!" she squeaked and then went into more gales of laughter.

"I'm gonna go home now," Joseph said to Lisa. "See ya tomorrow."

"Take me wit' you," Lisa said, her tone indicating a disenfranchised state rather than a plea from her heart.

"Why?" he asked.

"I hate it here," she answered.

"But we need you here," Joseph said as he put his arm around Lisa. "You know. To help create the happy, healing ambiance that allows MegaUnitedHealthyHealers/RadiationHut to care for everyone who needs help." He looked into her eyes. "Plus, you're the only one who can be trusted to keep an eye on her," he added, pointing his index finger at Gerry.

"What's the use?" she asked as she stepped away and started to pull Gerry back to her desk. "See youse tomorrow."

Tears were coming down Gerry's flaming-red face as Joseph turned to go to the door. He listened to make sure she was still breathing as he walked out.

***

The forty-minute, thirty-five-mile drive home went relatively quickly as he got off the parkway. The air-conditioner was going full blast as he listened to the news declaring that the heat wave would be lasting for the foreseeable future. He had seen at least two cars on the ride home that had pulled over because of the heat. He felt lucky that his car had made it. After turning off the parkway, he followed the main road that led past his town. He made a left onto a secondary road as the trees started to outnumber the telephone poles. Traffic dropped to scant few cars as he turned onto his block. The moment Joseph saw his house, his bladder notified his brain that it had to go wee-wee. He wondered why he always, suddenly, had to go to the bathroom when he knew he was almost home. Accelerating up the hill and passing his front yard, he saw Steph and the baby playing near the sprinkler. They were both smiling.

Joseph loved his new daughter, but he was still getting used to his new position in the lineup. She was the opening act and the headliner. Her material wasn't any better than his was, he thought. It was just that she was putting a new spin on it:

"Oh, look! She's spitting up. Hold on. Let Mommy get your nappy and clean you up. You're soooo cute."

Joseph knew he had been doing mostly old material for at least several years, but he felt it was quality material. Unfortunately, somewhere, it had lost its sweet naiveté:

"Oh, great. You're going to throw up. Here's a bucket. Just make sure you don't get any of it on the carpeting."

He had always had a good sense of humor, and he hardly ever worked blue. He couldn't remember exactly when he first heard himself saying things that were "over the line" while socializing, but Steph had noticed it often enough. It made her uncomfortable, and she let him know it. He figured she was just becoming more conservative as the years went on.

He pulled into the driveway, grabbed his bag and keys, and scooted rapidly toward the front door.

"There's Daddy," Steph said, holding Gabby up to look at her daddy.

"Gotta get to the bathroom," he said in a hushed voice as he reached for the doorknob. Locked! "Dammit! Why is the door locked?" he said to no one in particular. Steph looked up.

"I have the key," she said, pulling it out of her pocket.

"Why do you have to lock it all the time?" he asked with annoyance.

"We went out for a walk before," she answered, handing him the key.

He got the key into the doorknob on the fourth try and then turned it. The door wouldn't open. She had locked the deadbolt!

"Dammit!" he exclaimed as he felt a little urine get somewhere it was not supposed to be. "Why do you have to lock both the knob and the deadbolt?" he asked as he pulled out the key to put into the door handle lock.

"To be safe," she said as she started to towel Gabby off. He turned the key, and the door opened. He raced inside, leaving the door ajar. He got to the bathroom with little collateral damage. After putting himself back together again, he went back to the front. Steph had laid the baby down in the living room and was changing her diaper.

"Thanks for helping to locate my phone earlier," he said, trying to make up for his childish behavior.

"No problem," she said, smiling as she lifted Gabby's legs and tilted her up to clean her. "You're home early. Anything go wrong at work?"

"I was feeling like crap," he began. "Jess said I looked crummy too. I figured I should just come home and get some rest and get an early start tomorrow." He looked at the mess in the living room and then turned and saw the lumber in the dining room. "I'll get started on cleaning up all this stuff after I get cleaned up."

"Okay. I was going to make some chicken for dinner. What time do you want to eat?"

"I dunno," he said, starting to take off his jacket and tie. "Let me see how I feel after I'm done getting things cleaned up."

He turned and lumbered up the stairs. Once in the bedroom, he turned the air-conditioner on high, tossed his keys on the bed, and got out of his suit. Using his foot, he pushed around a pile of clothes that was on the floor. He picked up a pair of shorts and a faded blue T-shirt. After dressing, he turned back to the bed and saw the phone on the nightstand. He went over, picked it up, and put it in his suit so he wouldn't forget to take it tomorrow. As the temperature in the room dropped, he began to feel a little more alert again. Steph came up the stairs with Gabby.

"Can you play with Gabby for a few minutes while I get ready to go shopping?" she asked.

"Sure," Joseph said as he took their baby from her arms. He sat on the bed and stood Gabby up on his lap. He looked at her directly. "Mommy says someone was tearing up copies of old magazines. Do you know anything about that?" he asked.

His daughter, seeming nonplussed by her father's questioning, chewed on her fingers.

"Well, if you're not going to talk, then I'm just going to have to assume you plead nolo contendere."

Saliva started dripping out of the corner of her mouth.

"Your lack of response and flagrant slobbering force me to find you in contempt of court. You will be sentenced to tickling, which is to commence immediately." He then placed her on her back and started tickling her tummy. She began to squeal and laugh. Watching her smile filled him with happiness and let him feel more awake and alive.

"Don't be too rough with her," Steph called from the bathroom. "I just fed her, and I want her to fall asleep in the car while I do my errands."

"I won't," he said. "Don't worry," he reassured his wife as he stopped tickling Gabby. Once free, she rolled over onto her tummy and then got to her hands and knees. She spied Joseph's keys at the edge of the bed. Using the reaction time and unpredictable path of a mosquito on crack, she quickly scooted toward the edge of the bed. Joseph, using an outstretched-arms, soccer-goalie-styled dive, landed next to her just as Gabby's body weight was about to carry her and the keys off the bed and onto the hardwood floor. She squealed as he grabbed her and the clump of keys fell to the floor. Steph came back into the room.

"What was that?" she asked. Joseph held Gabby in his arms.

"Nothing," he said as he looked at his daughter. "I was just trying to demonstrate how gravity works to our little Ms. Newton." Gabby started to chew on her fingers again.

"What are you going to do while I'm out shopping?" she asked.

"Well," Joseph began, "I figured I would start with moving the wood out of the dining room and then cleaning the living room. After that, I'll either start translating the complete works of John Steinbeck into Old High German or take a nap. When do you think you'll be back?" He handed Gabby to his wife.

"Probably around four thirty. Maybe sooner if I can find everything I need to get."

"Sounds good," he said, kissing Gabby. He looked at Steph as he thought back to the conversation they had on the phone that morning. "I'm sorry for asking you to bring me my phone this morning. That was me being stupid."

"It's okay. Did you see the phone on your nightstand?"

"Yes. I already put it away in my jacket for safekeeping for tomorrow."

"Good," she said. They kissed good-bye. "Love you," she said, smiling. "Love your body, Larry," he replied.

She went out of the room and downstairs, carrying Gabby. *She didn't even acknowledge the Fletch reference,* Joseph thought. "She used to be *my* audience," he said aloud to the empty room. "I was the headlining act. Then the kid arrived. Now I'm just a has-been comic working the backroom who takes out the trash and shuts off the lights after the last drunk leaves." He pushed some clothes that were on the bed out of the way and decided to lie down to take a nap before tackling the work for the afternoon.

"Where did it all go wrong?" he asked as he tried to fall asleep.

After lying in bed for almost two hours, Joseph felt only slightly better. His legs felt stronger, but he still had no drive to get up. As he pulled himself out of bed to go to the bathroom, he slipped a little on a stack of papers next to his bed. One of papers stuck to the bottom of his foot as he dragged himself to the hallway and into the bathroom. Just as he got to the toilet and started to unfasten his shorts, his bladder decided it was time to start moving some inventory. He rushed to get his shorts undone and then quickly sat down. He was starting to feel like his daughter had better bladder control than he did. He sat on the toilet for a while, trying to make sure that everything that wanted to come out did. After washing up, he proceeded downstairs. Steph and Gabby had not yet returned. He saw the lumber in the dining room and his tools scattered about on the floor. The lumber looked heavier than it did in his memory. He thought about how many dings he had put in the walls when he first brought it home. He decided to wait until Steph got home so she could help him guide it down the stairs.

He went into the kitchen, looking for some energy. He walked past the table to the refrigerator. He took out a soda, twisted off the top, and put it to his lips. Throwing his head back, the cold, caffeine-sugar juice ran down his throat, producing a soothing, internal chill along with a mild, asphyxiating pain. After finishing almost half the bottle, he recapped it and looked around. There was a pile of mail on the table. He stared at it and then decided it would be wiser to let the mail stay there. If he picked it up, he might not be able to find where he had put it down later on.

He took his soda and lack of motivation to the living room where he turned on the TV and lay down on the couch. He flipped to the comedy channel and saw that two of his favorite comedians were having their stand-up specials on back to back. He had seen the stand-up specials for almost every major comedian at least three times each, but he loved listening to each routine over and over again. Each one had become a humorous mantra that he could do in his mind on demand. It gave him a sense of calm inside. As the theme song for the show came on, his blood pressure went down and his cares melted away.

After echoing the routines of two comedians verbatim, watching two episodes of a television show that he thought he had seen (but wasn't quite sure), and then watching the first hour of a movie that he had seen many times (but he really, *really* wanted to see the main character say the one line that *made* the movie), he saw Steph's car pull into the driveway. In rapid succession, he got up, took his soda to the kitchen, and put it in recycling. He then headed to the dining room and hurriedly started picking up the tools so he could ask Steph to help him take the wood downstairs. Sequentially tossing tools into his tool bag, he had picked up almost everything when he reached for something that he thought was a screwdriver. As he felt the end of the metal shaft slice his finger and then the warmth of what he knew was blood spreading over his palm, he realized it was not a screwdriver.

Without pause, he walked rapidly to the kitchen where he got a paper towel and applied pressure. He held his hand over the sink, not wanting to get blood on the counter as he had done the last time. He squeezed the paper towel between his left thumb and index finger as his right hand ripped off several more sheets from the roll. He folded one to do the main absorption and then wrapped the next two to keep the first one in place. He heard the locks on the front door open. Steph came in holding Gabby in one arm and carrying a sixteen-pack of paper towels in the other.

"Hi," she said. "I need some help getting the groceries out of the car." He turned to her with the red paper towels wrapped around his hand.

"I'll help you in a minute," Joseph started. "First, could you remind me where we keep the bandages?" Steph's eyes widened at the sight of Joseph's bloodied hand.

"Are you okay?" she said, with an urgency that prompted Gabby to start crying.

"It's just a flesh wound," he said in a British accent, not expecting any response from the audience but wanting to make himself feel better, knowing that his stupid move was going to wind up causing him more wasted time than he wanted to deal with. "Don't worry 'bout me. Just tell me where the bandages are, and I'll be fine."

"Upstairs in the bathroom closet," Steph said. Joseph walked closer to his wife and daughter on his way to the stairs. He looked directly at Gabby as he approached.

"Don't cry," he said, with a broad smile. "Daddy's okay. He still has at least seven other fingers and one opposable thumb that he can pick you up with after he stops the bleeding." Gabby started to smile as Joseph slowly backed up the stairs. He then looked back at Steph.

"I'll be down in a little while to clean up the rest of the tools."

After cleaning and drying the wound, Joseph kept pressure on his left hand for about five minutes before taking a look to see if he could start bandaging it. The first peek at it showed only a small leak. He continued to keep pressure on the cut for another minute by pressing his paper-towel-covered hand against the sink while he used his right hand and his mouth to open a few gauze pads, tear off a few pieces of adhesive tape, and prep some bandages with triple antibiotic ointment. Once they were laid out on the counter, he ran some hot water over a washcloth and then rubbed the bar of soap from the soap dish on the wet wash cloth. Slowly peeling off the paper towels, he saw that the bleeding had stopped. He gently dabbed the area with the soapy cloth and then blotted away any of the visible soap and water with some clean gauze. Once dry, he applied three separate bandages to keep the skin together, covered by two gauze pads for cushioning, which were secured in place by four pieces of adhesive tape. He looked at his work. He did not know if he should be proud of how quickly and efficiently he had set right his hand or if he should be kicking himself for how many times he had almost sheared off a part of his body. He remembered how his mother had always told him to not be so "rush-rush" when doing things. He couldn't help it, he thought as he gingerly tested out the dressing.

With his wound clean, dry, and intact, he went back downstairs. Steph was in the kitchen and had started making dinner. Gabby was lolling in her playpen. Joseph put the rest of his tools away and then looked at the lumber. He walked into the kitchen and over to the counter where Steph was cutting up some banana for Gabby.

"I don't want to try to move the lumber out of the dining room tonight. I want to give my hand a day to heal."

Steph looked up at him. "I can help you tomorrow," she said.

"Sounds good," Joseph replied. "Anything you need me to do?"

"You can set the table," she said. "It's almost dinnertime."

"Gotcha," he said, turning toward the cabinet with the dishes in it. He took out two plates, two glasses, and one sippy cup and put them on the table. Picking up a dishrag with his right hand, he wet it and then wiped down Gabby's highchair tray. He put her sippy cup on the tray and then got out utensils—two knives, two forks, and a rubber-coated spoon. He thought for a second about which setting should get the rubber-coated spoon.

"I think I'm going to go to bed after dinner," Joseph said as he walked back to Steph. "Ya know, so I can try to rest up for tomorrow."

Steph looked at him. "How did you cut your hand?" she asked.

Joseph saw the concern on her face. "I mistook a chisel for a screwdriver," he answered. "I should have been more careful, but I wanted to make sure that I cleaned up some stuff before you got back. I rushed too much."

"I wanted you to straighten things up, not maim yourself," she replied.

"Me neither," he said, sitting down at his place at the table. Steph nodded in agreement as she put down a bowl of mashed bananas on the table and went to the living room to get Gabby.

★★★

Light from a streetlamp shot through a slit in the shade just as a breeze puffed out the curtain, making it look like a fat guy was trying to get into Joseph's room through the window, stomach first. He had just drifted off to sleep. But that was a lie. He had been drifting between a light stupor and an uncomfortable semiaware state where the main sensation was his pajamas becoming less comfortable and more like plastic wrap. Each time he turned over, his T-shirt seemed to tighten in tourniquet fashion around his chest, shoulders, and arms. He decided to turn over in the opposite direction from the last time to unwrap himself. Joe was exhausted. He could lie in bed for days and feel no better than when he first hit the sheets. He needed sleep, but none was around. The sheep had gotten sick of being counted and decided to look elsewhere for work.

The sound of a garbage truck's brakes squealed faintly outside the window. He stared at the clock. It showed 2:27 a.m. He had been in bed for five hours. He had to get up in three. Steph was sleeping next to him. He thought about how lucky she was to be able to get real sleep. She deserved it though. She was the main caregiver for Gabby. He thought that he did his part as best he could, but he wasn't sure.

He thought back to his childhood. His dad never made dinner for his family or did homework with Joseph or his sisters. Then again, his dad had to work thirteen hours a day in the family business (wholesale drapery). His mom did not. She had been a registered nurse but decided to give it up to become a full-time mom. Joseph realized that mom was just another term for nurse without pay, as well as doctor, psychiatrist, tailor, designer, chef, and chauffeur. She had taught Joseph some of the most important things about being a doctor that were never taught in medical school or residency. She taught him about how an alcohol rub could help when a person was running a fever and that just listening to a person could help make him or her feel better. She died of breast cancer when she was fifty-nine—just before the millennium ended. One of the last memories Joseph had of spending time with his mom was sitting next to the bed that had been set up for her in the dining room. Together, they watched Chuck Knoblauch, then a Yankee, at bat in the playoffs.

"He retightens his gloves after each pitch," she said, mimicking Chuck's actions.

"Yeah," Joseph said, smiling at her and thinking how the radiologists had missed her breast cancer. She had always gone for her mammograms, but it was her masseuse who had picked up the mass in her right neck, near her clavicle. She lived for eighteen months after she was diagnosed. Three months later, they passed a law saying all mammograms had to be read by two different radiologists. She took one for the team on that one.

He heard the gun of the garbage truck engine for two seconds and then the squeal of the brakes.

His dad had worked hard. He used to squeeze fresh orange juice for the family every morning before he left for work. He had always reminded Joseph and his sisters that he was home for his kids every night and that he never missed a dinner. Joseph thought about how he and his sisters had taken the glasses of fresh juice and him being home every night for granted. His father had made enough money for all of his children to go to school and then get professional degrees. He did tell Joseph about the nightmare he had when his son told him he wanted to go to a private university for medical school even though he had gotten into a state school that would have been considerably less. Now Joseph was working thirteen hours a day and was on call 24/7 for his patients. He wished he could have squeezed orange juice for Steph and Gabby, but he was just making ends meet by working all the time. He didn't know how he and Steph were going to pay for college for their new baby (and maybe one more—possibly a son). They were both doctors, but

30

presently Joseph could see no way that they could pay for college, let alone professional school, for their kids. Maybe they could get scholarships, he thought. Maybe he could home school them. Maybe, just maybe, he could win the lottery. Joseph, however, thought it unlikely. He knew that he had already hit it big. His family was everything to him.

Joseph believed his priorities were well ordered. Among the creatures that roamed through his world, Steph had the top spot locked up. Second in the batting order was Gabby. The number-three slot was reserved for a baby to be named later. After that, it was a long road to the next most important thing. The top contenders for the spot would be either the 1978 Yankees or, if reincarnation technology progressed, the 1951 Yankees. He often spent time thinking about how much good fortune had come his way. He was forever humbled to be the one who was blessed to have Steph enter his life and become his wife. He sometimes imagined what the conversation would be like if he had a chance to ask the One Who Is why he had been chosen:

"Hi, God."

"Hello, Joseph."

"How's it going?"

"Okay."

"Can I ask a question?"

"Sure."

"Thank you. Look, I'm a simple guy."

"True."

"I've been told I have a nice smile. By the way, thank you for the dimples."

"I threw them in when your mother was praying that I give you ten fingers and ten toes. She's a nice person."

"Indeed she was. So I take it she's up there in heaven with you?"

"She runs the garden club and makes coffee and cookies for all who come."

"Wonderful! I wanted to ask about something else."

"I know. Go on."

"So aside from the dimples, I'm basically a pain in the butt."

"Okay."

"And I say stupid things. Not that I want to, but they just seem to come out."

"Agreed."

"And, quite often, I act like a child."

"Where are we going with this?"

"Well, since there are about 3.7 billion women in the world, why would you

bestow upon me Steph, who's the greatest woman in the world—except of course for Mother Teresa of Calcutta who was out of the running for obvious reasons?"

"Why do you think I did?"

"I'm thinking there might have been a mistake in the shipping department, and the angel you sent Steph to lead her to her husband was really supposed to take her to Derek Jeter, and I was supposed to get the new baseball mitt, but you couldn't have made a mistake because you are The Creator of Everything, right?"

"Correct."

"Well, why then?"

"Steph is patient, and you are not, so I sent her to teach you patience."

"Oh."

"And Steph is kind, and you are kind of obnoxious, so I sent her so you could learn how to be kind all the time."

"Is that all?"

"No."

"Please, go on."

"Well, you're an okay baseball player, but you're short while she is a languid, graceful, tall athlete."

"How does that matter?"

"In my free time, I do some scouting work for the Yankees. By the time your son is old enough to pitch in the Major Leagues, the Yankees will need another starting pitcher."

"And?"

"And while your genes are satisfactory for becoming a doctor, you just did not have the right chromosomes to make a guy that could get the Yanks to another World Series. Steph does."

"Makes sense. She is patient, and you need to be able to be patient and have control over your emotions to be a great pitcher. Right?"

"Yeah. Sure."

"That's what I thought."

"But it's mostly the short thing."

"Oh."

Some plastic garbage can lids hit the ground, and the sound interrupted Joseph's quasi-meditative state. His attention returned to his shirt, which was affixed to his skin with a slimy layer of sweat. His nights were epochs of irritating restlessness conducted in a wet, smelly cocoon. Authentic rest was rare. The dream to dream had never felt so distant. He peeled off his shirt and threw it on the floor. A breeze came in through the window, and it felt good as it passed over his body. It was hot in the room. He turned to look at Steph again. She had the covers pulled up to her face, hiding a long-sleeve turtleneck, long-sleeve pajama top, flannel pajama pants, wool socks, and the old college sweatshirt that she was wearing. Her knit cap had fallen off sometime around one in the morning. He hoped she wouldn't catch a cold.

The garbage truck made some crunching noises. The brakes released, and the truck travelled another twenty feet down the block, where the brakes squealed and the process repeated. Steph thought that Joseph drank alcohol too much, and sometimes he did too. He felt that alcohol helped to keep the electric fire in his head to an annoying but tolerable background static. He had had some trouble in college with knowing when to stop drinking. Since then, he had learned that he could not afford to abuse it. He had too much greatness in his life—Steph and the baby and the lives of his patients. Besides, alcohol kills brain cells. His MS did not need any help.

He would sometimes think about his child (and maybe children) getting MS, but only fleetingly. The first therapy approved to slow down the disease became available right when he was diagnosed. With the amount of research going on, he felt quite comfortable in knowing that treatments would continue to improve. Eventually, something would come along to make the disease inconsequential.

The garbage truck squealed to a stop and sounded like it was right outside Joseph's house. He heard the plastic lids of the new garbage cans that he had just bought being tossed down onto the pavement. He had gotten them at his favorite store, Home Depot. He liked walking up and down the aisles and seeing all the things that could be used to create stuff. Steph's parents always got him gift cards to Home Depot for his birthday. He thought about what nice people they were. He resolved to send them a thank-you note for raising such a lovely daughter.

The sound of the garbage truck moving away pulled Joe out of his mind, back to his body. His copious sweat made the sheets feel like sandpaper. He swung his legs over the side of the bed and went to the bathroom. He debated turning on the shower, but he knew it would wake the baby. He grabbed a washcloth, deciding to take a sponge bath. *SpongeBob SquarePants* came to his mind. *He gets to live in a pineapple under the sea where it's cool*, he thought jealously. Joseph started to let his mind go. He started to formulate a version of the show where he was the lead character. He saw his face flash across the screen as the children start to sing:

Who lives with a disease that no one can see?
JoeMan SpongeBath!
Flighty and tired and sleepless is he.
JoeMan SpongeBath!

He imagined marketing little figurines that have legs that sometimes worked or making an action figure where you could pull a string and it would say things like, "Where the hell did I leave my keys?" or "Oh crap, I missed another appointment!" or "I'm gonna punch you if you tell me, 'You look so good!'" He decided to call his agent when he got to work.

Sure. He knew he didn't have an agent, but it was fun to think about.

The cool water felt good as he squeezed the washcloth on his shoulders and let the water run down his back like tiny ice cubes. He thought about how he never liked the heat growing up. His dad always told the story of how Joseph had been found lying in a pool of his own sweat one summer night when he was three years old. His parents had central air-conditioning put in soon after. *Bless them*, he thought.

After drying off, he went back to the bedroom, put on a pair of boxer shorts, and lay on the bed on top of the covers. Steph was still out cold.

As he stared up into the darkness, he thought about not knowing what his disease was going to do to him.

It was quiet.

The clock showed 2:40 in bright-red numbers. He closed his right eye. The numbers were red. He closed his left eye. They were orange. The discordant color perception was left over from a case of optic neuritis he had had two years prior. He remembered when he would go jogging and got heated up, the vision in the center of his right eye seemed less clear when compared to the left. After finishing a run and cooling down, the vision would return to normal. That went on for most of that summer. He knew it must have been optic neuritis, but he didn't do anything about it until he mentioned it to a friend who was working in drug sales at the time. The conversation was still fresh in his mind.

"Why don't you start steroids?" she asked, incredulously.
"I dunno," Joe answered, turning his back on everything he had ever learned.

"You better," she urged. "Gosh. It's your vision. Wouldn't you treat one of your patients with steroids if they had the same complaint?"

"Yeah, I guess."

"What do you mean 'I guess.' I know you, and you would treat them! So go see your doctor and do something about your vision!"

And so he did. He saw an esteemed doctor about it. He was told that since he had been having symptoms for six months, it was too late to use steroids. Instead, he wanted to switch Joseph to another disease-modifying therapy. After the visit was over, Joseph took the script from the doctor and headed home. On the train ride, he started to think about what had transpired. It was Joseph's vision, and the doctor didn't even want to try a course of steroids! Joseph's stance, as an MS neurologist, had always been that if a patient came complaining of trouble with vision, walking, or anything special to their life then, steroids would be the next move, all other things being equal. It was then he realized that he had to be the doctor for himself. His mom had told him that doctors should never treat themselves. Maybe that's why he hadn't started the steroids right away, he thought. Regardless, the following week, he got hold of a five-day course of methylprednisolone, took it, and followed it with a prednisone taper. After that, his vision stopped getting worse after getting heated up. The difference in the intensity of red between his two eyes, however, persisted.

He started to wonder if he should have taken the steroids sooner but straightaway stopped himself. It didn't matter. He had learned that he couldn't play that game. He had done what he had done because he thought he shouldn't treat himself. However, after a friend who cared about him, using an objective eye, let him know that he had to do the right thing, he came to realize, in certain situations, a doctor can treat himself. So he learned and moved on …

He opened his eyes to the sound of two animals fighting. There was a high-pitched screech followed by the sound of an empty garbage can skidding across pavement. The clock read 3:31. Lying in bed was going nowhere at the speed of glue, so he decided to get up for the day. His head carried a dull, heavy ache on his shoulders. After standing and stabilizing himself, he lumbered his way to the bathroom, making sure not to wake Steph or the baby. The pile of keys that he kicked in the darkness had another idea. The metallic clanging caused Steph to rouse. He held still and listened to see if

Gabby started to cry in her crib. It was silent until Steph whispered, "Don't wake her! I just put her down."

I don't want to wake anyone! Joseph screamed in his head. *It's not my fault! It was the stupid, lazy keys' fault! Why the hell were they on the floor?* In a moment, he remembered that they fell off the bed when he was playing with Gabby. He guessed he could have put the keys on his nightstand before going to bed. He was not that much of a planner.

Waving his hands in front of his face, he groped for the door so he didn't slam into the corner of it like he did last week. Making it to the bathroom, he closed the door and put on the light over the sink. His reflection appeared in the mirror with the imprint of his pillowcase on his forehead. It underlined the scar that was healing from the door encounter. His otherwise pale image looked no better than the one he had seen at the office yesterday. He checked to make sure that his bandaged hand was still intact before sliding open the shower door. Once cleared, he turned on the shower and then went to use the toilet while the water heated up. He stood in front of the bowl as the stream mostly hit water. He knew the intermittent, splattering sounds would have to be cleaned up later. Turning to the shower, he held the sliding door firmly while moving one leg, and then the other, over the side of the tub. Once safely under the falling water, he stood. This was one of the best parts of the day for Joseph. He felt his head lighten. The tar that coated his mind seemed to slough off as he washed off the layer of slime from his body. He used to like to listen to the radio while in the bathroom, but that was before the baby. Now, he had learned to listen to the ringing in his ears.

After shaving and making himself smell pretty, he went back to his room. He tried his best to be quiet, but he wasn't, unless one considers hearing a baby rhinoceros playing chopsticks on a pipe organ to be quiet. Once clothed, as per routine, he kissed his hand and, with greatest care, touched it to the comforter overlying Steph's hip bump. At least he thought it was her hip. It might have been her head. Or it could have been a dummy that she put in the bed to make him think that she was still there, Ferris Bueller–like, while she had taken Gabby and went to her parents' house to get some sleep. He doubted it though. Her parents lived several hundred miles away, and he knew there were no flights leaving for North Carolina until 6:40 a.m.

He picked up his computer bag from the floor and groped his way downstairs. After turning on the light over the sink in the kitchen, he counted out his vitamins and then picked up a glass. The gallon container of orange was slick, but the better part of the juice made it into the glass. He mopped up most of the remainder from the counter with a rag. As for the juice that had gotten on the floor, he figured it could wait until later in the week when he got to cleaning up the urine in the bathroom. He had waited to clean up orange juice spills this way before and knew that he had at least three days before the ants would establish a base camp in the breakfast nook. Any longer than that, Joseph and his family would have to move to a new house. He knew that it would not be absolutely necessary to move, but it would just be easier.

On his way to the front door, he walked through the living room where a squeaky toy gave out a "heeh-uuh" sound as he stepped on and then off of it. He realized that he really had to straighten up the living room when he got home as he unchained the front door.

Once outside, he pulled the door closed behind him and heard it lock. He tested the door to ensure it was locked before starting to walk across the lawn to his car. The moon was full and bright. In its light, he could see the blades of grass clearly at his feet. His headache was gone. The air was cool and fresh. It was the start of a new day. Taking a deep breath, he reflected on what a lucky person he was.

He was finally done with schooling.

He was just beginning his career as a neurologist.

He was on medication to slow down his MS.

Most importantly, however, was his young family.

He had a wonderfully patient and caring wife. Together they were raising their beautiful, new baby. As he got to his car and reached into his pocket, he reflected on how lucky he was. He was comforted in knowing that the two greatest parts of his life were tucked inside a quaint, little home and locked safely away. Safe as safe could be.

Along with all of his keys.

Fourth

Immune Systems from a Neurological Point of View

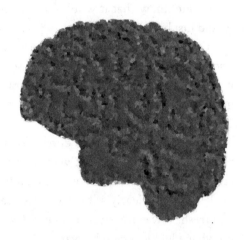

"The only true wisdom is in knowing that we know nothing."
That's us, dude!
—Bill quoting Socrates to Ted,
Bill and Ted's Excellent Adventure

In the previous two chapters, we examined two things. First, we saw how nerves work and how destruction of myelin causes them not to work. Next, we saw an example of the consequences of demyelination in how it can affect the thinking of a person who has MS. In this chapter, we will explore the part of our body, the immune system, that causes demyelination. In the next chapter, we will see a story about the internal conflict that arises when one part of a person's body, for no apparent reason, decides to attack another part of the same body.

IMMUNE SYSTEMS

On the whole, immune systems are great. They protect us from all sorts of invaders that are trying to attack us all the time. In fact, if we do not have a fully functioning immune system to protect our bodies from bugs, the infections that some bugs cause can kill us. Sometimes, the body's immune system starts to attack itself. This is called *autoimmunity,* and it is the cause of many diseases. If it decides to attack the myelin in the central nervous system, it causes MS. No one knows exactly why this immunological "mutiny" happens, but there is evidence that both genetics and the environment play roles in the development of MS.

GENETICS AND THE ENVIRONMENT

Across the world, the incidence of MS in the general population is about 0.01 percent (or 1 in 10,000 people).[15] The incidence between first-degree relatives (parent-child or sibling-sibling relations) where one of the relatives has MS is between 1 and 3 percent.[16] This is higher than the incidence of MS in the general population and tells us that genes are a crucial part of MS. There is a part of the human genome called the *human leukocyte antigen* (HLA) system. Many of the genes in this system (located on chromosome 6) are related to the immune system. The HLA gene *DRB1*1501* is a risk variant for developing MS.[17]

GENETICS AND TWIN STUDIES

When it comes to the role that genetics play in MS, some of the most useful data come from twin studies. There are two types of twins—fraternal and identical. Fraternal twins are, on a genetic level, the same as regular siblings (brother-sister, brother-brother, or sister-sister). Fraternal twins come from two (or more) eggs that were fertilized at the same time and went through their gestation in the same womb at the same time. Now, if MS were entirely due to a genetic cause, one would suspect that the incidence of MS in fraternal twins would be the same as for regular siblings (1–3 percent). However, the incidence of MS between fraternal twins (called the *concordance rate*) is about 5 percent. Why should this be? We have to consider what is different about fraternal twins as compared with siblings born at different times.

One of the most special things about fraternal twins, since they're conceived at the same time, is that they have many of the same exposures to the environment as they grow. Starting in the womb, they're exposed to the same intrauterine environment. After delivery, they're often in the same bedroom together. They take baths together, go to the same schools, have the same friends, catch the same colds, go to the same birthday parties, share clothes, and so on. While having these common experiences, they're exposed to the same viruses/bugs/environmental toxins more often than two siblings who are not the exact same age. This gives the hint that exposure to various things in the environment is a factor in developing MS.

Next we look at identical twins. These are people with the exact same genetic makeup. They come from the fertilization of one egg by one sperm that, at one stage in cell division, splits into two distinct embryos. The concordance rate of MS between identical twins is about 30 percent. That is substantially higher than the other rates (non-twin siblings and fraternal twins), so genes almost certainly play a role. However, the concordance rate is not close to 100 percent. If MS were entirely due to a genetic cause, a concordance rate approaching 100 percent would be expected in identical twins. It should be noted that even though identical twins have copies of the same set of genes, it does not mean that all of the same genes are expressed exactly the same way and exactly at the same time.

ENVIRONMENT AND THE WORLD AROUND US

While twin studies show us that genes are important in who gets MS, they are not the whole story. Another major factor that might play a role and give some more clues as to the cause of MS is the distribution of MS around the world. On the map in figure 7, the white line represents the equator and the white boxes indicate areas where the rate of MS is greater. As the map illustrates, there appears to be a relative lack of MS in the equatorial regions around the world and a higher incidence in the temperate climates.[18] There are multiple ways to interpret this arrangement. One way is to look at it and say, "Well, it looks like MS occurs more often in colder climates. People are more prone to catching a cold from a virus when they're in a cold climate. Maybe a person's chances of getting MS are increased if they get more infections."

That thought makes sense. When you go skiing, you see people who are coughing and sneezing more often than when you go to the beach in Jamaica. Maybe that's why there's a lower incidence of MS in warmer climates. It should be noted that, according to current knowledge, there is a *correlation* between MS and viruses. Two commonly associated viruses include Epstein-Barr virus and human herpes virus 6 (HHV-6).[19, 20] Remember that correlation does not mean *causation*. These are viruses that are seen both in people with MS and those without MS. However, people who do have

MS have a higher rate of harboring these viruses than people in the general population do.

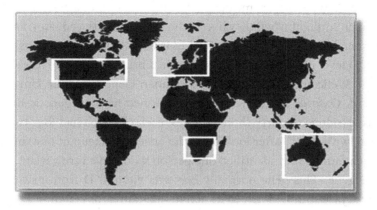

Figure 7. The geographic distribution of MS around the world.

GENETIC DRIFT

An alternative way to look at the incidence of MS around the world is in something called *genetic drift*. As humans have developed over the eons, we have moved all over the world. Quite often, we leave behind our genes as our calling card. Among the earliest documented cases of MS was that of a member of British nobility, Sir Augustus Frederick D'Este (1794–1848).[21] In his journal, he reported instances of losing vision or other functions when he became hot and recovery of those functions when he cooled down. In MS, this is called *Uthoff's phenomenon*, which many of us with MS know well. If we decide to say that some of the first representations of genetic material that predispose humans to MS occurred in people of English or Northern European ancestry, we can see how those genes might have traveled around the world (tip of south Africa, Australia, and North America). Yet, within those areas, there is still a higher incidence in the latitude that is farther away from the equator, which recapitulates the idea that MS is due to a combination of having the right gene(s) and being exposed to the right environmental factor(s).

Vitamin D

Getting back to the map, some people postulate that since a person does not get as much sunlight when they live farther away from the equator, and one of the crucial things that sunlight gives us is vitamin D, maybe having a low vitamin D level plays a part in the cause. In a paper written by researchers from the Wellcome Trust Centre for Human Genetics at the University of Oxford, Oxford, United Kingdom, published in 2011, genetic linkage analysis was done on forty-three families, each of which had four or more members with MS. [22] After looking at the genetic makeup of one member from each family, they identified one person who had a rare variant of the *CYP27B1* gene. This gene normally converts vitamin D from its inactive (25-hydroxyvitamin D) form to its active (1,25 dihydroxyvitamin D) form. After analysis of more than fifteen thousand people, it was found that the gene was strongly associated with MS and that vitamin D is almost certain to play a part in its cause.

Hormonal Changes and Gene Expression

Another interesting fact is that a person's risk for developing MS depends on where he or she is living before their early teen years. [23] If he or she moves from a lower risk/warmer area to a higher risk/cooler area, before the age of eleven or after the age of forty-five, their risk for developing MS is the same as the risk from where he or she came (i.e., lower). If he or she moves from a higher risk/cooler area to a lower risk/warmer area, at about the age of fifteen, then he or she keeps the same risk as the area from which he or she moved. One wonders what is special about the early teen years. Of course, puberty occurs around this time. Many genes that have lain dormant get turned on (e.g., genes that lead to the expression of the sex steroids, estrogen and testosterone). Possibly these hormonal changes can induce changes in the genes expressed in the immune system. At the same time, there are new behaviors expressed by the people of this age group. Close and intimate contact allows for the exchange of a whole variety of bodily fluids, which can carry a host of viruses and other pathogens. Based on these clues, [24] the cause for MS looks to be complex.

GETTING BACK TO THE IMMUNE SYSTEM

A question that often comes up is, "Doesn't the immune system also fix damage done to the body? And if so, why can't it repair the damage that it did to the myelin?" Well, there are several factors that go into the answer. The first is that in MS, demyelination is going on all the time in the CNS on a biochemical level. It is a continuous war that has no cease-fire. There are times when the war escalates (called *exacerbations* or *flare-ups* or *relapses*) and periods of détente (called *remissions*), but it never completely stops.

Next, the ability to repair the nerves in the central nervous system is very limited. This partly comes from the fact that there is a separation between the central nervous system and the rest of the body. This is called the *blood-brain barrier* (BBB) and only allows for transfer of oxygen, carbon dioxide, glucose, and a few other small items between the blood and the brain. In the setting of infection, this barrier breaks down, and other things, like WBCs, can get in and out of the CNS. Otherwise, the CNS can be viewed as an exclusive club that allows only the most select molecules to come and go as they please.[25] This separation may very well play a part in the development of MS.

During development of the immune system, some of the white blood cells have a very specific role. That role is to find out what things in the body are supposed to be there (called *self*). Anything seen by the immune system after this phase is over is considered *nonself*. Since the immune system, during normal development, does not get much of a chance to see the CNS, it is not as familiar with it as it is with the heart, liver, lungs, or any other organ that is not in the CNS. When the immune system finally sees the CNS (perhaps during a CNS infection that causes an immune response leading to a breakdown in the blood-brain barrier), it says, "Hey, we've never seen this CNS myelin before! It must be nonself. It should not be here!" and it starts to chew it up. This is not the whole story, however, since many people get infections in the CNS and do not develop MS, but it could very possibly play a role.[26]

In terms of repairing the damage, the trouble comes from having the right cells doing the repair job. In order for a nerve axon to be remyelinated, several things must be present. First, the axon must still be present. If a nerve has been demyelinated for a period of time, it also means that it has been idle for a while. When a nerve has not been used for a long period of time, it gets digested by the immune system and taken away. Second, if the axon is still present, the cell type that myelinates axons in the CNS (called an *oligodendrocyte*) has to do the remyelination. There is evidence that oligodendrocytes in the adult brain are still capable of remyelinating a nerve that has had its myelin stripped off, but the remyelination appears to be limited. This is where stem cells might be able to play a role in helping out MSers. If oligodendroglial stem cells could be placed at the area of demyelination while an axon is still present, there is a chance that they might be able to remyelinate it. But questions arise. Will the myelin be laid down properly to allow for proper conduction? Will the oligodendrocyte stop myelinating when the area has been repaired? What else might the oligodendrocyte want to put myelin on? Won't the MS disease process still be able to chew up the newly created myelin? These are a few questions that arise when thinking of possible ways to treat MS.

Promising research is going on for both remyelination and nerve regrowth. In a study, rats had the myelin in their spinal cords damaged and then had a compound called *IL-12*[27] administered to their spinal cords. The IL-12 turned on microglial and macrophage cells, as well as neural stem cells, which then led to remyelination that allowed for some recovery of function. Aside from remyelination, there is work going on to actually get the nerves that have been damaged in the CNS to regrow. LINGO-1 is a protein in humans that, when coupled with other proteins, inhibits the growth of neurons. Biogen Idec is currently working on a compound to stop the action of LINGO and thereby possibly allow neurons to grow again.

So, part of the immune system is the villain in MS, and we do not know exactly why it went bad. It appears that some inconspicuous triggers have taken advantage of some vulnerable genes, and that might lead to our disease. Thankfully, we now have therapies to slow down the whole process. Medical science has made breakthroughs that have allowed us to modulate the bad parts of the immune systems while still letting the good parts do their jobs to protect us. It's like when a good relationship goes bad. In the next chapter, this analogy is turned into a story. The central nervous system of an individual, Jeff, has a sit-down meeting with the immune system of Jeff. Both sides have issues that need to be recognized and they both need to get help.

SUMMARY

The cause of MS is unknown but it appears that it might be caused by a combination of a gene (or genes) and something (or things) in the environment.

[15] M. Pugliatti, S. Sotgiu, and G. Rosati, "The worldwide prevalence of multiple sclerosis," *Clinical Neurology and Neurosurgery* 104, no. 3 (2002): 182–191.

[16] C. J. Willer, D. A. Dyment, N. J. Risch et al., "Twin concordance and sibling recurrence rates in multiple sclerosis," *Proceedings of the National Academy of Sciences of the United States of America* 100, no. 22 (2003): 12877–12882.

[17] A. Alcina,* M. del Mar Abad-Grau, M. Fedetz, G. Izquierdo, M. Lucas, Ó. Fernández, D. Ndagire, A. Catalá-Rabasa, A. Ruiz, J. Gayán, C. Delgado, C. Arnal, and F. Matesanz. "Multiple Sclerosis Risk Variant HLA-DRB1*1501 Associates with High Expression of DRB1 Gene in Different Human Populations," *PLoS One* 7, no. 1 (2012): e29819. Published online 2012 January 13. doi: 10.1371/journal.pone.0029819 PMCID: PMC3258250.

[18] N. Koch-Henriksen, P. S. Sorensen, "The changing demographic pattern of multiple sclerosis epidemiology," *Lancet Neurology* 9, no. 5 (2010): 520–532.

[19] A. Ascherio and K. L. Munger, Department of Nutrition, Department of Medicine, Brigham and Women's Hospital and Harvard Medical School, Boston, MA 02115, USA, aascheri@hsph.harvard.edu, "Environmental risk factors for multiple sclerosis. Part I: the role of infection," *Annals of Neurology* 61, no. 4 (April 2007): 288–99.

[20] F. Blanco-Kelly, R. Alvarez-Lafuente, A. Alcina, N. M. Abad-Grau, V. de Las Heras, M. Lucas, E. G. de la Concha et al., Department of Immunology, Hospital Clínico San Carlos, Madrid, Spain, "Members 6B and 14 of the TNF receptor superfamily in multiple sclerosis predisposition," *Genes and Immunity* 12, no. 2 (March 2011): 145–8. Epub 2010 Oct 21.

[21] Stanley Finger, *Minds Behind the Brain: A History of the Pioneers and Their Discoveries* (Oxford University Press, 2005).

[22] S. V. Ramagopalan, D. A. Dyment, M. Z. Cader et al., "Rare variants in the CYP27B1 gene are associated with multiple sclerosis," *Annals of Neurology* 70 (2011): 881–886.

[23] J. F. Kurtzke. Neurology Service and Neuroepidemiology Research Program, Veterans Affairs Medical Center, Washington, DC 20422, "Epidemiologic evidence for multiple sclerosis as an infection," *Clinical Microbiology Reviews* 6, no. 4 (October 1993): 382–427.

[24] There are many clues that are not listed here. For a list of medically reliable data looking for the causes of MS, go to www.pubmed.com and put in "multiple sclerosis causes" in the search bar.

[25] And don't try tipping the bouncer. He'll take your money and then tell you he'll let you in when the girl/guy ratio gets high enough, but it never does, and you wind up going back to your friend's apartment, drinking warm wine coolers, and watching *Sanford & Son* reruns until you fall asleep.

[26] C. Coisine and B. Engelhardt, "Tight junctions in brain barriers during CNS inflammation," *Antioxidants and Redox Signaling* (February 21, 2011). [Epub ahead of print.]

[27] IL-12 is a chemical that immune cells use to speak with each other. "IL" stands for "interleukin," which translates as "between white (blood cells)."

Fifth

Immune Systems from the Other Side of the Desk

The following story is based upon the internal conflict that Jeff, a young man with MS, has. He is working his way up the corporate ladder at a very promising tuba manufacturing company. He has had MS for five years, and it has caused some trouble with his thinking and tuba playing. He knows that his immune system is doing the damage to his central nervous system. He cannot resolve the cognitive dissonance produced by the fact that two different organ systems, within his own body, are working against each other.

WITH OR WITHOUT YOU

The scene is set in lower Manhattan. Jeff's CNS, Woody, is waiting up for a prearranged meeting with Jeff's immune system, Sara, to discuss their issues.

This is Woody. He is a cerebral character—literally. He is Jeff's nervous system. He hates conflict and loves when things are logical and straightforward.

This is Sara. She is a macrophage—a cell from Jeff's immune system. She does her job well, and, like any white blood cell, she gets around.

Some might say that the story that follows is not realistic.
That's true.
When it rains in NYC, there is always some guy on the corner selling umbrellas.

Jeff's nervous system, Woody, sat at a table by the window in a diner on the Lower East Side of Manhattan. It was raining. Tiny rivers ran down the glass widow to the right of Woody and formed puddles on the sill. He took another sip of his coffee and placed it back on the saucer. He was listening to U2 on his pod. He softly sang along with Bono as he looked out the window. People scurried past, trying to get out of the most recent storm. It had been raining on and off for several days. It didn't make sense to Woody that no one was carrying an umbrella. His was on the floor by his superficial peroneal nerve, making its own puddle.[28] The waitress came over. She was chewing gum.

"Can I get you anything else?" she asked, with her pad and pen in her hand, looking at the multiple, sclerotic areas that covered the brain and spinal cord of Woody as he sat in front of a half-filled cup of coffee.

"I'm good," he replied. "Thanks."

"Ya look pretty bruised up," Kate commented. "Wild night out last night?" Woody shrunk back a little. Some sensory nerves fired and tingled down his spinal cord.

"Oh, no, nothing like that," he started, keeping his cortex down. "It's not that bad, really."

"Well, it don't look good," Kate replied, popping her gum and looking over her fiftieth customer of the day.

"A friend of mine has been acting out," Woody began while staring at his coffee. "She did this …" He motioned with some branches of his right median, radial, and ulnar nerves toward his brain and spinal cord.[29]

"Dat's some friend," Kate said, letting out some of her Brooklyn while rolling her eyes.

"Yeah. I don't know why she keeps doing it," Woody replied. He traced around the edge of his coffee cup with some sensory branches of his right median nerve.[30]

"Does it hurt where your 'friend' hit you?" she asked.

"Not really," Woody answered, avoiding eye contact. "It just kinda messes up how I function sometimes."

"'Just kinda messes up how I function,' he says. Dat's horrible is what dat is," Kate pronounced, looking at Woody. "What she's doing is abuse." She continued shaking her head.

"Yeah, I guess it is," Woody said, turning his cortex up to face Kate. "But we gotta make it work," he insisted. "She needs me as much as I need her."

"What's her name?" Kate asked, sounding like a CSI cop gathering evidence.

"Sara," he answered. "She's Jeff's immune system." Kate popped her gum and put her hand on her hip.

"Who's dis Jeff guy?" she continued.

"He's where I work. I'm his nervous system."

"Nervous system?" Kate asked skeptically. "You don't look nervous."

"No, I'm not nervous," Woody started. "I'm a nervous system. You know, brain, spinal cord, peripheral nerves." Kate remained quiet. "You know. I do thinking and make decisions. I send messages along my nerves to tell muscles to move. I tell Jeff when it's time to go to work and when to send birthday cards. Things like that." Kate turned her face and stared out the window. After about ten seconds, she turned back to Woody and lowered her brow.

"So, you do stuff, like, making Jeff move around?" she asked guardedly.

"Yep," Woody answered.

"And stuff like rememberin', like when *Da Price is Right* is coming on TV and stuff?" she continued, slightly faster.

"Yes," Woody reaffirmed, nodding his cortex. "I do his remembering and feeling and such."

Kate bobbed her head up and down as the concept of the nervous system started to crystallize for her. "Don't get too many nervous systems in here," she replied, looking over Woody. "Don't Jeff, like, need you, like—I don't' know—all da time?"

"Yeah, except for a few situations," Woody started to explain.

"Like what kind of situations don't he need you for?" Kate's eyebrows knitted together as she concentrated.

"Like when he goes for surgery and gets general anesthesia. Since he doesn't have to think or do anything, he doesn't need me."

Kate paused while she processed. "Like those shmegeges that Judge Judy has to deal wit every day, right?" she asked, seeking approval.

"Right," Woody said, acknowledging her viewpoint. "Today he's getting surgery for a busted leg, which he got when he tripped off a curb and a taxi hit him. He'll be under general for several hours, so I thought I could duck out and have a chance to meet up with Sara to discuss things."

"Who's dis Sara chick?" Kate pushed.

"She's Jeff's immune system," Woody answered.

"So Sara's the one dat's been beatin' you up, right?"

"So to speak," Woody said as he took some more coffee. He noticed the diner had just about cleared out.

"She doesn't have to be there for the surgery?"

"Nah. She's just one of hundreds of millions in her division," Woody explained. "If we decide to change anything, she'll let the others know."

"Well ya know, abuse ain't no good for nobody," Kate said pointing at Woody.

Woody turned away and looked out the window. "She wasn't like this when I first met her," he said. "She'd been good to me. She took care of me. She killed bugs—bacteria, viruses, fungal infections. Last week, she knocked out a case of salmonella that the guys in the gut were hit with."

"So what happened wit you?" Kate asked, her voice demanding attention.

"I dunno," he replied, looking back at the waitress like a second grader trying to explain why he lost his book bag. "She changed," he said, shrugging. "I changed. We all changed." Woody noticed the waitress's nametag. It read *Kate*. The *K* was worn down. He looked at her face. Early crow's feet were covered, thick with foundation. "By the way, Kate, you can call me Woody."

"Good to meet cha," she replied, switching her pen and pad to her other hand and offering her hand. Woody reached out to shake.

"Good to meet you too," he said.

Kate wrapped her hand around the outstretched nerves. The sensory nerves in Woody's hand fired.

"Ooh. Tingly," Kate said. "I never met a nervous system up close before." Woody nodded. "So, like you were sayin', how did youse all change?"

"It started back when Jeff was in college. He had kicked butt as a sophomore. I got the high score on the calculus exam for him." Kate put her pad and pen in her apron and leaned against the booth. "Muscles, skin, and eyes—they were all buff. They made some great plays in intramural football. Cardiovascular and pulmonary systems were coming into their own. All systems were go." Kate noted the sides of Woody's brain were sparking with activity.[31]

"When he started third year, Jeff got his first real girlfriend."

Kate nodded her head. "What was she like?" she asked, returning to CSI mode.

"A beautiful brunette with class and refinement," Woody recited, describing the picture of her that he held in his mind.

"Hadn't Jeff dated in high school?"

"We went to an all-boys high school. Cognitively, we were as sharp as a switchblade," he said with aplomb. "Socially, however, we were as dull as a ball of lint."

"Uh huh," Kate affirmed.

"We knew a lot, but we were not very developed on the emotional front. He had his friends but never a steady relationship that went anywhere. He hadn't learned what it meant to be in love," he continued as Kate noticed increased activity in the center of Woody's brain.[32]

"So how did you learn to socialize?" Kate asked while glancing at the pale area where her wedding ring used to be.

"Alcohol," Woody answered without a pause. "Our friends called it a social lubricant. It was rampant on campus. I didn't like how it impaired my functioning, but when we found that we could interact with girls on another level after having a few drinks, it was like we had discovered a hidden universe," he said as his right parietal cortex lit up.[33] "It was only then that I discovered that putting our knowledge of biology into action could be fun." Kate raised her penciled-in eyebrows. "We never went *all the way*. Jeff had gone to a Catholic high school. He had his mores set. He did just about everything else, though."

"Couldn't you control Jeff's actions?" Kate impugned.

"Not so much," Woody answered.

"Didn't you tell me that's your job?" she leveled at Woody.

Woody's cortex nodded. "Not long after the relationship started, things started changing," he said, squirming a little in his seat. "Jeff couldn't pay attention anymore. He kept on getting distracted."

"By what?"

"By every little thing that entered his sensorium," he said, noting Kate's brow furrowing again. "For example, if we were reading, and the ears heard a mosquito flying around, Jeff's mind told the eyes to forget about reading and start looking for the mosquito. So every time Jeff got distracted, he would immediately stop whatever he was doing and start thinking about the distraction."

"Was that the way it had been before?" Kate asked, pulling a chair over to the side of the table.

"No!" Woody answered, with frustration in his voice. "He couldn't concentrate anymore!"

Kate sat on the edge of the chair. "But aren't you in charge of the body?" she pressed.

"Yes and no. My frontal lobes make the judgment calls along with the mind. They normally work together in a 'checks and balances' fashion to steer the ship. But something happened the spring of junior year that damaged my frontal lobes, and I lost most of the control over Jeff's mind that I had had." The front of Woody's brain was lit up with activity.

"So the mind was runnin' the show, and you couldn't control it?" Kate asked.

"And it went wild! It took me and the rest of Jeff with it," he said as he started waving his upper extremity nerves in the air. "We no longer cared about the things that had always been the most important to us—like doing well in school and acting like a gentleman and helping out others! We had totally changed." Woody finished and slumped back against his seat. He turned to look directly at Kate.

"And ya wanna know the most concerning thing about it?"

Kate nodded intently.

"We couldn't have cared less about our lack of concern," he said as the electrical storm in his cortex quieted.

"And Jeff never did that before?" Kate asked.

"Never. At first, I thought I had gotten to a stage in life where everything was all wine and roses. We were all having fun. For the first time in Jeff's life, we were using parts of the body that had never been used before. I hadn't realized that the frontal lobes had gotten damaged and that I was acting like a child. It was like flying a fighter jet full throttle, seeing just how high you could go," said Woody as he leaned back in his seat with his upper extremity nerves pulling an imaginary yoke.

"Until?"

Woody turned his cerebrum toward Kate.

"Until someone got hurt," he said, and then sat upright again.

"Who?"

"Jeff's girlfriend." Woody hung his cerebrum while a fire kindled and then raged in his frontal lobes, limbic system, and splanchnic nerves.[34]

"Was it bad?" Kate asked, expecting the worst.

"When you lose control of a fighter jet while going vertical at top speed, the only thing you can hope for is that the crash won't destroy too many lives."

"What was the body count?"

"After his girlfriend broke up with him, Jeff was decimated emotionally. He had been the cause of the crash. The mind was realizing that it was out of control in the actions that it took. He had mistreated friends, but many stood by him, misleading him into believing that he was acting normally. I had no handle on his learning anymore. I assume his girlfriend and her girlfriends had been hurt emotionally as well, but they haven't spoken since."

"So what did ya do to clean up the mess?" Kate asked.

"Well, after realizing that our whole personality had somehow changed, Jeff's mind and I spent a lot of time figuring out how to get things back in order. We—me, GI, Muscles, Bones, Immune, Heart, and Lungs—decided on a stricter regimen. More exercise. More studying. Better eating habits. Less booze. We tried out for the football team."

"What position?" Kate asked, thinking about Tony, the football player she dated in high school.

"Wide receiver."

"How did he do?"

"Crummy. Once we started practicing with the team, I realized something was wrong. Jeff would be running down the field, and when we looked back for the ball, I didn't have good control over his eyes. The ball would bounce in Jeff's vision with each step that he took," Woody said while bobbing his cerebrum up and down. "I couldn't tell the hands where to go to catch the ball. It made Jeff look like a spaz. We never played a down."

"And da grades?"

"I was able to focus better without Jeff having a girlfriend, but I still wasn't me," Woody lamented, turning to look at the rain again. "I had headaches every morning when I woke up and never felt rested. Jeff's mom told us to start taking vitamins. We took them."

"Did they help?"

"A little, but not really," Woody answered, turning back to Kate. "The rest of the body was doing well, but I felt out of it all the time. I just couldn't focus. None of us could pay attention."

"And so what did ya do?"

"I just kept my cortex down and moved on. When we went to business school, we felt like blithering idiots." Woody stared down at his cold coffee.

"So how was the work in business school?" Kate asked, with a voice anticipating more misery.

"Hard as hell. I just felt like every time I tried to learn something, I would forget it. I would start reading a page of text, and then the mind would start wandering." Woody let his cerebrum wobble aimlessly like a bobble head. "I told the eyes to look at the words, which they did. We saw words and sentences, but when we tried to comprehend what they were saying, they would never become a memory because Jeff's mind was thinking about the car that just drove by the window and how it was red like his car was in college and how everyone wanted him to take them to the store and how fun it was when they took road trips to the other college on the west side to go and party, and before I knew it, the eyes had finished the page, and I had no memory or understanding about what we had just read."

"So how did you make it through business school?"

"I don't know."

They sat in silence for a moment, and then Kate spoke.

"And you think Jeff's immune system is the cause."

"Well, I know she made all of the lesions that you can see. The brainstem lesions affected his eye tracking and the coordination of his movements. The swelling that she causes, which you cannot see, does most of the trouble in my frontal lobes. That's what affected Jeff's attention the most."

"But why are you able to concentrate so good now?" she asked, brow furrowed, lips pursed.

"Because when I get out of the confined space of Jeff's skull, the pressure on me is reduced. My frontal lobes, limbic system, hypothalamus, and most of the nerves that have not been directly attacked by the immune system can function again."

"So, it's like you're thinking outside the box, but your box ain't a box, but a skull, right?" Kate synthesized.

"Well said," Woody said.

"So why da heck did she beat you up like dat?" Kate asked as she started to get up.

"I dunno," Woody said as his spinal accessory nerves fired.[35]

"Did you and Jeff treat her right?"

"What do you mean by 'treat her right'?

"Did you give her what she needed—ya know—exercise, vitamins, a good diet?"

"Yeah. At least I thought we did," Woody said, tilting his cerebrum back and forth.

"And you never spoke with her about it before?" she said as she put her pad and pen in her apron.

"Not until now."

Kate looked at the table. "Should I bring another setting?"

"That would be good," Woody said as Kate made her way back to the kitchen. "And a glass of water," he added. "I know she likes water."

"Gotcha," Kate said as she went behind the counter.

Woody turned to look out the window. The rain was constant. The gutters were full with runoff. The street was empty except for some trucks and a taxi. The cab slowed and pulled to a stop in front of the diner. He saw Jeff's immune system paying the cabbie through the sliding window. The door to the cab opened. Sara got out. She was the way he remembered her—before the lesions started. Inviting. Warm. Willing to wrap herself around you and protect you. It had been nice. She opened the front door to the diner. Woody stood.

"Sara," he said, waving some peripheral nerves, motioning for her to join him at the table.

"Hello, Woody," she replied, with minimal inflection in her voice. Her surface was dynamic.

"Like your outfit."

"They had a lot of turnover at the PlasmaHut, so I picked up some extra branes," she said. "No offense."[36]

"None taken," he answered.

She looked robust as she sat down across from Woody. "How have you been?"

"Hard to say," Woody replied. "I have good days and bad."

"Have you seen your doctor?" she asked. Woody paused. He picked up a spoon.

"No," he said in a terse monosyllable. No embellishment. He was waiting.

"So I guess you haven't started any medication yet," she said. Her tone was somewhere between disappointed mother and annoyed witch.

He stared at her. *I wouldn't have to take any medication if it weren't for you,* he thought to himself.

"No," he replied as he added more sugar to his coffee and stirred. Slowly.

"Look," Sara began. "We both know you have MS—"

"What do you mean 'you'?" Woody interrupted. "You know that you're the one that's doing this to me!" His frontal lobes lit up like Times Square. "It's *we*! *We* have MS!"

Sara smiled and extended an adhesion molecule to the menu.[37] "I'm just doing what I do," she answered, without meeting his glare. "I see an antigen. I make an antibody. I phagocytose an antigen.[38] That's my job."

"But why myelin? Why me? I've been with Jeff as long as you have."

"I might not be as smart as you," Sara started, "but I wasn't the one who insisted on keeping to myself during development. Remember when Jeff was a fetus?" she began. "All the other parts of the body were out there for me to meet. I could touch them and remember them. We all became friends."

Said the immunological vamp, Woody thought.

"But you were a real touch-me-not in your ivory tower, surrounded by your tight junction mote. Your blood-brain barrier allowed no one to cross— like a night club bouncer protecting your precious neurons with their cell bodies and axons and myelin." She paused as a smile-shaped, invagination crossed her membrane. "That delicious myelin." Woody saw Sara release some chemokines. He knew he should have gotten a nonsecreting table.

"Why not Pancreas or Thyroid?"

"I have issues with them too, but they don't put up barriers like you do. I like a challenge."

"Barriers! You're putting up the biggest barrier by not realizing that for whatever reason, you went from a normally functioning immune system to Miss I'll-Eat-Any-Antigen-Even-if-I-Destroy-the-Body-I'm-Protecting!"

"That's how I roll," she responded as she pushed a small polypeptide chain away from her surface.[39]

"I know how you roll," replied Woody. "First you roll. Then you diapedese.[40] Then the next thing I know, you're all over my guys like a white blood cell on lice."

"Stop! You're making me hungry. Where's the waitress?"

Woody looked up. Kate had just come out of the kitchen with a glass of water. "Here she comes," Woody said. Kate walked up and placed the water on the table in front of Sara.

"Can I get you anything?" Kate asked Woody as she looked over Sara.

"Just sugar please," Woody responded.

"You want it in normal saline?"[41]

"Yeah. And gimme an amp of D50 on the side.[42] We're gonna be here for a while."

Kate nodded. She turned to Sara. "How about you?"

"I'll just have some omega-3 fatty acids and Echinacea," she replied. Woody's amygdalae lit up.[43]

"You know that you get pumped up on Echinacea, and the stronger you get, the worse it is for me. Right?" he said while staring at Sara. She held his glare. The rain beat against the window. Kate cleared her throat.

"I think you two gotta start listening to each other," Kate started.

Sara twisted to look at Kate. "Who do you think *you* are?" Sara asked indignantly.

"Me?" Kate started, leaning into the table. "I'm the voice of reason, honey. I've been talking with your alleged 'friend' here. He started telling me about your relationship and how it was all wine and roses until your boss, Jeff, starts dating a girl. Suddenly, you become Miss Hannibal-the-Cannibal immune system, and you're all like "O-M-Glycoprotein! I'm here to clean up this place, and I don't care if I throw the myelin out with the mucus!" Sara crenated slightly as Kate waved her hand in front of her.[44] "Then you started whackin' your friend like some kind of cerebral piñata." She stuck her face up against Sara's main food vacuole. "My momma taught me that that's no way to treat someone you love." Woody looked smugly at Sara.

"Meanwhile," Kate continued as she turned to Woody, "Mr. Brainiac here has to realize that yes, while she might be doing the nasty with every Thumb, Dick, and Fanny that she comes across, you're the one who has to get to the doctor and find a way to help both of youse out. It's called communication, and it can solve just about every problem. But what do I know? I'm just a waitress. I'll be back with your food."

Kate went back to the kitchen. Woody and Sara sat in silence. Outside, the rain had lightened up, but the rivers still ran down the window.

"Okay," Sara began. "I have acted a little over the top, but I'm just doing my job. And if I don't do my job, Jeff goes down. Hard. Sepsis isn't pretty for anybody." [45]

"I'm not asking you to stop working entirely. I know you gotta do what you gotta do. But can't you pull back a bit?"

"That's not how I function. It's an all-or-none phenomenon. Like you, with your action potentials."[46]

"Look. You're right. With the action potentials in my nerves, it is an all-or-none phenomenon. That's how nerves are built. We're simple. We turn on. We turn off." Sara stared at Woody and pinocytosed some water.[47] "But you. You're so much more subtle. You have shades and nuances. You can regulate how active you are. I've seen you."

"It's not that easy," Sara said. "My response depends on the situation. What I see very much dictates what I do."

"Yes, but not entirely," Woody said as his processing speed went from high beta to gamma frequency.[48] "They have these medications that help to dampen how aggressively you go after an antigen."

"No. No. No. I'm not going to let you turn me into some kind of gorked-out septic system catching some of Jeff's infectious garbage but missing most of it. I'm a highly skilled system able to detect, locate, and execute invaders," she said. Markers started exocytosing on her membrane.[49]

"No. I'm not talking about suppressing you," Woody pleaded. "They have medications that can modulate your responses."

"I don't like it."

"Look, Jeff takes antibiotics, right?"

"Yeah."

"And they help you to overcome an infection when it gets too big for you to handle on your own. Right?"

"Yeah."

"Well, the medications they have for MS now are still letting you fight, but they help keep you away from hurting me. And you don't want to hurt me, right?"

"Yeah. But why does it always have to be me?"

"Like I said, I'm just a bunch of nerves. We fire. Sodium goes in. Potassium goes out. Game over. You. You're complex. You're more special than that. You've got chemokine messengers. You've got immunoglobulins that adapt and change! You've got a tremendous array of cells! You can show responses anywhere from slight inflammation to frank anaphylaxis! You are special. You're an immune system. You're Jeff's immune system." Kate came back with two Petri dishes and put them down on the table.

"Sugar for the nervous one and omega-3s for the hell ... thy one."

"What about the Echinacea?"

"We're out. I added some vitamin C and cranberry juice instead," Kate said with authority. "It'll help you to keep Jeff free from urinary tract infections without getting you so pumped up you start playing another round of Wak-a-Lobe with your date." She looked at the two systems at the table. "How are things going? Did ya make any progress?"

"Better," Woody answered. "We started talking."

"That's a start. Would you like anything else for now because my shift is about to end and I wanted to close out your tab." Woody and Sara looked at each other. Sara motioned no.

"I think we're good. We'll take the check."

Kate reached into her apron, ripped off the bill, and laid it on the table.

"It's been a pleasure," she said, and walked to the kitchen, pulling the tie on her apron loose and disappearing through the doors. Woody took a deep breath.

"She made sense," Sara said.

"She was nice," Woody said, nodding as he took out his cell phone.

"Should we make an appointment with the doctor?"

"Not yet. In a little while. I just need some time ..."

Woody put his phone away and turned to the window. The rain had stopped, and people were out on the street again. He saw a door to the side of the diner open, and Kate went out wearing a blue overcoat and a wide-brim rain hat. She carried a closed umbrella in one hand and a burgundy purse in the other. She looked up and then down the street and stepped onto the sidewalk. She immediately mixed in with the other people and was gone.

"She is a wise lady," Woody said.

"Did you see the psoriasis she had?" Sara asked.

Woody turned back to look at Sara. "No. Where?"

"On the back of her arm. Above the elbow."

Woody swung his cortex back and forth. "Why didn't you go after Jeff's skin?" he asked.

"Maybe I will," she said.

Woody saw some antibodies appear on her surface. She started rearranging some of the variable regions on the new antibodies.[50]

"I don't remember seeing you with those before," Woody commented. Another indentation ran across Sara's membrane.

"Sometimes I wonder which of us has the better memory," she said as she began to actively transport some fatty acids from her Petri dish. Woody helped some glucose to diffuse across his membranes.[51]

"As long as we both remember that our goal is to keep Jeff going, it doesn't matter who has the better memory. Right?"

"You never can lose, can you?" Sara insisted.

I can and I do, thought Woody. *I just don't like it.*

They sat in silence while they finished their plates. After a few moments, a young man walked up to the table.

"Are you two done?" he asked, with a big smile. Sara and Woody looked at each other and then the back at the waiter.

"Yeah," Woody said.

"Is it okay if I clear up the table for you?" he asked energetically.

"Sure," Woody said. "We just want to talk for a few more minutes."

"Great!" he answered, becoming happier and bouncier with ever word. "I want to make you folks happy."

Woody looked at the boy. "Do you know Kate very well?" he asked.

The rosy-cheeked boy smiled. "Sure do. My wife and I were having troubles. She sat down with us one day and lectured us about communication."

"Did it work?" Sara asked.

The boy scratched his chin and thought. "It was hard at first," he started, "but after a while, we realized some things."

"Such as?" Sara asked.

"Well, number one, if we were going to be able to communicate with each other, first we needed to learn *how* to communicate with each other."

"What does that mean?" Woody asked as his medial temporal lobe and angular gyrus started firing.[52]

"The first thing we learned was that we had to listen to each other. Second, we learned that nothing should be assumed. No one can read any one else's thoughts. We had to let the other know what each of us was thinking."

"I'm sending messages out all the time, but I don't hear any answers coming," Sara said with a shrug.

"I send out signals all the time too!" Woody replied. "I've got stress hormones running amok, trying to dampen what you're doing to Jeff!"

"That's why we keep sending out more inflammatory cells! We think Jeff is under attack!"

The boy paused and thought, thinking back on his own experience. He nodded to himself. "It sounds like you're not even talking the same language," he began. Sara and Woody looked at each other. "How can you expect to communicate if you don't understand what the other person's words mean?" They shrugged. The boy looked at Woody. "You're a nervous system, right?"

"Yeah."

Then he looked at Sara. "You're a monocyte, right?"

"Close," Sara said, blushing. "I'm a macrophage. My mom was a monocyte."

"I knew you were from the myeloid family," the boy continued. "I could tell from your pseudopodia."

"Excuse me ..." Woody interrupted.

"Oh, sorry," the boy apologized, smiling impishly. "Well, you speak different languages. You're all electrical impulses," he said, pointing at Woody. "And you're all chemokines," he said, glancing at Sara. "If you two are going to have a real dialogue, you need to see a doctor that specializes in your disease—like a neurologist." They looked at the boy and each other. "You two have MS, right?" Sara and Woody nodded. The boy had a big grin on his face. "I could tell. You have marks all over your brain and spinal cord, but your peripheral nerves are clean."

Woody looked at the boy's nametag. It said Babe.

"Well, Babe. How is a neurologist different from a regular doctor?" Woody asked.

"Well, all doctors know something about every part of the body. Neurologists focus on the nervous system."

"Okay, so we need to see a neurologist," Sara said.

"Yes, but make sure he or she specializes in MS," he continued. "They've discovered so much that you want to make sure you find someone who knows what he or she is talking about."

"You seem to know a lot for a busboy," Sara commented, looking at the happy young man.

"Thanks," Babe said, his smile growing bigger. "My wife and I do a lot of reading. And listening. And talking. But mostly listening. That's how we learn."

"Hey! Inski!" a tall, dark-haired man shouted from the other end of the diner. "Geddovaheah! Ya gotta mop the back room before the dinner crowd starts comin'!"

"Right away, Mr. Sharko!" Babe shouted back. "Listen," he said, turning back to Woody and Sara. "I gotta run. I'm sure once you find a good MS doctor, things will start to get better for you," Babe said as he gathered up the dishes. "But the thing to remember is what Kate taught my wife and me," he said, placing the coffee cup on the plates and backing away from the table. "Listening to a person is so much more important than talking." He nodded, turned, and scurried through the kitchen door.

Sara and Woody looked at each other.

"He was interesting," Woody said.

"He made sense," Sara concluded.

"Just like Kate," Woody added. Sara took out her cell phone and opened her browser.

"I'll start checking out some MS doctors if you pick up the bill," Sara offered.

Woody nodded his cortex. "You got it," he said as he reached for his wallet.

Sara noticed that Woody's limbic system was lighting up. "What are you feeling?" she asked.

"Well, for the first time in a long while, I think I'm feeling some hope that the two of us might be able to make things work out okay."

Sara nodded.

"I know a quiet club nearby," Woody offered. "Serabella's Cellar. They let in all types. Ya wanna go?"

"And do what?" Sara's voice had lost its edge.

"Listen?"

"To each other?" Sara asked.

"And maybe get to a better level of understanding. Jeff has a few more hours under anesthesia," Woody said as he left a twenty on the table and picked up his umbrella. "Listening should be good," he said as he stood.

Sara smiled as she slid out of the booth, smoothed her brane, and walked with Woody, closely, to the door.

Fin.

---

[28] The superficial peroneal nerve travels down the lateral (outside) aspect of the shin.

[29] The median, radial, and ulnar nerves innervate the arms and hands.

[30] The median nerve carries sensation from the palmar surface of the thumb, index, and middle fingers.

[31] The lower parts of the sides of the brain, called the *temporal lobes*, are where memories are stored.

[32] The posterior pituitary releases a hormone called *oxytocin*, which is intimately related with the feeling of love and is located in the middle of the brain, closer to the front than the back.

[33] The right parietal region of the cortex deals with spatial relationships.

[34] The limbic system handles emotions, and the splanchnic nerves innervate the gut.

[35] The spinal accessory nerve innervates the sternocleidomastoideus and trapezius muscles, which shrug the shoulders.

[36] The skin of a cell is called a membrane. Sometimes, when cells are speaking to other cells, they abbreviate *membrane* as *branes*. This can sometimes offend certain cells, specifically in the brain—especially the cells that are in charge of helping the mind form the *ego*.

[37] Adhesion molecules allow cells to bind to other cells (and menus).

[38] Phagocytosis is how certain immune cells move molecules, like an antigen, into themselves to be digested.

[39] A polypeptide chain is a chain of amino acids that are thin and long, like a strand of hair.

[40] Cells in the immune system are very pliable. They can squeeze between cells that are not joined by tight junctions. When a WBC squeezes between cells to move from one space in to another, it is called *diapedesis*.

[41] Normal saline is what dextrose (sugar) is diluted in when given to a person who cannot take sugar by mouth.

[42] D50 is 50 percent dextrose. Basically, it is like a shot glass of sugar.

[43] The amygdala (pl. amygdalae) is part of the limbic system. The limbic system is the part of the brain that mediates emotions, aside from having other important roles.

[44] When a cell crenates, it shrinks.

[45] Sepsis is when an infection in a person gets out of control and cannot be handled by the immune system by itself. It usually requires intravenous antibiotics and is quite often fatal.

[46] An action potential is an electrical potential generated in the cell body of the nerve that causes the electrical impulse to travel along the nerve cell membrane.

[47] Pinocytosis is how a cell ingests fluid.

[48] Beta frequency is the frequency range the brain works at during waking consciousness. Gamma frequency is 30–100hz and is the frequency attained in multidomain processing when sensory input (sights, sounds, etc.) are integrated with other spheres of cognition like memory and spatial relationships.

[49] Exocytosis is when a cell releases intracellular contents (fluid or proteins) that can either stay on the cell surface or be expelled into the extracellular space.

[50] Variable regions are the part of the antibody that can get rearranged and produce a new antibody to attack new invaders.

[51] Active transport and diffusion are other ways cells can move things into and out of the cell body.

[52] The medial temporal lobe and angular gyrus are some of the parts of the brain used in understanding speech.

Sixth

THE NEUROLOGICAL EXAMINATION FROM A NEUROLOGICAL POINT OF VIEW

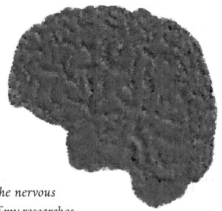

I have selected the study of diseases of the nervous system for the object of my life and goal of my researches.
—Moritz Heinrich Romberg,
neurologist
(1795–1873)

Now just relax while I hit you with this hammer.
—Vince Macaluso,
neurologist
(1968–until I forget my anniversary)

Almost all of us humans have been going to see doctors ever since we were little kids. Our first doctor is usually our pediatrician. As we get a little older, we meet the dentist and then the eye doctor if we have trouble seeing the blackboard in school. For young women, they usually see a gynecologist for the first time in their early teens. Once we are adults, we need to see our primary care doctor. For those who are in good health and are lucky, their primary care doctor could be the last doctor they have. However, this is not the case for the vast majority of people. When it comes to the world of multiple sclerosis, the neurologist is called into action. When a person has a new onset of symptoms like tingling, dizziness, visual difficulties, urinary urgency, trouble with coordination, weakness, or anything that is weird feeling, they might see their primary care doctor,

GYN, or eye doctor first. If any of those doctors see findings consistent with possible MS, a call is made to the bullpen, and the neurologist starts warming up.

Since people don't usually meet a neurologist until some trouble starts brewing, the word that reflexively follows "neurologist" in most people's minds is "uh-oh." This is a normal response because most people do not know exactly what a neurologist does. They know it has something to do with nerves or the brain, but that's about it. A person usually does not see his or her nerves and hopefully never sees his or her spinal cord or brain, so when the topic of a neurologist comes up, there's bound to be some anxiety. What follows is an explanation of what a neurologist does at an office or hospital visit with a patient. The "… from the Other Side of the Desk" half of this chapter-couplet is based on my experience in learning, as a patient, what a neurologist does.

NEUROLOGY

Neurology is a fascinating specialty of medicine. It deals with the entire nervous system. When you go to see a neurologist for a neurological problem, the experience can be different from what you have experienced at the doctor's office before. At first, it seems the same. The receptionist gives you paperwork to fill out, and then you wait for a while until she puts it into the computer system. Then you're taken into the doctor's office or the doctor comes out to meet you. When you get into the office, the first thing the doctor needs to do is get your history. This includes finding out the following:

- ➤ why you came in for the visit
- ➤ how long you have had your problem
- ➤ what makes your problem better or worse
- ➤ what other medical issues you have
- ➤ what medications you are on
- ➤ if you have had any surgeries
- ➤ if you have any allergies
- ➤ if you take any medications (including vitamins, minerals, herbs, or anything else you put into your body on a regular basis)
- ➤ if you smoke or have ever smoked

> ➤ if you use or have ever used any other drugs (including alcohol)
> ➤ what your family situation is
> ➤ if your family members have any chronic disease
> ➤ if you are married, single, separated, divorced, living with someone, or living alone
> ➤ if you have any kids
> ➤ what your work status is (student, firefighter, horse whisperer, unemployed, etc.)

The next part of your visit will be the neurological exam. It is a screening exam of the entire nervous system. The exam allows a neurologist to detect almost any abnormalities in the nervous system. Based upon your history and physical findings, the neurologist can then order tests to help in making a final diagnosis of what ails you.

Before starting the neurological exam, however, the neurologist might also examine the heart, lungs, and abdomen and then take a look at and feel (palpate) the arms and legs. This is a screen to look for any other signs of systemic disease that could affect the nervous system. If a person mentions anything specific during the history, a little more time is spent looking at that area (e.g., looking in a patient's ears with an otoscope if he or she has any balance or hearing troubles).

THE NEUROLOGICAL EXAM

Traditionally, the neurological exam[53] is divided into eight parts, but it is not always split up this way.[54] The parts include the following:

1. Mental status
2. Cranial nerves
3. Motor system
4. Reflexes
5. Station
6. Gait
7. Coordination
8. Sensation

MENTAL STATUS

This is a screening test to look at how a person is thinking, feeling, and speaking. It evaluates how he or she views their relationship with the world around them. While each doctor has his or her own questions, the goal is to see if there are any areas of cognition that are grossly abnormal. It begins as soon as we meet a new patient. We take note of the person's appearance. Are they neat? Well groomed? Disheveled? Odiferous? We notice what the person's speech is like. Is it clear or is it dysarthric?[55] Is the speech logical or does he or she make comments that do not follow reason ("My cat threw up all over my living room so I had to get my car painted a different color.")? Does he or she have normal volume in their voice? What about the prosody (rhythm and intonation) of the speech? How does he or she appear? Alert? Sluggish? Happy?

Then we start asking questions as a screen of cognitive functioning. The questions are geared to look at the major areas involved in cognition, which include the following:

- abstract thinking
- attention
- calculation
- comprehension
- expressive language
- judgment
- memory—both remote and recent
- naming of objects and colors
- orientation
- repetition

Some of the questions involve having the patient do certain tasks (the cognitive sphere being tested is in parentheses):

➢ Starting with the number one, add three and keep on adding three (e.g., "one, four, seven …") until I stop you. (calculation, attention)
➢ Touch your left ear with your right hand. (left/right confusion)
➢ Repeat after me, "Around the rugged rock, the ragged rascal ran." (repetition, bucco-oral coordination)

> ➤ The patient is shown how to alternately hit the front, then the back of their hand on the exam table. He or she is then told to do it. If he or she can do that, then the patient is shown how to hit the palm, then fist, then back of the hand on the table, about five or six times.[56] (attention, memory)
> ➤ Spontaneous word production is tested by asking him or her to say as many words as he or she can think of starting with the letter F in one minute. (frontal lobe function)

If we have any concerns about cognition, we proceed with more neurocognitive testing as indicated.

CRANIAL NERVES

The cranial nerves are the nerves that control the muscles in the head, face, and neck. There are twelve of them. When we are in medical school, we commonly use the mnemonic "On Old Olympus's Towering Top, A Finn And German Viewed Some Hops" to memorize the names of the nerves. [57] Tables 2 and 3 list the twelve cranial nerves. It tells the general function of each nerve and also shows how each nerve is tested during a neurological examination. Each doctor performs cranial nerve testing according to how she or he learned the exam during their training, so your experience might differ from the testing listed in tables 2 and 3.

MOTOR

In this part of the exam, the doctor is looking to evaluate the system that does the work when you move—the motor system. First, we look at the general structure and development of your muscles. We palpate the muscles to pick up spasms (which feel hard) or flaccidity (which feel mushy) and look for fasciculations.[58] We will also move your arms and legs around to see if everything moves freely. Then we start testing your strength. We ask you to push and pull against us in a number of different muscle groups. Usually the deltoids, biceps, triceps, wrist extensors, wrist flexors, and hand muscles are tested in the upper extremities. In the lower extremities, we test the iliopsoas, quadriceps, hamstrings, gastrocnemius, anterior tibialis, and the extensor hallucis longus muscles. Depending upon what problem or problems you came in for, other muscle groups might be tested. The strength of each muscle group gets a score according to a defined scale as shown in table 4.

Table 2. Function and testing of cranial nerves I–V.

Cranial Nerve	Name	Function	Testing
I	Olfactory	Smell	Hold coffee grounds or mint under nose and ask what the patient smells
II	Optic	Vision	Check visual acuity with vision chart, check peripheral vision; look into the patient's eye with fundoscope to look at the head of the optic nerve and check pupillary functioning
III	Oculomotor	Helps to control movement of the eyes by innervating 4 of the 6 extraocular muscles; also involved in eyelid opening and pupillary functioning	Have patient follow finger in all directions (up, down, left, right) looking at how the eyes move; shine light in eyes to evaluate pupillary function
IV	Trochlear	Helps to control Movement of the eyes by innervating 1 of the 6 extraocular muscles	Have patient follow finger in all directions (up, down, left, right) looking at how the eyes move
V	Trigeminal	Does sensation over face. It is also the sensory part of corneal reflex and helps with jaw movement	Test pinprick and touch over all parts of face to see if sensation is the same between each division of the nerve or between the sides of face

Table 3. Function and testing of cranial nerves VI–XII.

Cranial Nerve	Name	Function	Testing
VI	Abducens	Helps to control movement of the eyes by innervating 1 of the 6 extra-ocular muscles	Have patient follow finger in all directions (up, down, left, right) looking at how the eyes move
VII	Facial	Facial movements and taste from the anterior 2/3 of the tongue	Have patient smile and wrinkle forehead then have the patient taste salty or sugar water on the front of tongue
VIII	Vestibulo-cochlear	Balance and hearing	Have patient close eyes while the doctor rubs fingers together near each ear and then asks the patient if it sounded the same in both ears
IX	Glosso-pharyngeal	Taste from the back of the tongue, gag reflex, salivation and speech	Have the patient taste salty or sugar water on back of tongue; have patient say "Ahhh' and then gag them with a tongue depressor
X	Vagus	Motor, sensory and autonomic functions of viscera (gut, heart rate, glands)	Have the patient say 'Ahhh' and then gag them with a tongue depressor
XI	Spinal accesory	Shrug shoulders and turn head	Have patient shrug shoulders and then turn head against resistance
XII	Hypoglossal	Moves the tongue	Have patient stick out tongue

Table 4. Motor system grading.

Grade	Action
0	No movement of the muscle at all
1	A twitch or flicker that you can see in the muscle group but no movement of the joint
2	When the muscle can move the joint through space but not against gravity
3	When the muscle can move the joint through the full range of motion against gravity
4	When the muscle can move the joint through the full range of motion against gravity plus added resistance but is not full strength
5	When the muscle demonstrates full strength

REFLEXES

Remember when you were a child and you went to your pediatrician and he or she would tap on your knees with that little, orange hammer? Well, we neurologists are different. Our hammers are more elaborate and have names like Queen's Square Reflex Hammer, Babinski-Buck Hammer, Dejerine Hammer, and Troemner Hammer. Most are big and impressive. Some are shiny and have our names engraved on them. We often proudly display them by threading them through the buttonholes on our lab coats. Part of our

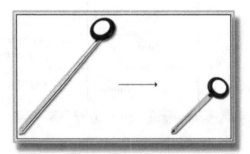

Figure 8. Neurology reflex hammer.
This high-tech, overpriced neuro hammer can be collapsed to less than half its original length, allowing neurologists to carry it in their pockets for use at a moment's notice.

training is learning how to subdue most types of bears armed with nothing except our neuro hammer and a winning smile.[59]

That having been said, neurologists are a highly skilled group of individuals who know the exact technique for hitting people with hammers and causing the least amount of discomfort possible. Most importantly, however, is that the information we get from a patient's reflexes (or lack thereof) is often the most useful part of the entire exam. Reflexes do not lie. Reflexes can be a huge help in figuring out where in the nervous system the lesion is located.

There is also a grading system for reflexes, but the scoring is a little more subjective:

Table 5. Reflex grading.

Grade	Action
0	No muscle contraction noted
1	You can feel the muscle twitch but you can't see the extremity move
2	"Normal" movement of the extremity
3	Increased movement noted
4	Clonus – when the movement continues with alternation between contraction and relaxation, ranging from several "beats" to "sustained" where the reflex will not stop until all stretch is taken off the tested muscle group

STATION

After getting hammered, we then invite you to stand.[60] First, we note the way you get to a standing position. We look at your posture and how far apart your feet are placed. Of course, not all patients can stand, but if at all possible, we will try to see how much weight a person can support on his or her legs.

If you can stand on your own, then we see how well you can do when you stand with your feet together and your eyes closed. If you start to fall over, someone *will* catch you. If you cannot remain standing with your eyes closed on a narrow base, it is called Romberg's sign.[61] There are several things that go into standing:

1. Visual cues letting you know where you are in space
2. Input from your legs letting your cerebellum know where the ground is
3. The balance center in your brainstem/cerebellum

Two of these things need to work to keep you standing. By having you stand with your legs together (thereby narrowing your base and limiting the input from your legs) and then taking away vision by having you close your eyes, we have stressed the system. If you fall, it could indicate trouble with any of the systems listed above.

Gait

Next thing in the exam is checking how you walk. We ask that you walk back and forth several times in the exam room. We note how high you lift your legs with each stride (called *clearance*). We look to see if you plant your heel first and then roll to the front of your foot and then push off well with your toes. We look to see if your feet are in line with the stride or if you swing one or both legs around with each step. We look to see if the hips are stable or if there is any hip-drop. We also watch to see if there is good arm swing.

We then ask patients to walk a little on their heels and then their toes. Then we ask the patient to walk with one foot in front of the other, touching heel to toe. This is called *tandem walking*.

Coordination

In this part, neurologists want to see if the patient can make coordinated, smooth movements. We put our finger up and then say, "Touch your nose with your finger, then touch my finger, and then touch your nose again." After the patient touches the examiner's finger, the examiner moves the finger to a different spot. After the patient touches his or her nose, he or she has to reach out to touch the finger again in the new spot. We do this three of four times depending upon how the patient's arm, hand, and finger are moving. We look to see if everything travels smoothly or takes a shaky path to get to the endpoint (ataxia) and then see if it hits the finger precisely or misses it (dysmetria).

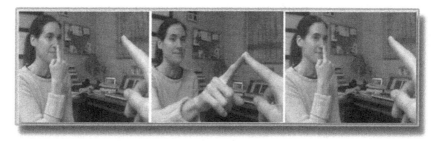

Figure 9. Finger-to-nose testing.

We then test coordination in the legs. We do this by having the patient take the heel of one foot and place it against the knee of the other leg. Then we have the patient run the heel down the shin to the foot and then slide it back up. We look to see if the heel stays on the shin and if it stops when it gets to the foot.

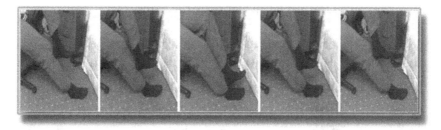

Figure 10. Heel-to-shin testing.

SENSATION

In this part of the examination, we test out the different modalities of sensation. Primary modalities include light touch, pinprick, vibration, and joint position sense. They are primary because they are exactly what you are feeling. We lightly stroke the skin over your hands and feet for light touch. We poke you with something sharp (like a safety pin) for pinprick. We place a tuning fork on your fingers and toes to see if you can feel vibration. We have you close your eyes and then move a finger or toe up or down to see if you can tell which way it was moved.

There are also tests for things called *secondary modalities*. These are primary modality sensations which then get interpreted by your brain to figure out what you are feeling. The secondary modalities include the following:

- Stereognosia. With the patient's eyes closed, a three-dimensional object (like a coin) is placed in the patient's hand, and he or she has to figure out what it is.
- Extinction. With the patient's eyes closed, the examiner touches one part of the patient's leg and then asks the patient to open his or her eyes and point to where he or she was just touched. The patient is asked to close his or her eyes again, and this time the examiner touches two different areas on the patient's legs at the same time. The patient is then asked to open his or her eyes and show where he or she was touched. If he or she points to both places that were touched, that is normal. If he or she only points to one place, then extinction is said to be present.
- Graphesthesia. With the patient's eyes closed, the examiner traces a letter or number on the palm of the patient's hand, and then the patient has to say what was written. N.B.—make sure that you leave the cap on the pen when you write the letter.

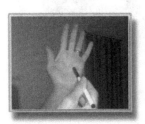

Figure 11. Correct way to test graphesthesia.

Figure 12. Incorrect way to test graphesthesia.

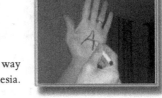

Based on what your doctor finds out about you and your nervous system during your office visit, he or she might order various tests to confirm or deny what he or she thinks is going on. The doctor might also start treating you with various therapies or drugs. The most important part (I believe) is explaining what was found and teaching what those findings mean for you. A full neurological exam takes a long time to complete. Every doctor has her or his own version of the exam. The first time you go to see a neurologist, the exam is longer because more data is needed to reach a diagnosis. When you go for follow-up, the exam can be more focused on the specific condition being treated.

SUMMARY

The nervous system is extremely complex. The neurological exam appears weird if you do not understand what is going on.

If you have any questions about what your doctor is doing, you should ask your doctor about it.

PERSONAL NOTE ABOUT THE NEUROLOGICAL EXAM

When I first learned the neurological exam in medical school, I found it to be fascinating. Knowledge, logic, and reasoning are needed to solve the problems of: 1) what the trouble is; 2) where the trouble is; 3) what's causing the trouble; 4) why the trouble showed up now; and 5) how I can help a person get through the trouble.

I know one of the reasons I decided to go into neurology was because of the thinking required to solve each mystery that each neurological patient presented. I have enjoyed reading mystery novels since the age of ten. I started with the Hardy Boys and then went to Agatha Christie's Hercule Poirot and Edgar Allen Poe.[62, 63] During the summertime, my favorite show was the 1984 TV series *The Adventures of Sherlock Holmes,* produced by Grenada Television. It starred Jeremy Brett as Holmes and David Burke (followed by Edward Hardwicke) as Watson. This was a turning point in my life. Sherlock Holmes fascinated me. With a paucity of information, he was able to build an explanation for what had led to the crime and, just as importantly, who did it.

The Holmes character defined how I pursued knowledge from that point on. Brett's interpretation of the Holmes character validated my quiet, often solo, early teen years. He would show consternation when opinion collided with fact. He would remand himself from a situation so he could allow his thoughts to flow freely and interconnect in the most logical way possible. He would show a brilliantly enlightened visage, for a fraction of a second, after hearing or finding a fact that allowed a conclusion to be drawn. This would be followed by rapid eye movements, fine twitches at the corners of his mouth, and an appropriate but perfunctory expression of gratitude for whoever had offered up a crumb of information from which he could then create a cake. It was then I learned that listening carefully and thinking fast were things to be admired. Every little thing counted.

In high school, I took an elective in English that dealt with the evolution of the mystery novel.[64] The course concluded with us reading Robert B. Parker's stories about his detective, Spenser.[65] His detectives were social creatures who always had a sarcastic bite. His books were light with dialogue and kept things moving. It was one of my getaways from the harsh lifestyles of med school and residency. However, as my medical experience increased and I realized that I had to think again (as I had been taught in high school), I found myself reverting to my original love, Sherlock Holmes. Holmes is the pinnacle of sleuthing. Holmes is brilliant. He has a vast knowledge of almost all things, and what he doesn't know, he looks up as needed. When presented with a new case, he does two things. First, he listens to the facts as presented. Second, while he is listening, he is acquiring more information. Why is the person coming to me now? How is he or she dressed? What is their mood? Why is there discoloration of the shoe on the left and not the right? These are the primary clues—plain only to those who observe them.

The greatest similarity between Holmes and a neurologist, however, is seen in the one case where Holmes was not the first to solve the case. Irene Adler, in *A Scandal in Bohemia*, outwitted Holmes. Without giving away the ending, Irene figured out Holmes's plan to obtain a certain picture that she had in her possession. When Holmes arrived to make his move and solve the case, he wound up not with what he was looking for, but only with a picture of Irene and a note. The note let him know she had been one step ahead of him and that no trouble would come to his client. While Holmes is pompous, he remained cerebral. He decided to keep the picture—not for romantic reasons, but as a tribute to the one woman whose intelligence, for that moment, rose above his. He knew when he had been beaten and, equally important, what he could learn from it. For the neurologist, disease is our Irene Adler. The crime and situation can look the same as those before. We listen and notice. We have "Ah-ha!" moments when the pieces fall into place. We do our studies and start our treatments. It might appear as if the solution has been made manifest. Often, success is ours.

However, the person, the body, and the disease dictate the rules, and they might be, at any moment, one step ahead. And sometimes, just like Sherlock, when we thought the match was ours, we are left holding not the winner's cup, but instead a picture of Irene.

The following is a poem about a patient who had a rapidly progressive course of a disease that initially appeared to be MS but then turned out to be something much more aggressive and eventually fatal.

BEAUTIFUL N.

N. wanted to be beautiful like everybody else.
She tried doing it like *everybody* did in her small town.
In her small country. But no one told her that she might die.
Because no one has ever proven that silicone kills.

Sure there were cases of some people who got sick,
but so many people get it done, and no one really died.
And the data are poor and often inconclusive,
so it is mostly safe, and hardly anyone ever gets hurt.

There was another friend's friend who became depressed
after getting the silicone injections, but she was already depressed,
wasn't she? Yes, depressed, so the depression
must have killed her more than the silicone did.

And sure you might have heard about someone
whose implant ruptured, and they hardly ever rupture.
But, you know, when they tried to replace it,
her body rejected it like a properly vaccinated child does the measles.

But N. was different because she got only a little sick after
the first round of injections. Like with a flu shot.
But her money ran out and another round of injections,
later on, would be needed to make her beauty complete.

And so I asked her sister at her third hospital stay,
Was her walk kind of funny before the injections?
Because maybe she had the MS before
she had any silicone invade her body at all.

No, you say?
And she did not have any abnormal speech either?
Not until a few months after the second round of silicone, you say?
Hmmm …

Yes, her first MRI looked exactly like MS
with Dawson and his fingers.
And enhancing ring lesions.
Both open and closed.

You say she responded to the steroids the first time,
but not completely.
Yes, that can happen in MS.
And many things that look like MS aren't.

And the second relapse?
She went downhill with zero response to steroids.
Yes, that also happens in MS.
But how many times must a zebra smile before we realize it is not a horse?

So now she comes a third time.
Her lesions have spread like Vulcan's flames.
Let's try plasma exchange.
She does well. Curious. Off to rehab then.

Discharged from rehab—indeed!
Outpatient exchanges—two.
She was very good at follow-up. Almost perfect, in fact.
Put that one in the left-hand column. Well done!

R-r-r-ring.

Hello?
You say now she's staggering? Delirious?
Eight weeks since her last exchange?
Another relapse already? Bring her in.
I think Irene just called.

Doctor.
She's here.
In a wheelchair.
With her sister.

She just moans? All day? Since last week?
Her left leg is in extensor spasm. She can't talk.
She moans. And stops. Then moans again.
Admit her.

In the hospital, her desperate, rhythmic wailing fills the halls.
Doctor, the other patients can't sleep, her vitals are good,
and she has no symptoms of pain, but the moans won't stop.
Nurse, please start steroids and this opiate, now and around the clock.

You're her aunt? And her brother?
And her cousins? A pleasure to meet you all.
You take shifts with her so she's never alone?
Families and their love is some of the best medicine.

You say she can still drink the supplement
when you put the straw in her mouth.
Excellent!
She's lucky to have such a supportive family!

No, I'm not giving up!
"The harder you work, the harder it is to surrender."
Yeah, my name is Vince too.
I'm hitting with everything I've got.

I pull into the hospital. Four o'clock. Every morning.
What day is it? They all begin to become the same.
I hear her and then see her.
Her cries tear through the frustrated wasteland of my mind.

Doctor, now her entire left side is out.
What else do you want to give to stop that horrible sound?
Nurse, is that the right question?
That's the only thing that lets me know that the clock is still going!

79

Change the steroids. The lesions grew.
Exchange the plasma. The cries continued.
Try IVIG. The good leg went down.
Give her the poisons and tell her immune system to *go away!*

But she did not get better—just quieter.
The EEG showed chaos, and the head CT the same.
The spots that appeared to be MS last year had grown
and destroyed everything in their way.

Does MS usually kill in eighteen months?
No.
So what did she have?
I don't know.

Perhaps, with some samples,
we can discover if antibodies had formed
to the injections she had had
in the pursuit of some material beauty.

But why, Doctor?

So that maybe the singular life of Beautiful N.
can be a story that lets others see
that one's beauty cannot be seen,
but instead
manifests as benevolence
that is shared with another.

---

[53] Doctors learn the neurological exam during medical school. If they become neurologists, they celebrate the length and intricacies of it each time they meet a new patient. Over time, we, as neurologists, develop our own version of this exam that we learn from both textbooks and our dedicated teachers. For those who are interested in learning more about it, I would recommend: B. M. Patten, Source Department of Neurology, Baylor College of Medicine, Houston, Texas 77030, USA, "The history of the neurological examination. Part 1: ancient and pre-modern history—3000 BC to AD 1850," *Journal of the History of the Neurosciences* 1, no. 1 (January 1992): 3–14.

[54] Here is a great website that has a great description/demonstration of the neurological exam: http://edinfo.med.nyu.edu/courseware/neurosurgery/.

[55] Dysarthric speech is speech that is difficult to understand because the distinct sounds of the words are not being formed properly.

[56] These are called the *two and three step Luria maneuvers*, and they test frontal lobe functioning.

[57] The **A** stands for Auditory nerve since the eighth cranial nerve mediates the sensation of hearing. However, it also plays a crucial role in the carrying fibers from the cochlea (part of the inner ear), which mediates balance. Because of this, the proper name of the eighth cranial nerve is the Vestibulocochlear nerve.

[58] Fasciculations are twitches of the muscle fibers near the surface of the skin that can sometimes be seen or felt.

[59] Most residency programs offer training in handling brown, black (both American and Asiatic), giant panda, sloth, sun, and polar bears. For your more exotic bears (e.g., your Qinling panda, spectacled, and grizzly-polar bear hybrid) you're gonna wanna do a two-year fellowship at one of your more "bear-focused" university programs such as Cornell, Brown, and Kutztown University of Pennsylvania. For post-fellowship training, the most revered, and only program is at Leningrad Politeknika in Russia. Go polar bears! When choosing a fellowship program, however, one must be careful. Programs claiming to have courses in koala bear warfare are scams. This is because 1) koalas are not bears, they are arboreal marsupials and 2) there has never been a documented instance where a koala "bear" was able to be subdued using a neurohammer. Reports that Dr. Cöktöestensengen, from the Phlegmenspüten Clinic in Håågendasenseyesenkremen, Norway have been proven to be false after his daughter, Möõñênstâren, reported that her father, after having gone barënhoppën had in fact returned home and pummeled her Paddington Bear doll beyond all recognition with a soup spoon.

[60] Neurology humor.

[61] Moritz Heinrich Romberg, neurologist (1795–1873).

[62] Christie, via Poirot in *The Mysterious Affair at Styles*, introduced me to "These little gray cells," (i.e., the neurons of the brain) that could solve mysteries.

[63] My eighth-grade English teacher, Mr. Roger Vose, set upon my class the absurdly brilliant works of Edgar Allen Poe. Of all Poe's works, *The Purloined Letter* was the one that left its calling card in my memory. It taught me that sometimes the hardest thing to see is that which is sitting right in front of your face.

[64] Mr. Robert Sabatelli taught this course and was one of the many teachers at Regis High School who made me think. I believe this is the greatest gift a student can receive from a teacher. Mr. Sabatelli's passion was history, but he used the same immersive approach when teaching about the mystery genre. His course began with Poe and Holmes, touched on Émile Gaboriau's *Monsieur Lecoq*, and then went through Dashiell Hammett (*The Maltese Falcon*), Raymond Chandler (*Farewell My Lovely*), Ira Levin (*A Kiss Before Dying*), and John le Carré (*The Spy Who Came in from The Cold*). We concluded with Robert B. Parker's detective, Spenser, in *God Save the Child*. The crux of the class focused on how the basic elements (problem, presentation of clues, red herrings, discovery,

gathering together of main characters for the *j'accuse* moment and resolution) remained constant but how the specifics changed with the culture and time period. At the time (being a student in an all-boys high school), I did not like the detectives that came after the 1960s. Those detectives were spending way too much time talking with other people (including women) and not spending enough time obtaining facts! It was not until I had had my first real girlfriend that I realized that talking with others and exchanging ideas was the essence of being human.

[65] Since the conclusion of the course in 1985, I wound up reading every novel written by Robert B. Parker.

Seventh

The Neurological Examination from the Other Side of the Desk

For this "...from the Other Side of the Desk" section, there are two parts. The first part is an example of what a neurological exam is like from the points of view of a patient named Pat, Pat's parents, and a doctor. While the exam follows the form of a real neurological exam, the characters' thoughts and words, while being based on many doctors, patients, and families that I have worked with, are completely fabricated—especially when the doctor thinks that he could have been a stand-up comedian.

The second part is an entirely different story. It is about a patient, Mike, who like me was treated in a most inhospitable fashion by not just one, but two alleged experts in the field of MS. I have tempered Mike's remarks substantially for several reasons but mainly because I try to see the good in all people. If I have a negative encounter with someone, I try to assume that they were having a bad day. Unfortunately, I came to learn that for one of the doctors, what happened was his usual modus operandi. The other doctor was older, and I think he was just trying to run out the clock on his career at the hospital where he worked. It taught me that every person who comes to me for treatment deserves to be treated first as a fellow human being and then as a person who is looking for help from a neurologist. If I ever start feeling otherwise, I have promised myself to hang up my stethoscope and walk away.

NEUROLOGICAL EXAM IN THE ROUND

The following scene takes place in the doctor's office after the doctor has obtained the history from the patient, Pat. The physical exam is beginning. Pat's parents are in the room. Pat is sitting on the exam table after having removed both shoes and socks. In the scene, the reader can see the thoughts of each character, but the only dialogue is between the doctor and the patient.

Mental Status

Doctor	Okay. Let's get started. I have to check Pat's mental status. First I'll ask Pat's name. It seems stupid, but I have to ask. "Tell me your name."
Pat	What does he think I am, an idiot? "Pat."
Pat's mother	Nailed it!
Pat's father	This guy gets paid for this?
Doctor	Now I'll find out if Pat is oriented to place. I'll ask if Pat knows where we are right now. "Tell me where we are."
Pat	Good thing I printed out the directions on QueryBlip last night. "Fifteen seventy-five Hyperbole Avenue, Putzville, New York."
Pat's mother	Oh, Pat's so smart. I would have just said New York.
Pat's father	An address? Sure, Pat can tell you that. But go ahead and ask where all the money in my wallet went.
Doctor	I have to ask Pat what the date is. I know it's the twenty-ninth, but I'll take anything from the twenty-eighth to the thirtieth. "Can you tell me what the date is today?"
Pat	Of course I can. I've been waiting for this appointment for a month and a half. "March 29, 2012."
Pat's mother	Oh, no! It's the twenty-ninth! It's Lizzie's birthday. I thought it was tomorrow. I have to get her a gift!
Pat's father	Isn't it the twenty-sixth? Oh crap. If it's the twenty-ninth, that means I forgot to pay the car insurance.
Doctor	Okay. Now that I know that Pat's oriented properly, I can check short-term memory. "I'm going to tell you three things. I want you to say them back to me now and remember them for later. The things are: ball, house, justice. Now repeat them."

Pat	I'll pretend I'm playing ball in the house with that justice lady who's blindfolded and holds the scales.
	"Ball. House. Justice."
Pat's mother	My memory isn't that great anymore. What did he say? Ball—hey, a ball would be a good gift for Lizzie. Hose. Justin.
Pat's father	How could I forget to send in the check? Oh wait. I just switched insurance to that one with the lizard. I don't have to pay until April. Wait. What did he say?
Doctor	Now let's test some language. I'll hold up a pen and ask Pat what it is.
	"What's this?"
Pat	I feel like I'm in first grade.
	"A pen."
Pat's mother	Pat nailed it!
Pat's father	What the hell?
Doctor	Now let's check the arcuate fasciculus and ask Pat to repeat something.
	"Repeat after me, 'No ifs, ands, or buts.'"
Pat	Is this really necessary?
	"No ifs, ands, or buts."
Pat's mother	No ifs or buts.
Pat's father	Heh, heh, heh. He said butts.
Doctor	Now let's go back to short-term memory.
	"What were those three things I asked you to remember?"
Pat	I'm playing ball in the house with the scales lady.
	"Ball. House. Justice."
Pat's mother	I know bell was one of them. Hey, I could get Lizzie some bell-bottom jeans.
Pat's father	What three things?
Doctor	Let's test attention some more.
	"Start with the number one and add three to it."
Pat	I stink at math.
	"Four."
Pat's mother	Pat was always so good in math.
Pat's father	One plus three? Really?
Doctor	"Now keep on adding three to each answer you get, until I tell you to stop."

Pat	"Seven, ten, thirteen, sixteen, nineteen, twenty-one ..." Stop. I think that's right. Oh, no. Wait! Can I go back? "Twenty-four, twenty-seven, thirty, thirty-three, thirty-six, thirty-nine."
Pat's mother	Nailed it!
Pat's father	Seven, ten, thirteen, fifteen, seventeen ... Wait. It was supposed to be threes, right? Twenty, twenty-three, twenty-six, twenty-nine ... the twenty-ninth. Did the lizard say that I could skip the first month or did I have to pay on the twenty-ninth? Oh crap.
Doctor	Pat missed one. "You missed one, but you did pretty well."
Pat	Stupid! Stupid! Stupid! He's just trying to make me feel better. I'm such a moron. "It was the nineteen plus three, right?"
Doctor	"Yep."
Pat	I hate math.
Pat's mother	Wait. Nineteen plus three equals ... nineteen, twenty, twenty-one, twenty-two ... wait do you include the nineteen? I should really carry a little calculator with me ...
Pat's father	I need a drink.
Doctor	Now let's move onto the frontal lobes. "Okay, for this next test, I want you to tell me all the words that you can think of in one minute that begin with the letter F."
Pat	This is interesting. "Okay."
Doctor	"Go."
Pat	"Face, fort, fat, fork (pause) ...
Pat's mother	Pat is so good in English.
Pat's father	Well there's ****. ******. ********. *******. ********.
Pat	"Are curses allowed?"
Doctor	"No curses or proper names."
Pat's mother	Pat should know better than that. Why would Pat ask a question like that?
Pat's father	Awww, that's not fair. Okay. Fornicate. Flatulence. Fart. Fat. Fatty-fat.
Pat	"Fact, flat, fish, four, fun, flea, fever, fellow, fell, fall, falling."

Doctor	"Good."
	Now let's go back to memory.
	"What were the three things I told you to remember?"
Pat	Ummm … playing ball …
	"Ball."
	In the house …
	"House."
	With the lady with the scales …
	"Justice."
Pat's mother	Potty mouth Pat. It's my husband's fault. He curses all the time. What was I thinking when I married him?
Pat's father	Fellatio. Did I say fornicate? Oh, we're done with the F words.
Doctor	Pat did that well.
	"Good."
	Now, let's test for constructional apraxia. I'll give Pat a pen and paper to draw a clock on.
	"Now draw a clock for me that shows quarter past six."
Pat	Does he want me to draw a digital clock or one of those old-timey clocks with the hands on them?
	"Which type? Digital or one of those old-timey clocks with the sticks on it?"
Doctor	Old-timey clock? Smart-ass kid.
	"Oh, yes. The type of clock that has a face and hands."
	(Pat draws a clock showing a quarter past six.)
Pat's mother	Pat was always a good artist.
Pat's father	What the hell?
Doctor	Clock looks good.
	"Good job."
Pat	Oh goody. Maybe I should tell him I was top of my class in second grade.
	"Thanks."
Doctor	Now let's test for interference. I'll draw two interlocking pentagons for Pat to copy.
	"Now copy these interlocking pentagons."
Pat	Crud. I hated geometry more than regular math.
	"Okay."
	(Pat copies the interlocking pentagons.)

Pat's mother	Aren't pentagoms used in devil worship?
Pat's father	Pentagrams! Whoa. Anarchy. Sex Pistols. This doc is cool!
Pat's mother	Or are pentagoms the shapes with six sides?
Pat's father	*Cuz Iiiiiiiiiiiiiiiiiiiii wanna beeeeeeeeeeee, anarchyyyyyyyy!*
Pat's mother	But if pentagoms have six sides, how many sides does a polygom have?
Pat's father	I wonder if he listens to the Clash. *Shariiiif don't like it. Rock the Casbah! Rock the Casbah!*
Pat's mother	No. It's the other way. Polygoms have six sides. Pentagoms have five sides.
Doctor	All right. Almost done with the mental status exam. Let's check memory one more time.
	"Tell me those things I asked you to remember one more time."
Pat	Ball.
	"Ball."
	House.
	"House."
	Justice.
	"Justice."
Doctor	"Great!"
	Let's go to the cranial nerves.

CRANIAL NERVES

Doctor	Need to check the baseline visual acuity.
	"Read the smallest line of numbers on the eye chart that you can see with your right eye."
Pat	Good. Something that I know how to do.
	"Four-two-eight-seven-three-nine."
Doctor	Now the other eye.
	"Good. Now read it with your left eye."
Pat	Okay.
	"Four-two-eight-seven-three-nine."
Pat's mother	Pat always had good vision.
Pat's father	I hope there's nothing wrong with Pat's vision. I need someone to run the trucks at work.
Doctor	Pat's got 20/20 vision.
	"Good."

	Time to look into Pat's eyes. Let's open the door slightly and turn off the lights.
	(The doctor opens the door slightly and turns off the lights.)
	"Now look at the clock on the wall while I look at your eyes using my ophthalmoscope."
Pat	Oh crap. I hate this. I just had an onion bagel. I hope my breath doesn't smell.
	"Okay."
	(The doctor looks into Pat's right eye.)
	How much closer is he going to get?
Pat's mother	Pat has such pretty eyes.
Pat's father	It looks like he's trying to kiss Pat.
Pat	My eyeball is drying out.
	(The doctor looks into Pat's left eye.)
Doctor	The fundi look good.
	"Your eyes look good."
Pat	Doesn't really matter. I'm blind now.
	"All I see are spots."
Doctor	I hate it when I have to do something to a patient that doesn't feel good.
	"Sorry. Your vision should clear up pretty quickly."
	Now I need to make sure that there are no abnormal eye movements.
	"Now, follow my finger."
Pat	I wonder if he's going to see anything when I look to the left.
	(The doctor moves his finger slowly in front of Pat's eyes.)
Pat's mother	Pat was having that abnormal eye flicking last week.
Pat's father	Pat mentioned seeing two things sometimes. I wonder if Pat's too tired.
	(The doctor notices nystagmus in the left eye when Pat looks to the left.)
Doctor	There's nystagmus.
	"Do you see one finger or two?"
Pat	He saw it. I see two fingers.
	"Two."
Doctor	Nystagmus with the diplopia. Possible left internuclear ophthalmoplegia.

"Okay."

(The doctor jots his findings down in Pat's chart.)

Pat's mother	I think he saw something.
Pat's father	What's going on?
Doctor	Let's check for red desaturation as a sign of optic neuritis. (The doctor holds a bright red magic marker in front of Pat.) "Does the tip of my pen look red?"
Pat	I guess he's testing my ability to see colors. "Yep."
Pat's mother	I have no idea what he's doing.
Pat's father	I'm lost.
Doctor	"Now close your left eye. Does the red cap appear the way it was when you looked at it with two eyes?"
Pat	I wonder why he's asking that. "It's the same."
Doctor	That's good. "Good."
Pat	That's good I guess.
Doctor	"Now switch eyes. Does it appear the same?"
Pat	Looks the same "Yep."
Doctor	That's good. "Good."
Pat's mother	Good!
Pat's father	Shouldn't everything be the same in both eyes?
Doctor	Let's check out the trigeminal nerve. "Does it feel the same everywhere that I touch you on your face?
Pat	He went fast. I think it felt the same. Just shut up and go on before he finds something else wrong. "Yep."
Pat's mother	Pat has always had such nice skin. I'm glad I got Pat that aloe vera cream.
Pat's father	Why is he stroking Pat's face?
Doctor	Pat's face looks symmetrical, but I have to make sure it moves properly. "Smile and show me your teeth."

Pat's father	What? He's a dentist too?
	(Pat smiles a big smile.)
Pat's mother	Pat always had a nice smile.
Pat's father	Maybe he could take a look at my teeth later.
Doctor	Smile is symmetrical. Now check forehead wrinkling.
	"Raise your eyebrows like this."
	(The doctor wrinkles his forehead.)
Pat	Does he want me to keep smiling while I raise my eyebrows?
Pat's mother	Pat always loved making goofy faces.
Pat's father	My God. Pat looks like a clown.
Doctor	Everything looks good.
	"Great."
	Now let's see how the hearing is.
	"Repeat what I whisper in your ear."
	(The doctor whispers in Pat's right ear.)
	"I like the New York Yankees."
Pat	I hate the Yankees. I like the Mets.
	"I like the Mets."
Pat's mother	Pat always had great hearing.
Pat's father	What kinda doctor whispers to a patient?
Doctor	The hearing in the right ear appears okay but Pat likes the Mets.
	"Your hearing is okay, but I think I have to do a dementia workup now."
Pat's mother	Why did he say that?
Pat's father	Huh?
Pat	Damn Yankee fan.
	"You're soooooo funny ..."
Doctor	I try to lighten the mood when I can.
	"Okay, let's try the other ear."
	(The doctor whispers in Pat's left ear.)
	"The Mets need better pitching."
Pat	He's right.
	"You're right."
Pat's mother	I guess that sports have something to do with the nerves in the brain.
Pat's father	What is he right about?

Doctor	I need to check the glossopharyngeal and hypoglossal nerves. I'll put the tongue depressor in Pat's mouth, look to see how the uvula moves, and then check for gag reflex.
	"Open your mouth, stick out your tongue, and say 'Ahh.'"
Pat	Good thing I brushed my teeth.
	"Ahhhhh."
Pat's mother	Good thing Pat brushes every day.
Pat's father	I forgot to brush my teeth this morning. My memory is shot. Maybe I should see this guy.
Doctor	Let's test the sternocleidomastoideus and trapezius muscles, which are innervated by the spinal accessory nerve.
	"Shrug your shoulders like you're saying 'I don't know.'"
Pat	That's easy.
	(Pat shrugs shoulders.)
Doctor	Strength appears okay.
	"Good."
Pat's mother	Pat doesn't have to shrug. Pat's too smart.
Pat's father	I can do that. I do it a lot at work.
Doctor	Okay. Let's go to the motor system testing.

MOTOR SYSTEM

Doctor	Let's start with the deltoids.
	"Okay, let's test your strength. Put your elbows up like this."
	(The doctor raises his elbows out on each side, like a pair of bird wings.)
Pat's mother	Pat is very strong.
Pat's father	My shoulder has been hurting me.
Pat	I feel like I'm playing Simon Says.
	"Okay."
	(The doctor pushes down on Pat's elbows.)
Doctor	There's some weakness in the left deltoid.
	"You're a lefty, correct?"
Pat's mother	Why is he asking that?
Pat	"Yep."
Doctor	"Have you noticed any weakness in your left arm?"

Pat	Hmm. My left arm has been a little weaker recently.
	"Yep."
Pat's mother	No.
Pat's father	Pat's probably still sore from yesterday's basketball game.
Doctor	Let's test Pat's biceps.
	"Now pretend you're lifting weights."
Pat	"Okay."
	(Pat holds arms flexed. The doctor pulls and pushes Pat's arms.)
	Hmm. Biceps and triceps are weak on the left.
Pat	Hmm. My left arm is weaker than my right.
Doctor	Let's test the hand muscles.
	"Spread out your fingers and don't let me squeeze them together."
	Interossei are weak on the left.
	"Now squeeze my fingers."
	Grip is also.
Pat	Wow. Maybe that's why I keep on dropping things from my left hand.
	(The doctor writes down his findings.)
Pat's mother	What is he writing in Pat's chart?
Pat's father	What's he writing in Pat's chart?
Pat	I guess he's writing down that my left arm is weak.
Doctor	Now I'll test Pat's leg muscles.
	"Okay, now brace yourself on the exam table and lift your knee up like this."
	(The doctor flexes his leg at the hip.)
Pat	"Okay."
	(The doctor pushes down on each of Pat's knees.)
Doctor	Left iliopsoas is a bit weak.
	"Have you had any trouble going up stairs?"
Pat	Wow. Maybe that's why my left foot catches when I go up the stairs.
	"My left foot has been catching sometimes."
Pat's mother	Pat has tripped a few times on the stairs. I wonder if ...
Pat's father	Pat's back probably got hurt when Chris came over to move the stuff out of the basement. That's why the leg and arm are weak.

Doctor	Let's test the quads and hamstrings.
	"Kick out your right leg. Now pull it back. Okay, now on the left."
	Weaker on the left. Now I'll test the anterior tibialis and extensor hallucis longus.
	"Now point your toes up."
	Left is weak.
	"Okay. Good job."
Pat	Crap. My left leg is weak too. That's not good.
Pat's mother	How can Pat be weak? Pat's young and strong.
Pat's father	Pat's just weak from a sore back.
Doctor	Time for reflexes.
	"Okay. Let's check your reflexes."

REFLEXES

Doctor	Let's see what the reflexes show. I can't tell a patient to relax because then they tighten up like a drum and then I can't get a good reflex exam.
	"Okay, Pat. Do you know what a ragdoll is?"
Pat	Sure.
	"Yeah. I've seen them."
Doctor	"You know how they just lie there on the bed and do nothing. They're just limp and lifeless."
Pat	Sure.
	"Yeah."
Doctor	"I want you to pretend that you are a ragdoll. Let everything go. Like this."
	(The doctor lets his head drop and shoulders slump.)
Pat	I'm so tired anyway; I feel like a ragdoll.
	"How's this?"
	(Pat slumps while sitting on the exam table.)
Pat's mother	No, Pat! Sit up straight. You always have had good posture.
Pat's father	That's what Pat's mother does when I ask if she wants to have sex.
Doctor	Perfect.
	"Perfect. Just let it all go. Do you feel relaxed now?
	(Pat nods.)
	"Good. Now I'm going to hit you with a hammer."

Pat	I guess he's kinda funny. I mean, at least he's not a tool like my other doctors.
	"Ha ha ha. You're soooo funny."
Pat's mother	That's not funny. That's my child. Pat's sick, and Mr. Doctor Man is making jokes. I wonder if I should ask Pat's father if we should leave.
Pat's father	I wanna go out drinking with this guy.
	(The doctor checks Pat's reflexes. Pat's leg kicks out quickly and strongly when the doctor tests Pat's left patellar reflex.)
Doctor	Reflexes are definitely increased on the left.
Pat	Whoops!
	"Sorry. I didn't mean to kick you like that."
Pat's mother	Do it again! But harder this time!
Pat's father	I wonder if he ever got kicked in the nuts.
Doctor	If I had a nickel for every time I was kicked …
	"No worries, Pat."
	… the insurance companies would say that it counts as part of the copay.
	(The doctor takes his keys out of his pocket.)
	I need to check for Chaddock's reflex.
	"Now I just want to scratch the side of your foot with my key."
	(The doctor kneels down and starts to pull the teeth of the key along the side of Pat's foot.)
Pat	This just went weird.
	"Okay …"
Pat's mother	Now's your chance, Pat. Kick him in the face!
Pat's father	Didn't the stripper at Micky's bachelor party do something like this?
	(The big toe on Pat's left foot goes up, and the big toe on the right does not.)
Doctor	That's a sign of upper motor neuron lesion.
	"Okay …"
Pat	Strange how my big toe went up on my left foot but didn't on my right.
Pat's father	No! It was at Joey's party.
Doctor	Okay. Done with reflexes.

STATION

Doctor	Let's stand Pat up.
	"Pat, come down off the table and stand right over here."
Pat	Sure.
	"Sure."
	(Pat gets up and stands in front of the doctor.)
Doctor	Pat's standing up straight. Shoulders and hips appear aligned properly. Pat's feet are about shoulder width apart. Looks good. Let's see how the cerebellum, inner ear, and proprioception are working.
	"Now, stand with your feet together and then close your eyes."
Pat's mother	What's Dr. Wackjob going to do now?
Pat	This should be interesting. My balance hasn't been so great recently.
	"Okay."
Doctor	I'll watch Pat's belt buckle so I can follow Pat's center of gravity in case Pat starts to fall over
Pat's father	Why is the doctor staring at Pat's crotch?
	(Pat's eyes close. Pat sways slightly but remains standing in place.)
Pat's mother	Oh my God! Pat's about to fall down! Somebody catch Pat!
Pat's father	Pat's swaying. That's the way I looked last week down at Murphy's pub.
Doctor	Pat swayed a little but did not fall over. Romberg's sign is not present.
Pat	I wonder what the doctor is looking at while I have my eyes closed. Does he see the spot on my shirt? I should have worn my other top.
Doctor	Okay. Now I'll check for weakness in the upper extremities. Pat will probably have a drift on the left since the motor exam showed weakness in the left arm.
	"Good job. Open your eyes. Now stand with your feet apart, put your arms out in front of you with palms up, and close your eyes."
Pat	I wonder why the doctor wants me to do that.
	"Sure."

	(Pat's arms go out at chest level with palms up.)
Pat's mother	What the hell is he doing now?
Pat's father	What the hell is he doing now?
	(After a few seconds, Pat's left arm rotates inward slightly and drifts down several inches.)
Doctor	Pat has some drift in the left arm. Goes along with the left-sided weakness.
	(The doctor holds Pat's hands in the position that they moved to after Pat's eyes closed.)
	"Open your eyes."
	(Pat's eyes open.)
Pat	Wow. It felt like they hadn't moved at all after I closed my eyes. What's that mean?
Doctor	"See how your arms moved? It's another sign of some weakness in the muscles in your left arm. We'll find out why it's going on."
Pat's father	After Murphy had his stroke and sold the bar, we used to kid him because he spilled beer on himself if he held it in his weak hand. Pat couldn't have had a stroke! Could he?
Pat's mother	After Mother had a stroke, her arm moved just like that. Oh no. My baby had a stroke!
	(Tears well up in her eyes.)
Pat's father	Aw, jeez. The wife's starting with the water works.

GAIT

Doctor	Let's see how Pat's walking is.
	"Walk across the room like you're going for a stroll."
	(Pat walks back and forth. The tip of the left foot drags slightly.)
Pat	My feet are dragging. Mom gets so mad when I drag my feet.
Pat's mother	That must be why Pat's feet have been dragging and wears through shoes so quickly.
	(Pat's father searches for tissues in his jacket pocket.)
Doctor	I wonder how long this has been going on for.
	"Is it okay if I take a look at the soles of your shoes?"
Pat	Weird.
	"Okay."

	(The doctor picks up Pat's shoes that were taken off at the start of the exam.)
Doctor	The tip of the left shoe is more worn than the right. "Are these new?"
Pat	"Yeah. I wore through the last pair after about two months. My mom got me those last week."
Doctor	"For how long have you been wearing through your shoes?"
Pat	"I dunno. Since last year maybe. Right?"
Pat's mother	Oh God, I feel horrible! I shouted at Pat for that, but it was because of a stroke! My God! I am the worst mother in the world! (She starts crying.)
Pat's father	Crap. The floodgates just opened. (Pat's father hands Pat's mother a wad of tissues from his pocket. The doctor notices Pat's mother crying, gets a new box of tissues out, and offers them to Pat's mother.)
Pat	Why is she crying? I feel fine. "Don't mind her. She cries at the littlest thing." (The doctor acknowledges Pat and turns to Pat's mom.)
Doctor	"Are you all right?" (Pat's mom nods while holding the fresh tissues to her face.) "There are some things we've seen on Pat's exam, but we don't know what their cause is yet. Hang in there and we'll talk about everything after the exam is over. Okay?"
Pat's mother	Just nod yes. (Pat's mother nods.)
Pat	"Don't worry, Mom. I'm fine."
Pat's mother	Don't tell Pat that I think the symptoms are due to a stroke like my mother had. (She nods again.) But I know it's a stroke.
Pat's father	I think Eamon's kid had a stroke. His face was drooping on the right side, but then it got better. I think they called it Bell's palsy. Is that the same thing as a stroke?

	(Pat's dad holds his wife's hand.)
Pat's father	I better hold onto some of these tissues in case I lose it. Maybe Pat's got a Bell's palsy stroke. Hope it gets better. Pat's the one that I need to run the trucks.
Doctor	Okay, let's get back to the exam.
	"Okay, let's have you walk one foot in front of the other, touching heel to toe."
Pat	I haven't done this since I was a kid.
	"Okay."
	(Pat starts walking.)
Doctor	The doctor notices that Pat leans more toward the left while walking tandem but does not fall over.
Pat's mother	Good thing I always told Pat as a child to never walk on the curbstones like that because people get hurt doing dangerous stuff like that.
Pat's father	I know I couldn't do that. Never could. Probably a genetic thing. Ge-ne-tic. Gin-n-tonic. God, I really need a drink.
Doctor	"Great! We're almost done."

COORDINATION

Doctor	"Pat, why don't you get back up on the table."
	Gotta lighten the mood a little.
	"Okay. Now this time, the questions *are* harder but the dollar value is *double*."
Pat	Huh?
	"Huh?"
Pat's mother	Huh?
Pat's father	Oh boy, maybe we can win our copay back!
Doctor	I know I passed on a great career in stand-up comedy for medicine, but I coulda been one of the greats.
	"Just kidding."
Pat	Oh.
	"Oh."
	(Pat smiles.)
Pat's mother	He's more like a game show host than a doctor.
Pat's father	Oh.
Doctor	Now we are going to test Pat's coordination.

	(The doctor stands in front of Pat and holds up his index finger.)
	"Okay, touch my finger with your right index finger."
Pat	Okay.
	"Okay."
	(Pat reaches out and touches the doctor's index finger.)
Doctor	Nice and smooth and Pat hit the mark.
	"Good. Now touch your nose."
Pat	Okay.
	(Pat touches nose.)
Pat's mother	Why is he doing the drunk-driving test on Pat?
Doctor	Perfect. Now let's try the left side.
	"Great! Now do it with your left hand."
Pat	Okay.
	(Pat reaches for the doctor's index finger, but the hand oscillates slightly on the way to the doctor's finger and again on its way to Pat's nose.)
	"I've been having some trouble with the coordination in my left hand."
Doctor	"When did that begin?"
Pat	"About the same time as the walking trouble did."
Doctor	"Gotcha."
	Now I'll have Pat do heel-to-shin testing.
	"Now take the heel of your right foot, put it on the knee of your left leg, slide it down your shin to your foot, and then slide it back up again."
Pat	Interesting.
	"Okay."
	(Pat touches heel to knee and goes down and back up shin smoothly.)
Doctor	Perfect.
	"Now do it with your left foot going down and up your right shin."
Pat	Right.
	"Right."
	(Pat's left foot is less accurate and follows a slightly ataxic route when going from the knee to the foot and back up.)

Doctor	There's ataxia in the left leg.
	"All righty. One last thing. I want you to hit your right palm against your left palm and then turn your right hand over and hit the back of your right hand against your left palm like this.
	(The doctor demonstrates by alternately hitting both sides of his right hand against his left palm in a regular rhythm.)
Pat	That's interesting.
	"Like this?"
	(Pat alternately hits the right palm and then the back of the right hand against the left palm. The alternating movements are rapid and smooth.)
Doctor	Perfect. Now for the left hand.
	"Okay. Now try alternately hitting your left palm and back of the hand on your right palm."
Pat	Okay.
	"Okay."
	(Pat alternately hits the right palm and then the back of the right hand against the left palm, but the alternating movements are irregular in tempo. Sometimes the same side is hit twice in a row.)
Doctor	Dysdiadochokinesia is present on the left.
	"Okay. We have just one more thing to do. We have to test your sensation."

SENSATION

Doctor	Let's start the testing of sensation with pinprick.
	"I'll test your sensation to pinprick with this tongue depressor."
Pat	I wonder how he is going to test pinprick?
	(The doctor breaks a tongue depressor in half, leaving it with a spiky end.)
Pat's mother	My God. He's making a weapon!
	(Pat's mom reaches into her purse for her mace.)
Pat's father	I bet you could kill a guy with something like that.
Doctor	I'll just touch lightly over the face, arm, and leg on the right.

	(The doctor touches the pointy ends of the spikes over Pat's face and body on the right.)
	"Does this feel pointy?"
Pat	It's pointy. Cool. I bet I can do that with a pencil and stick Chris with it.
	"Yes."
Pat's mother	Hmm. Maybe I can do that with a pencil to Pat's father when he snores.
Pat's father	Cool! I'm gonna try that on Murphy at the pub this weekend.
Doctor	Now, I'll just touch lightly over the face, arm, and leg on the left.
	(The doctor touches the pointy ends of the spikes over Pat's face and body on the left.)
	"Is it the same on both sides?"
Pat	Yep.
	"Yep."
Pat's mother	Or when he wants to have sex.
Doctor	Great! Pinprick sensation is normal. Let's try light touch over the face, arm, and leg.
	(The doctor lightly touches Pat's face and body with his fingers.)
	"Does this feel the same on both sides?"
Pat	Yep.
	"Yep."
Pat's mother	Pat has such soft skin.
Pat's father	Is he trying to make a pass at Pat?
Doctor	Normal light touch sensation. Now for vibratory sensation.
	(The doctor taps a tuning fork and touches it to Pat's wrists and ankles.)
	"What do you feel now?"
Pat	Feels funky.
	"Vibrations."
Pat's mother	I like that song "Cool Vibrations" by the Beach Boys.
Pat's father	Maybe If I got Pat's mom a vibrator she would want to have sex with me more.
Doctor	Compare sides.
	"Is it the same on both sides in your hands and feet?"

Pat	Yep.
	"Yep.
Pat's mother	Or is it "Good Relaxations"?
Pat's father	I think Vibe-o-rama is having a sale, but I know I could probably get it cheaper online.
Doctor	We're done! Now I have to put all of this together and then explain what it means to Pat and the family.
	"Great! We're done! Now we can talk about what we saw and figure out what our next steps will be."
Pat	Great! Sounds like a plan!
	"Great! Sounds like a plan!"
Pat's mother	Oh, thank God that Pat doesn't have to suffer anymore and that we can learn what's going on and then make a plan about what to do.
Pat's father	Great! So after that, we'll go home, I'll pay the lizard, go to the bar to see Murph, and then see what they have on sale at Vibe-o-rama. Sounds like a plan!

The following is a short story about Mike—a young gentleman who had some double vision and was being evaluated for possible MS. He is sitting with his parents, Paul and Rebecca, in the doctor's office.

MIKE GOES TO THE DOCTOR

So there Mike was, sitting in a funky chair in the neuro-ophthalmologist's office, playing with the tools on a tray. He figured since he was in medical school, he had license to play with medical toys. His folks had brought him to the doctor's office and were sitting in chairs by the wall. The appointment was scheduled for eleven o'clock, but the nurse said the doctor was running behind. The lights were fluorescent and too bright for the room. His dad was wearing his sunglasses. He normally had glasses that would turn dark when in the sun, but he wore his regular sunglasses today. Mike's mom, who had been a nurse, was in her pre–cry mode. She was not crying, but the edges of her eyelids were pink, and she was all set to go when the doctor finally got to a life-altering diagnosis. After Mike finished playing with the toys, he decided to chat a little bit with his dad to try to alleviate some of the tension in the room.

"So how's it going, Dad?"

"You know you're going to be fine. People that have MS and get sensory symptoms first do better. Plus, I read in the *Wall Street Journal* that a company reported that their third-quarter earnings were good because they almost have a cure. So you'll be all right."

Sounds good, Mike thought. "What disease are they almost about to cure?" he asked.

"Well, you know. MS."

"But I haven't even been diagnosed yet. I just saw the eye doctor last week about the double vision I was having. He said he wanted me to see a neuro-ophthalmologist about it." The doctor Mike had seen, after he first came home from his first year at med school, was his ophthalmologist, Dr. Richie. Dr. Richie had been his dad's best friend growing up. Mike knew that MS was a possible cause of double vision in a young person, and his dad's friend had called him after seeing Mike to let him know what he had found. His dad had taken that as gospel and had proceeded to inundate Mike with "good news about MS." Mike had been trying to be objective about everything since he was trying to become a doctor and objectivity, he thought, was important for a doctor. Also, he realized the other things that could cause double vision (brainstem tumors, strokes, and the like) could be much worse. He was getting used to thinking that MS would be the best news he could hear.

"No. I'm not saying that it is definitely MS, but Dr. Richie sounded like he knew what he was talking about. But you're right. We have to see what this guy says. Then your aunt says that she found the most famous doctor in MS that we can see. She says he's the best." Mike listened and digested what his father had just said.

"Maybe I should subscribe to *Tombstone Monthly* at the same time," Mike taunted with a small smirk on his face. "You know. Just to stay one step ahead."

"Look. No. I'm not saying you're going to die. It's just that she wants to make sure you get the best care."

"Yeah," Mike agreed while looking down at the tools. He knew his folks and aunt loved him, but he thought they were going overboard. "I still think we should have a diagnosis first."

"But the guy she found didn't have an appointment available for three months, but she was able to get one for next week!"

Mike nodded. Then he thought about his mom, who was sitting next to his dad. He just thought about her, mainly because he knew that if he were to look at her, she would turn into a pool of tears. He dared not ask how she felt or what she was thinking about since he had not brought nearly enough rolls of paper towel to keep her dry. He decided to start with a question and then go from there.

"See the hockey game last night?"

"No. Who won?" his mom asked.

"Toronto," he answered, turning to look at her. "Broke their three-game losing streak."

"That's good," she replied. "I always liked Toronto. They're based on the other side of Lake Ontario across from where I went to nursing school."

Mike's dad jumped in about what a good game it was. They spoke about hockey for an hour.

Then they waited for an hour and a half in silence.

Then the doctor came in while staring at Mike's chart.

"Hello. I'm Dr. Obnoxiously Tardy," he said. At least that was what Mike thought he had heard. He was tall, about six two, but his shoulders were slumped.

"Hi," he replied. "I'm Michael, and these are my folks, Paul and Rebecca Tompkins." They stood and shook the doctor's hand.

"So, you're having some double vision?" he began as he looked through the page of his chart. He kept flipping the page back and forth like he was looking for some valuable data that had surfaced since the form was filled out three hours ago but was now somehow missing.

"Yeah," Mike replied. "When I look to the left, I see two of each thing. It began last month, at the end of my first year of med school, when I was studying for my final in neuroanatomy."

"Okay. When you say that you 'see double' what do you mean?" he asked, sounding like he wasn't convinced that Mike knew what the word "double" meant. Or maybe it was the word "see," which can be confusing since it has so many homophones—see, sea, c, cee, si, she (if you're drunk), ci (if you're French), and pomegranate (if you're an incorrigible miscreant who does not want to even acknowledge that he and his staff kept a family of three waiting expectantly for two and a half hours without even a hint of regret).

"I see them side by side with the medial image slightly higher than the lateral image."

"Hmmmm," he acknowledged. "Is it painful?"

"No. But after a while, it gives me a headache."

"Uh-huh. Okay," he said as he went over to the tray of toys. He picked up the red glass and put it over Mike's right eye while having him look to the left. "Do you see two images?"

"Yep," he said.

"Which one is closer to the wall, the red one or the regular one?"

"The red one."

"Okay. All right. Follow my finger," he said. He then held Mike's head from the top with his other hand. It was not so much of a hold as it was a sensation of someone trying to push him down through the floor, into the basement of the building. As the neuro-ophthalmological exam continued, Mike started to smile.

"Why are you smiling?" Dr. Miserable asked in an unpleasant voice.

"Because I just learned this exam in med school last semester," he replied. The doctor did not reply, so Mike tried to keep a straight face. But the smile just kept on coming back. He tried to tell himself that if he was going to be a doctor, he had to learn how to take serious things seriously. This guy was a doctor. He was being serious. He made Mike feel like he was the village idiot for giggling while he was being analyzed. Mike's parents remained silent, trying not to show any emotion. Mike was trying to not get any spittle on Dr. Serious while holding back his laughs.

Mike went inside himself. *Yes,* he thought. *Double vision is an abnormality that can portend a serious disease. But shouldn't a person be allowed to laugh if their spirit was telling them to laugh?* Mike thought he was being told to laugh by his laughing center (ventromedial frontal lobes) because he was having a confluence of thoughts creating an absurdity at a strange time in his life. He had just finished his first year of med school. He was having trouble with learning like he never had before. He had managed to learn the neurological pathways that were being tested now, except this was the first test where his brain knew the right answer but his body was showing something different.

Why was his body acting that way?

That was the unknown. That's why he was laughing, he realized. He was uncertain about the cause of the double vision. He knew the problem was most probably in his brainstem, but what was causing the problem? Multiple sclerosis? A tumor? A vitamin deficiency? Stroke? Infection? Trouble with his thyroid? Another autoimmune disease that he blew off learning about in pathology class because he had never heard of it and it was weird and had no cure? He started to realize that the smiling was not from being happy but from being scared.

At the end of the exam, Dr. No Smile said that he needed to get an MRI to see what the cause of the double vision was. "To rule out multiple sclerosis," he said.

"Might it be a brain tumor?" Mike asked.

"Yes, but we'll have to see." He looked at his folks. His dad was hidden behind his sunglasses. His mom was the big story. Her eyes looked normal.

"And the MRI is done to rule out multiple sclerosis, right?" she reiterated like the nurses did that Mike had seen in the hospital when he had his "Introduction to the Patient" class. She was in top form. Go, Mom!

"We have to get the MRI to make sure it is not MS," Mike reiterated to his folks. They nodded. While the doctor was writing the prescription for the MRI, Mike decided to ask a professional question of his soon-to-be colleague.

"If I do have MS," he began, "would you recommend that I focus on any special area of medicine to either go into or stay away from?" The doctor finished writing for the MRI and then looked up.

"You might develop a tree-mor," he said, pronouncing the word "tremor" in the way most affected people do. He shrugged and then added, "So you should probably stay away from surgery and go into a medical specialty." Mike nodded and thanked the doctor for the excellent care he provided. He felt like someone had taken over his voice box and started to say stupid things. He realized he should shut the hell up before he offered his firstborn as compensation for the care he had received. The doctor shook hands with Mike and his parents and quickly left. *I guess he's in a hurry to club some baby seals*, Mike thought. They walked in silence to the front desk. Paul paid the bill in cash. He was not going to leave any paper trails of Mike's ailment that could be used against his son.

★★★

The day after the MRI, Mike and his dad were watching football on the TV in his parents' bedroom. The Giants were playing the Eagles. Paul was on the bed, and Mike was sitting on the couch. The Giants had turned over the ball three times, and it was only the second quarter.

"How are you feeling about all of this?" Paul asked.

"I would feel a lot better if they could hold onto the ball," Mike answered, his eyes on the screen.

His father thought for a second and then responded. "No. I mean the MS."

Mike turned to look at his father. "We still don't have a diagnosis."

"What did the MRI show?"

"I don't know. They printed out a copy of it for me to take, but I don't know what I'm looking at. I mean, I know the anatomy, and I don't see anything vastly abnormal, but I haven't done a radiology rotation yet."

His father nodded. They both turned back to watching the game. The Eagles ran the ball up the middle and were stopped for no gain.

"When do you do the radiology rotation?" Paul asked.

"Not until next year," Mike responded. "I have some electives then."

"So maybe you don't have it," his dad continued.

"Maybe, but the other causes are no walk to the park either," Mike replied.

"So what else could it be?" Paul asked, still staring at the game.

"It could be an infection or a tumor or a metabolic problem or a vitamin deficiency or just about anything else." The Giants were back to receive a punt. "Good thing the Eagles are playing as lousy as the Giants."

"Does it bother you?" his dad asked.

"Sure it does. The Giants paid that new guy a lot of money, and they still can't score."

Paul was quiet.

"I'm glad you're not letting this MS thing eat you up like it is with your mother."

Mike turned to his dad. "What's going on with Mom?"

"She can't sleep. She has been tossing and turning all night."

Mike looked at his dad's face. There were bags under his eyes. "How have you been doing?"

"I can't sleep either."

Mike turned back to the TV but focused on his dad.

"You look like you're fine, but you say you're having trouble in med school like you never had in college. I watch you, and you look the same as you always have. Maybe you're just under a lot of stress at school."

Mike took in the words and let them percolate for a minute. The Giants ran the ball up the middle and got nowhere.

"Overall, I feel fine, but I don't feel like the *me* that I was, back, early in college and high school."

"None of us do," Paul said, resting his face in the small, yellow pillow that he was propped up on. "We all get older."

"Yeah, but I don't think the changes that go on with aging occur as abruptly as what's happened to me," Mike said, glancing at his father and then back to the screen.

"Does anything make you feel better?"

"Staying cool," Mike said without equivocation. "That's one thing I hate about going to school in the south."

"Do you take your vitamins and get exercise?"

"I take vitamins every day. Exercise is about twice a week." The Giants completed a twenty-five-yard pass, but there was a flag down.

"How are you eating?"

The Giants got called for holding.

"I eat well. I don't drink any alcohol anymore," Mike answered and turned to his dad to see if he had any emotions about the holding call. Paul's face was still half buried in the pillow. He turned back to the TV.

"Is the work load too much?"

"Well, there's a tremendous amount of work, but no more than I had before," Mike said, staring at, but not really watching the TV.

"It's just that I don't care about getting a top grade anymore. Or even a good grade." The Giants tried a run up the middle again and got a yard.

"That's no good," his dad said as he brought his face up to watch the game.

"I know, but I just feel so lethargic in the heat," Mike said, looking at his dad. "I want it to be over with so I can move back here and be a doctor."

"Well, the appointment with the specialist that your aunt got is scheduled for tomorrow," Paul said as he turned toward Mike. "Maybe he can help." The Giants lined up for third down.

"I hope he's better than the last guy," Mike said.

Pass play.

"Maybe he can help out," his dad added.

Incomplete. The Giants' offense started to jog off the field.

"*Can you believe it, Dick?*" the announcer began. "*The Giants are bringing out the special teams again for the seventh punt of the game, and there's still 2:30 left in the second quarter!*"

"I hope he can," Mike said refocusing on the game. "He's a specialist." The Giants lined up for the punt. The long snapper shot the ball over the head of the punter. "That should mean something."

The punter picked up the ball and kicked it off the side of his foot out of bounds.

"Well, Bob. Heh, heh. Sometimes the word 'special' doesn't necessarily mean 'good.' Heh, heh, heh."

***

They were all up early, showered, shaved, and fed. Mike's dad was known to be a fast driver, and that morning was no exception. In fact, he was so fast that they had already gone over the Betheva Bridge before Mike's mom remembered that they had left Mike's MRI films on the kitchen table. After one major and several minor traffic violations went unnoticed, they retrieved the films and eventually got to the doctor's office. Two minutes early.

"That's why you should always plan on being ten minutes early," Mike's dad said. "Grandpa always said if you're not ten minutes early, you're late."

Mike carried the films as they walked into the building. They stood in the cramped, dirty elevator as they rode up to the doctor's office with a woman holding the hand of a little girl. Mike looked at the little girl, who smiled at him. He smiled back as the doors to the elevator opened. The girl's mother pulled her out, causing a whiplash action, and Mike saw the look on the girl's face go from smiling to terrified in an instant. He heard the girl crying after the elevator doors closed. Mike kind of felt the same way. One moment he was a med student, and the next he had a major neurodegenerative disease. Both he and the girl were hit with something that they had not expected. Both can be frightening. The girl's nursemaid elbow could be treated by supination of the forearm while the elbow was held at a ninety-degree angle. Treatments for MS were a little more involved.

They got off the elevator and walked down the hallway to the doctor's office. They filled out papers and started to settle in, but the receptionist came out right away and took them into the exam room. Mike exchanged glances with his folks. They smiled and thought that such prompt attention boded well. Once in the exam room, they took their seats. Mike did not see an exam table. Aside from the wood chairs that they were seated in, which had yellowed, vinyl cushions, there was one cold-looking wooden chair, a window with a radiator under it, and a hanging fluorescent light.

"Pretty simple surroundings," Mike said as he sat, placing the films at his feet.

"I guess when you're the best, you don't need to have much else," Paul commented. Looking out the window, Mike could see the bridge that they had driven over to get to the office. It was hazy outside. It was warm in the office.

"That was some pretty fast driving, Dad."

"Your father drives too fast," Rebecca said quickly.

"Oh, your mother ..." Paul added as he rubbed his hands together. "She—" Mike's dad was cut off as a man who appeared to be in his early sixties entered the room. He had on a white shirt that was open at the neck and corduroy slacks. He appeared out of breath. His belly showed him to be about eight months pregnant. His discolored and worn wingtip shoes gave evidence that his water had broken sometime during the Nixon administration.

"Hi. I'm Dr. Neal Burdorg," he said. Paul walked briskly over to him with his hand extended.

"Hi. I'm Paul Tompkins. This is my wife, Rebecca, and our son, Mike. He's the patient."

"Oh. Hi," Dr. Burdorg said as he shook hands with Rebecca and Paul.

"I want to thank you for seeing us on such short notice. We've been told that you're the best."

"Well, not if you speak with my wife," Dr. Burdorg replied. There was some weak laughter, and then the doctor turned to Mike. "So you have MS?"

"Well, the last doctor we saw sent me for an MRI, but we decided to come to you after we had it done."

"Who did you see?" he asked. Mike looked at his father. Neither one wanted to remember the name of the doctor.

"His name escapes me," Paul began. "He worked out of the Melman Center."

"Oh. That was probably Moe." Everyone nodded and agreed. "So. Tell me your story," the doctor said as he sat in the chair. "Oh. Are those your films?"

"Yes," Mike said as he handed the heavy manila envelope to the doctor. "It began last month, at the end of my first year of med school, when I was studying for my final in neuroanatomy. I was trying to memorize the cranial nerves. It was then that I noticed that I saw two corners in the corner of my room when I looked up and to the left." The doctor had taken the films from the jacket and was holding them up to the fluorescent light, one by one.

Shouldn't the best MS doctor have a light board to view films on? Mike asked himself. He also thought it interesting how the expert decided to look at the films first and not do the physical exam first, as Mike had been taught. *I guess things change when you become an expert,* he concluded.

The doctor continued to stare at the films as he held them up to the light. He held them up, one at a time, in his right hand. He had his back arched against the back of his hard wooden chair, holding the film up to the light. *What does he see? What is he looking for? Has he picked up something that he heard about once in some remote island in the South Pacific? Is he trying to come up with a way to tell me that I only have two weeks to live?* Mike wondered. *Had he fallen asleep while being able to maintain a posture that allowed him to hold film up to light using a technique that he had mastered throughout the years of his training under other MS experts and was now able to achieve a perfect center where both images and arm were balanced upon the lordotic spine slung over the back of the wood chair while the traction from his amniotic-fluid-soaked shoes prevented him from sliding out of his seat altogether?*

"Is it MS?" Mike asked.

The doctor, moving nothing, replied succinctly. "You know what they asked Shoeless Joe, right?"

Mike paused and looked at his shoes while he tried to make the leap from medicine to baseball. Shoeless Joe—1919 Black Sox. He lifted his head and turned back to the doctor.

"It ain't true, is it?" With that, Mike figured the doctor had seen enough and now wanted to examine him. Dr. Burdorg then slid the films back into the manila jacket, reached down to look at his pager, stood, and excused himself. Mike looked at his parents.

"I guess he got a page. He'll examine me after he gets back."

"I wonder what he saw on the MRI," Rebecca said.

"Dunno. I stared at them myself, and I couldn't find anything. What do I know," Mike said as he smiled. "I'm just a med student." The door opened, and the receptionist came in.

"Okay. You're done. You can come out into the waiting room while I get your bill ready." Mike stared at his mother as she began to shake her head. She began to mutter something, but then Paul cut her off.

"Okay," he said as he started to walk out into reception.

"What the hell was that?" Mike asked, picking up the films.

"That's what you get when you go to an expert, I guess," Rebecca replied. They walked out and watched as Paul paid the bill in cash as before. They left the office and waited for the elevator in silence. The silence continued on the ride down to the lobby and the walk across the parking lot. Once back in the car, Rebecca started talking.

"What did he ask you back there?"

"He asked if I knew what they said to Shoeless Joe."

"Who?" she asked.

"Shoeless Joe Jackson. He was one of the eight players that threw the 1919 World Series," Mike answered.

"So what did they say to Shoeless Joe?"

"The legend says that a little boy came up to him after Joe came out of the courthouse and said, 'It ain't true, is it, Joe?'"

Mike's mom muttered "Oh" and then asked another question. "What does that have to do with MS?"

"It must mean that he doesn't think you have it," Paul replied. "That's good news, right?"

Mike sat in the backseat. He didn't know which was more shocking—seeing two people who were allegedly doctors act like they were not qualified to hold a dinner reservation much less a medical degree or how Dr. Burdorg could be regarded as being an expert.

"Dad, who told Aunt Ann that guy was an expert?"

"Your uncle's business partner, Mr. Flosnagen."

"He's the guy that runs that brokerage firm, right?" Mike asked.

"Yeah," his father affirmed.

"You don't have your money with him, do you?"

"No. Why?" Paul asked, glancing at Mike in the rearview mirror.

Mike looked at his mom.

"I don't know if I trust Mr. Flosnagen's judgment."

"Why not?" his father asked as he started to merge onto the expressway. "Look. The doctor said you don't have MS! You should get into a racket like that. "He was with you for five minutes, and he makes six hundred bucks. You're going to have a good living when you become a doctor."

Mike thought about doing that to other people.

Then he threw up in his mouth a little.

Not me, Mike promised himself. *Not me.*

Eighth

MRIs and MS from a Neurological Point of View

I am putting myself to the fullest possible use, which is all I think that any conscious entity can ever hope to do.
—Douglas Rain/HAL
2001: A Space Odyssey

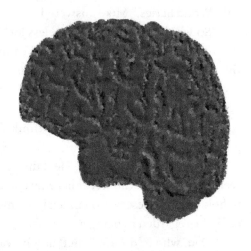

When a person goes to see a neurologist for evaluation of a problem, and after the history and neurological examination are done, a person will often be sent for tests to help confirm or deny what the doctor believes is causing the trouble. Testing commonly includes things like blood work, electrophysiological testing, and imaging. The imaging method of choice in multiple sclerosis is currently MRI. Prior to the advent of MRI technology, however, imaging of the brain was challenging. X-ray imaging cannot produce good resolution images of the brain since the brain is a soft tissue in the body unlike bone, which is dense and hard. In the early 1900s, Dr. Walter Dandy developed X-ray imaging techniques of the brain called *ventriculography* and *pneumoencephalography*. These modalities produced images of the spaces in and around the brain by injecting filtered air into the ventricles or into the space around the brain, respectively. The images allowed Dr. Dandy to surgically treat many patients and his work advanced the sciences of neurosurgery and neuroradiology. The procedures, however, were painful and came with significant risks. Also, these techniques could not show the brain "stuff" (gray matter and white matter) itself. In the 1970s, CAT (computed axial tomography) scans were developed, which were able to produce images that gave a slightly better picture of the brain. Strokes, bleeding, and tumors were able to be better localized within the brain, but the resolution was still poor. The major advance in imaging that has helped doctors to diagnose MS is MRI technology.

MRI machines are wonderful in that they can give us pictures of parts of the human body while we are still using them. It used to be that if doctors wanted to see what was going on in the brain of a person who was sick with a neurological disease, the only thing that could be done was to wait until the patient passed away and then remove the brain, preserve it, cut it up into painfully thin slices, stain them with certain dyes, and then look at them under a microscope. Now, with an MRI machine, we can look at the structure and some of the functioning of the brain while it is still being used. This is a much more satisfying option both for the patient and the doctor. MRIs can produce a good picture of the brain and can show us what specific areas of the brain (gray matter and white matter) are being affected. It can also show us what the abnormalities (commonly called *lesions*) within the brain look like. Lesion size, shape, and enhancement with gadolinium are clues that can help doctors to develop a list of diseases that might be potential causes of the person's neurological problems. In medicine, this list is called a *differential diagnosis*. In the case of MS, there has been developed a set of criteria (called the Revised McDonald Criteria[66]) that can help lead to the diagnosis of MS when used in conjunction with proper neurological history taking and examination. MRI by itself, as of the writing of this book, *cannot* diagnose MS.

HOW MRI MACHINES WORK

MRI stands for magnetic resonance imaging.[67] Here is a simplified version of how it works. The machine is basically a strong magnet attached to a computer. [68] Do you remember in grammar or high school when the science teacher sprinkled iron shavings

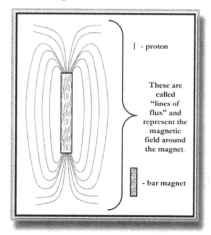

Figure 13. Bar magnet and lines of flux. The figure-eight energy field generated by a bar magnet.

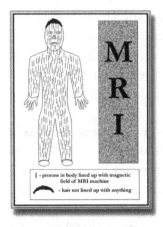

Figure 14. Protons lined up.

on a piece of paper and then put a magnet underneath the paper? All of the filings lined up into a figure eight. That was because all of the protons were lining up with the magnetic field of the magnet (see figure 13). When you go into the MRI machine, almost all of the protons in your body align themselves with the magnetic field (see figure 14). Actually, only the protons that are staying relatively still can become magnetized. Often, the MRI technician will tell you to lie as still as possible while in the machine. The protons that move, like the protons in your blood, cannot become magnetized. Because of this, the inside of the blood vessels do *not* send a signal back to the MRI receivers. If the computer does not get a signal back, it assumes nothing is there. On certain MRI sequences, the inside of the blood vessels appear black. These are called *flow voids.* [69]

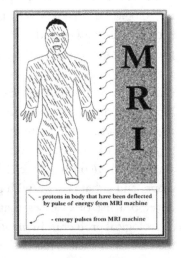

Figure 15. Energy pulse hits protons.

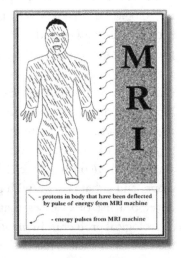

Figure 16. Protons return energy.

Once all of the stationary protons are lined up, we have to do something to the protons to be able to see them. What happens next is that the machine starts making all sorts of buzzing, banging, and clicking noises. With some of the noises, pulses of electromagnetic energy (using frequencies in the TV/radio range) are "thrown" at your body. This knocks the protons in your body out of alignment with the magnetic field. Each tissue in your body (brain, myelin, cerebrospinal fluid, etc.) contains a different amount of protons. This is important because this is what is going to help make the picture that gets laid out in the MR image.

THE CONSERVATION OF MASS AND ENERGY

Now for a quick review of something you might have learned about in high-school science class—*the laws of conservation of mass and of energy.* These laws state that if you add a certain amount of energy (like heat or electromagnetism) to something (a human body, glass of water, your pet snail), the same amount of energy has to come back out after you stop adding energy. So at first in the MRI machine, the protons are lined up in a magnetic field (see figure 14). Next we hit the protons with energy that causes them to get knocked out of alignment (see figure 15). Then, as soon as that pulse of energy is over, the protons have to go back into alignment since they are still in the magnetic field (see figure 16). When they do that, they send back the energy that they just absorbed; this way the amount of mass and energy remains the same.

NOW FOR HOW THE PICTURES GET MADE

The sensors in the MRI machine pick up the amount of energy that was sent back from each of the different tissues. They then send the information to the computer, which can then start to format (or draw) a picture of whichever part of the body it's looking at. The computer samples the amount of energy that is returned at different times after it stops "throwing" electromagnetic energy at us. The first time the returned energy is sampled is called *T1* (Time 1), and the second time is called *T2* (Time 2). These are the images that you and your doctor review together. T1 images show things differently from

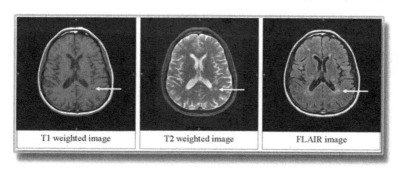

Figure 17. Different MRI sequences.
Comparison of T1, T2, and FLAIR MRI sequences through the same cut of my brain.

T2. For example, on T1 weighted images, the pure cerebrospinal fluid that is inside the ventricles and surrounding the brain appears dark while on T2 it appears bright. In figure 17, you can see the difference.

> <u>Key Point</u>
> Since every tissue in your body contains a different concentration of protons, every tissue is going to absorb and then release a different amount of energy back to the MRI machine.

The third panel in figure 17 is an image from an MRI sequence called *FLAIR*. FLAIR stands for FLuid-Attenuated Inversion Recovery. In this sequence, the lateral ventricles are dark like in the T1 image because the signal coming from the pure cerebrospinal fluid (CSF) is being attenuated. However, note the oval at the head of the arrow on the T1 image. It's dark. On the T2 image, the oval is bright just like the CSF in the ventricles on the T2 image. So is the oval just another space filled with CSF or is something else going on? If we then look at the oval at the head of the arrow on the FLAIR image, we see that it's bright! This is telling us that there's a difference between the fluid that's in the oval area and the "pure" CSF fluid that's in the ventricles. This difference comes from the different signal characteristics of the immune cells, which are in the lesions that are in the brains of those of us with MS. If you look at the other bright white dots on the FLAIR image, you can now compare them with the T1 and T2 images and tell if you're looking at pure CSF signal or if the signal characteristics indicate that something else, like inflammation from an immune response, is going on.

MRIs can take anywhere from twenty to ninety minutes to complete. They take longer than other scans (like CAT scans and X-rays) because the computer needs as much data as it can get. This is one of the reasons why the banging has to go on for such a long time. The more data the computer in the MRI machine gets, the better the picture.[70]

GADOLINIUM

Sometimes, about halfway into the MRI, we are pulled out of the machine and get an injection.[71] The enhancer they are injecting us with is something called *gadolinium*. Gadolinium is basically a whole bunch of extra protons that are being put into our bloodstream (see figure 19). Normally, our blood and CNS do not party together. The blood usually just leaves off oxygen and sugar, picks up carbon dioxide, and then goes on its way. However, if we have a lot of disease activity going on, the barrier between the CNS and the blood (called the "blood-brain barrier" or "BBB") can get broken down and other stuff (like gadolinium) can get into the brain from the blood. When this happens, the area with active inflammation and demyelination going on can light up like a lightbulb on the MRI (since the gadolinium has extra free protons that can absorb and release more energy). This indicates that there is more active disease going on in that spot (see figure 20). We, both doctors and patients, do not like to see gad-enhancing lesions because that means that a person's MS is pretty active and needs to be slowed down. Please note that just because no enhancing areas are seen on an MRI,

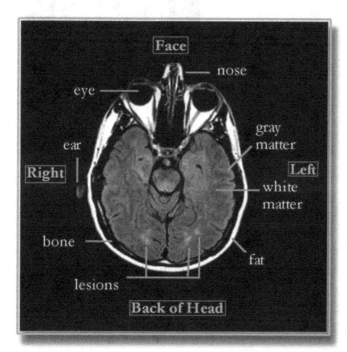

Figure 18. Brain MRI with labels. In this axial, FLAIR MRI image of my brain, you can see that my right ear appears different from the gray matter, the white matter, the subcutaneous fat, and the fluid that is in my head.

it does not mean that the disease is not going on, it just indicates that it is not very active. As of now, we have no cure for MS and can only slow it down with the available therapies.

WHAT GOES ON WHEN YOU GET AN MRI

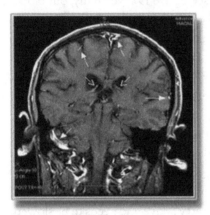

Figure 20. Blood vessels containing gadolinium. In this coronal T1 weighted MRI, the thick arrows on the edge indicate blood vessels with gadolinium inside. The thin arrows in the middle indicate gadolinium in the choroid plexus, which makes the cerebrospinal fluid (CSF). Also note that there are no bright areas within the brain itself anywhere from twenty-to ninety minutes

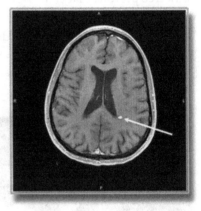

Figure 19. Enhancing MS lesion. This is a gadolinium-enhanced, axial T1 weighted MRI with an arrow pointing at an enhancing MS lesion. The bright areas at the top and bottom are high signal coming back from the gadolinium that is in blood vessels.

The process of getting an MRI differs from location to location, but overall it's pretty much the same. Here are some things that usually go on. When you arrive at the MRI place, they give you a screening form to make sure you do not have any devices or implants that can be affected by the strong magnetic field. The list will include questions like this:

— Are you pregnant?
— Have you ever had any surgery or operation?
— Have you ever had any eye injuries (metallic slivers, foreign bodies, etc.)?
— Have you ever worked in a machine shop?

- Have you ever been injured by a metallic object or foreign body (e.g., BB, bullet, shrapnel, etc.)?
- Have you ever used silver dressing?
- Do you have a cardiac pacemaker or defibrillator?
- Do you have an aneurysm clip or clips (location)?
- Do you have a cardiac stent?
- Do you have a neurostimulator?
- Do you have a spinal cord stimulator?
- Do you have a heart valve replacement?
- Do you have an implanted drug infusion pump?
- Do you have a cochlear implant or implanted hearing device?
- Do you have a permanent Holter monitor?
- Do you have a Swan-Ganz catheter?
- Do you have an eyelid spring wire?
- Do you have a hearing aid?
- Do you wear a nicotine, medication, or other metal-containing patch?
- Do you have any type of prosthesis, artificial limb, or implant?
- Do you have any external or internal metallic objects like EKG lead wires or body piercings?
- Do you have any metallic breast tissue expanders?
- Have you had a GI endoscopy done in the last thirty days?

Many of the metals used in surgery are not magnetizable (nonferromagnetic) and can go into an MRI machine, but make sure the radiologist knows about it. He or she is the person who makes the call.

You should go to the restroom before the scan begins since it can take anywhere from twenty to ninety minutes. Depending upon what type of MRI you're getting, you might either be in an open or closed machine. You should make sure to let your doctor know if you're claustrophobic when you're given a prescription for an MRI. If you're claustrophobic and your doctor thinks that you really need to have the study done in a closed machine, you might need some medication to relax you so that you can get the study done.

When you get called in for your study, you will be asked to go into a changing room. They usually give you a box or a locked room where you can leave your valuables. The MRI technician will ask you to remove anything metal that's on your body. This can include but is not limited to shoes, belts, jewelry, eyeglasses, watches, cell phones, PDAs, prosthetic limbs, barrettes, rings/piercings, dental bridges, and retainers. As you get dressed before going for the MRI, just think, *Might this thing that I am putting on be attracted by a magnet?* If you have any questions about whether something can go in the MRI machine with you, ask the people at your MRI facility.

When you're ready, you're brought into the room with the MRI machine. A closed MRI usually has a round tube in the middle with a gurney that slides in and out of it. The tech will (hopefully) offer you earplugs. If not, ask for them. The machine is usually quite loud. There has been development of MRI machines where the noise-making parts are housed in a vacuum, thus rendering the machine quiet, but these currently are a minority. You then lay down on the gurney, and sometimes a cage is swung over your face. These are the receivers of the energy that gets returned from your brain. Some people feel constricted by it. I just close my eyes and try to go to sleep. Since I can't be on my cell phone in the MRI machine, I view it like a forty-minute mini-vacation where I can get away from it all and no one can bother me.[72]

Once you're in the machine, the tech will go to their booth and communicate with you via a speaker in the machine. He or she will tell you when the test is about to start. Here are a few things to be aware of before the test begins:

1. Make sure that you're comfortable. If there's something like a piece of clothing that you're lying on that is folded weird under you, let someone know and try to straighten it out before the test begins.

2. The less you move the better the images will be. Of course, you have to move for some things, like breathing. You also have to swallow occasionally. That's fine too. These movements are minimal and should not degrade the images. If they do, then the tech will tell you if they need to repeat a sequence.

3. There is usually a jet of cool air blowing through the space where you're lying. It's a good thing because in a closed MRI you're in a tight space where you and the machine can heat up the air pretty easily.

4. The sounds that the MRI machine generates quite often have a repetitive, regular rhythm. Whatever you do, *do not* break out into a musical number. You might have seen an excellent production of *West Side Story* the night before, but if you start humming the intro bars to "America," first your fingers will start doing miniature snaps, then your shoulders will start to make tiny movements to each syllable of "Am-MER-eeee-ca," and since your head is connected to

your shoulder girdle, these movements will make the MRI images look like a plate of refried beans.

When the testing begins, things are going to start clicking and humming and brrrrrrraaaaaaaaaaaaaping and banging. This is the way the MRI normally sounds. You should start to realize how lucky you are that you're wearing earplugs. Enjoy your time alone. No parents bothering you about coming home late. No boss to think about. No kids to chase down. After you've had a couple of MRIs done, you might be able to fall asleep in the machine.

If your doctor ordered gadolinium to be used in your scan, about halfway through the process, the gurney will be slid halfway out of the machine. Don't worry. The machine is not broken. It's just that they only need to get you halfway out so they can place an IV in your arm. Hopefully, the radiologist or tech can get the IV placed after one stick, but it doesn't always happen that way. Sometimes, multiple attempts have to be made before they can find a blood vessel. If you know you're going to get gadolinium with your MRI, make sure you're well hydrated. I drink a Gatorade along with several glasses of water the day before and again three to four hours before the MRI. This helps to increase your intravascular volume (so your vessels bulge more) and often makes it easier for someone to start an IV on you. Of course, speak with your doctor to find out what hydration technique is best for you. After the IV is placed, the technician or other health-care professional will inject you with gadolinium. After the injection is complete, the IV catheter gets removed and you go back into the machine for another round of clicking and humming and brrrrrrraaaaaaaaaaaaaping and banging. Soon after, if the images look good, the technician will come back into the room and let you out of the machine.

Once out of the machine, you can go to the changing area, get your valuables, start listening to all the phone messages you got, and then check out at the front desk. Quite often, I'll have my patients pick up a CD copy of their images on their way out so they can bring them when they come in for follow-up. This way I can show them what their brain looks like. You can ask your doctor if he or she wants you to do that or if they have direct access to the images via a web portal, VPN, or some other system so you can review them together.

I feel that reviewing the images of a brain with a patient is an important and personal matter. If I'm looking at a picture of a brain, I'm looking at a picture of the thing that makes that person who he or she is. When I got my first MRI, it was initially an existential experience. Eventually, I came to realize that an MRI was a structural, and not a functional, test. Thankfully, I've come to realize that what my brain looks like does not reflect who I am.

SUMMARY

MRI technology uses electromagnetism, like the kind found in TV and radio, to look at the soft tissues in our bodies. This has been proven to be very helpful in diagnosing MS.

---

[66] C. H. Polman, S. C. Reingold, B. Banwell, M. Clanet, J. A. Cohen, M. Filippi, K. Fujihara et al., "Diagnostic criteria for multiple sclerosis: 2010 revisions to the McDonald criteria," *Annals of Neurology* 69, no. 2 (February 2011): 292–302, doi: 10.1002/ana.22366.

[67] One of the greatest websites about MRI imaging is The Whole Brain Atlas. The website is http://www.med.harvard.edu/AANLIB/home.html.

[68] By "strong magnet," I'm talking about a *really* strong magnet. You know how Mom stuck the picture of the hand-turkey you drew in kindergarten on the refrigerator with a little magnet? With the magnetic field that the MRI generates, the refrigerator would get stuck to the MRI machine's magnet.

[69] To see where the blood is in blood vessels, the computer can run a different sequence called an *MRA* (magnetic resonance angiogram). What the MRI machine does is take a picture of the area in question. The computer then takes away the parts of the picture that it made from the energy from the stationary protons (all the stuff that does not move), and it is left with a negative image of where the moving protons must be. This image then represents blood that is flowing in the blood vessels.

[70] This is the same reason that your digital camera makes better pictures when you use a higher resolution.

[71] "Just when I thought I was out, they pull me back in." Michael Corleone, *The Godfather, Part III*.

[72] Of course, I am lying in a tube, so the activities are limited. I usually pretend that I'm lying by the pool with a towel over my head on the Fourth of July and the banging sounds are fireworks.

Ninth

This is the story of when I had my first brain MRI. I play the part of me, my mother plays the part of my mom, and the MRI technician is played by Ms. MRI-tech lady. The part of Fish, as always, is played by the incomparable Abe Vigoda.

MIND, MEET BRAIN

I was staring at the fish tank in the dim waiting room of the MRI place. The fish were floating and swimming and kissing the top of the water with their lips going "bloop," trying to snag particles that might be food. A bright yellow one came to the top and sucked something into his mouth. It must not have been what he expected since his next move was to spit it out and wander off in another direction. Lucky fish. He didn't have to get an MRI to see if he had MS. Then again, he had to live in a fishbowl. But it didn't seem that bad. He appeared not to have any responsibilities. He didn't have to take neurobiology and pathology and gross anatomy and biochemistry. He didn't have to go to work. He swam and ate and checked to see if there was anything new at the treasure chest by the guy in the deep-sea diver outfit. Then again, if someone forgot to feed him, he'd die. Okay, the benefit-cost analysis for being a fish indicated that it was better to be a human.

At least for now.

The clock on the wall said 10:15 p.m. I turned and looked at my mom. She was sitting, reading a magazine. I walked over and sat down next to her.

"What are you reading?" I asked.

"Looking for some recipes for dinner this week," she answered, turning her head to look at me. "How are you doing?" she asked as she put her hand on mine.

"Fine. I guess." I paused and thought. *How am I supposed to feel? I feel the same physically as I did before I went to see the doctor. We still don't know what we're dealing with. MS would be better than a brain tumor causing my symptoms.* I had localized the lesion causing my diplopia to the left medial longitudinal fasciculus. It was an area of the nervous system that controlled a lot of stuff that I considered crucial for a full and meaningful life—like maintaining consciousness. I figured that I either had MS or a brain tumor. I didn't think a brain tumor could be removed from that area without causing a whole bunch of damage.

"I hope it's MS," I said. Mom's eyes were slightly red but no tears. She nodded and looked at her magazine. She was handling it well. Or at least that was her game face. She always had a good hold on her spirituality and sense of self. We sat for a few moments in silence. I know she was trying to think of what she had done that caused her son to get MS. She always tended to implicate several things when there was a disease that didn't have an apparent cause:

#1 Overhead power lines. "They're overhead and everywhere you look," she would state while waving her arms, and then let her thought die out.

#2 Aluminum cans. This came from the fact that her mother died after having Alzheimer's disease. She heard something on the radio about how heavy metal buildup in our bodies can cause neurological disease. She then thought back about how my grandmother always stored half-eaten cans of foods in her refrigerator, covered with aluminum foil. Double whammy. Mom taught my sisters and me to have the dull side of the aluminum foil facing the food and the shiny side on the outside. She never gave a specific reason. I guess the dull side looked less aluminum-foil-like than the shiny side.

#3 Vaccinations. "There's something in the preservatives that can possibly trigger something like cancer or Alzheimer's or MS," she would say with the all-knowing talk radio going in the background in our kitchen. She always had a pot of coffee going while ironing and folding clothes and listening to the talk radio. It was usually around ten at night that she would be doing her housework/medical research. That was my mom.

"We're ready for you now," the forty-something-year-old, blue-scrub-clad MRI-tech lady said, opening the door to the next room. I looked at Mom.

"See you later," I said, with resignation.

She blinked several times, keeping the tears from running down her face.

"I'll be here," she said, with a smile.

Moms are great, I thought as I walked toward the bright hallway going to the MRI machine. My sneakers squeaked on the linoleum tile while the MRI-tech lady started talking at me.

"I'll need you to take off all metal on your body and put it in this basket. Take off your shoes and belt, and you can leave them in the changing room." I took out my wallet, keys, and some change and put them in the basket. I walked into the changing room.

"Do you have any piercings or implants?" she asked.

"No," I answered. I was going to use a line from *Fletch* to lighten the mood, but it just didn't seem right. I don't know why it didn't because I always try to keep things light, but I felt a transformation creeping up in me. I was getting ready to go into a machine that was going to generate pictures of the part of my body that I had been using to feed myself ... make friends ... turn eight years old ... play baseball ... become self-aware ... realize that there was a whole world around me that I shared with five billion other people ... go to high school ... work hard ... make more friends ... do chores because that's what you do when you grow up in a family ... study ... like girls, but never really have a girlfriend ... go to college ... have a great experience that went in the dumpster after losing my first real girlfriend ... get into medical school ... and to be the editor of the medical school newspaper when school started after this, my last summer vacation, was over. But this moment was different. I was about to meet, via a picture, the part of me that had made the decisions my whole life. The part of me that generated and felt every emotion. The part that learned, categorized, and integrated every piece of information that had ever met my sensorium. I was about to meet that which would have the final say on whom I would marry. I was about to meet *me*.

Sure, I had seen and felt and studied and weighed and poked and dissected other people's brains the past year in med school, and they were amazing. But now my brain was to be put on exhibit. The MRI-tech lady running the machine would be the first to ever see my brain. That seemed more invasive into my private life than being seen naked. We are all born naked. Our brains, however, are kept in a secure box never to be seen with the eye until something absurd happens. If the brain stops working properly, then we have to look at it. I stepped back into the hallway.

"Do you need to go to the bathroom?" she asked.

"No. I'm good," I replied, with no intonation in my voice. She opened the door to the MRI room. It was brightly lit and almost cold. This was now a movie. I looked at the machine—a big, white machine with a hole in the center. It reminded me of a scene from *A Space Odyssey*. She walked over and pressed a button on the machine causing the gurney to slide out. She opened the cage that would close over my face after I lay down on the thin, tan cushions on the table. She led me over to the table, and I sat down on the edge for a brief second to see what the support of the table felt like. It was solid, so I swung my legs up and lay back. My head fit into a U-shaped holder at the top of the gurney. The head holder made my head feel like it was separate from the rest of my body. I remembered when I played football in sixth grade and a seventh grader was making fun of me while I had my helmet on. He grabbed my facemask and started swinging me from side to side. I became terrified as soon as I realized he had total control over my life—that he could snap my neck like a plastic spoon and I couldn't do anything to stop him!

I was not terrified now, but another thought entered my mind. As MRI-tech lady placed some cushions on either side of my head to keep it fixed, I had to trust that the geniuses who developed MRI technology had thought of everything. Not just the scientific aspects. The existential stuff too. I was thinking about the fact that the machine was going to be able to show me the organ that was thinking about being imaged. It would add another layer of awareness to my existence. M. C. Escher suddenly became hyperfluorescent in my mind—"He who wonders discovers that this in itself is wonder."[73]

A pillow was placed under my knees, which felt better than lying flat. She put my arms at my sides and wrapped wide Velcro straps around me.

"Do you feel all right?" she asked.

"I feel like a burrito," I replied, again without intonation.

"We'll get started soon," she said and pressed the button to slide me back into the machine.

As the different parts of the tunnel came down through my visual field, I was reminded of the rocket launch video I saw as a kid. I pictured the big U-S-A letters scrolling past me as I continued my journey into this part of my life. The technology that I was about to experience was so many times that of what the astronauts had when they were in their rocket back then. But at the same time, if it were not for them, I probably wouldn't be able to have my journey now. Newton was right. I thought it interesting that I needed to stand on the shoulders of giants not only to see farther but to look inside myself as well. The gurney stopped moving. The pod bay door was shut. The mission was about to start..

"Okay," the voice said through the speaker. "We are going to start the first sequence." I wasn't sure if this was a one-way conversation. She didn't ask for a response. The machine started making some clicks and a hum. There was a cool jet of air shooting down from above me. I made myself not move. Then I realized doing that was like concentrating on relaxing. I needed to realize that the Velcro wrap was not going to let my body move and my head bumpers would keep my head fixed. I released the tension in my head, neck, and body. I was supported on all sides. Safe.

My eyes were going crossed since there was nothing to fixate on in the white tunnel. I closed them. The humming and clicks got louder. I could feel that the tail of my shirt was slightly bunched up under my left lower back at the belt line. I could not change that now. Just deal with it—like the astronauts did. The clicks stopped, and then the banging began.

And continued.

For a long time.

It was low pitched like someone knocking on your door with a brick. The banging stopped and was replaced by some high-frequency machine-gun fire. Magazine after magazine after magazine of gunshot ripping through my white-tunnel world. I realized that when deprived of any other frame of reference, the brain's clock will regard a single stimulus as persisting for eternity. I let the sound drill into my head.

Then silence.

Then more clicks.

More banging.

Machine guns.

I noticed that the second round was not as loud as the first. Either my brain was adapting or I was going deaf. I chose the former and this time listened to the machine guns. I was starting to hear a second pattern of sound behind the first. It was like the initial sound waves had harmonized and their quasi-sympathetic vibrations had generated another song. I started to notice an itch on my nose. I couldn't scratch it. The itch intensified. The fact that I couldn't move allowed me to conclude that either the nose itch would go away or I would die. I thought back to when I had first laid in the machine and how far away that place was. My brain had never been seen before, but

I knew that pictures were coming up in front of the tech while I lay there. I noticed briefly that the folded shirttail issue had resolved. I felt like I was the astronaut in the spaceship and the tech was one of the crowd at the launch pad watching the ship do its job. The astronauts had no frame of reference either. They were going to a place that was different. My only reference now was the time since the shirttail issue and the nose-itch situation. The song continued. The nose itch started to lessen. I listened to the music and felt the itch fade away. The sound stopped.

"Okay, we'll slide you out and give you your gadolinium."

The gurney started moving back out of the machine. "How are you doing?" she asked.

"Okay," I replied, quietly. She wrapped the tourniquet around my arm, cleaned the bend at my right elbow, placed the IV, injected the gadolinium, took out the tiny IV catheter, and wrapped a bandage around my arm.

"We have one more long sequence and two short ones. Then we'll be done."

I nodded.

One long. Two short.

Roger, Houston.

She slid me back into the machine.

I wondered how my mom was doing.

The air kept blowing over me.

Silence gave way to my old friends.

Clicks.

Hey, where you guys been?

Banging.

Remember back when I had a shirttail folded under my low back?

Machine guns.

Yeah. That was like forever ago.

I knew they wouldn't answer me.

David Bowie's "Major Tom" came to mind.

What if I were just lost to the universe.

No one around.

Floating in an ill-defined space.

Like in a fishbowl.

No responsibilities.

A little food.

Some oxygen.
My brain brought me here.
I didn't want to come.
I'm glad I did.
Mom's here.
It will be all light.

Tech-lady's voice woke me up.

"Okay. We're done." I heard her come back into the MRI room, and the gurney started to slide out. *Riiiiiiip* went the Velcro wraps. She unsnapped the cage, and I sat up. The world looked the same. I felt different. I went back to the little room and collected my stuff. I walked back out to the waiting room. Mom was still reading. I passed the fish tank. They were still swimming. She didn't see me walk up.

"Hi," I said.

"Oh, honey. I didn't see you there. How did it go?"

"Swimmingly," I said.

"What happens now?"

"She's going to print out the films, and then we bring them to the doctor."

"Okay. Did you want to get anything to eat?"

"Sure," I answered, going up to the window to pick up the films. MRI-tech lady picked up the films off the printer, put them in a jacket, and handed them to me.

"Thanks," I said, with a tiny spark in my voice.

"You're welcome," she replied as she looked to call in the next patient.

I opened the door for my mom, and she went out.

"I'll get the car and bring it around," she said.

"Okay," I answered. I looked at the fish tank one last time and saw the yellow fish. He was doing the same thing. Treasure chest. Swim. Bloop. I turned, went out the door, and walked out to the parking lot. It was cooler out than when we had arrived. The clock on the bank read 11:45 p.m.

I drew one of the sheets of film out of the jacket. I held it up to the ring of light cast by the streetlamp and looked at one of the saggital cuts. Like a baby seeing his reflection in a mirror for the first time, my mind froze, and I stared. I saw a saggital image of my brain. It looked like every other brain I had ever seen on MRI.

Quite dehumanizing, I thought.

Hold on a second, chief, I thought back at myself. *I'm unique. I'm not just like everyone else. It's just a picture of what my brain looks like. It does not indicate how my brain was functioning. My mind is who I am.*

But it's the brain that makes the mind, no?

Yes, in combination with all the nerves and experiences and people in my life. I looked at several other images and saw a few white dots in the white matter of my frontal lobes.

But your brain is getting shot up.

I love the people around me, and they love me.

Even when you act like a baby?

People love babies, don't they?

They love babies but not necessarily the things they do.

Why?

Because they know that they'll eventually grow up and act properly.

We don't always act properly, do we?

Nope.

So I've regressed to being a baby?

Intermittently.

But most of the time, I'm me though, right?

Yeah, but when you stop being you and start getting impatient with people and stop thinking of others, then you become a baby, and people don't want to be around you as much.

But they still love me because they know I'm a good person.

Yeah. But how long are you gonna play that game before someone you love puts up their hands and says they're outta here because they didn't sign up to be a babysitter.

But that's not my fault. It's the damn disease that's messing up my frontal lobes and causes me to act like a baby.

How do they know that? They only know what they see by your actions.

I say please and thank you.

You also told your girlfriend that she was the mother of a dog.

That was just once, and she knew I didn't mean it.

Is that what her actions told you?

No.

I wouldn't have stayed around either if I were treating me like that.

My mother's car pulled up to the sidewalk. I put the sheet back in the folder and opened the car door.

I guess we need some help.

Tenth

WHAT MRIS LOOK LIKE FROM A NEUROLOGICAL POINT OF VIEW

It's okay, Vin.
Size doesn't matter.
—Lauren Macaluso speaking to Vincent
Macaluso when she saw the disappointed look on
her husband's face while he looked at the MRI images
of his atrophied brain after having had MS for twenty-five years.

While getting a brain MRI done is an existential experience for some, it's a much more objective and well-defined entity for others. In this chapter, we're going to learn the basics of reading a brain MRI. Please note that all of the MRIs in this book are mine. This decision was made after I, Vincent Macaluso, MD, sat down with me, Vince Macaluso, Guy, and reviewed my rights as a patient. Many of these rights fall under HIPAA (Health Insurance Portability and Accountability Act) regulations. These regulations, among other things, protect confidentiality and security of US residents' health-care information, including things such as MRI images.

Be it known that, while I am allowing me the use of the pictures of my brain that I have reviewed, I reserve the right to bring action upon myself if any picture is used or described in a fashion that is demeaning, defamatory, or derogatory or brings financial, emotional, or personal hardship upon me or my family, including, but not limited to, my wife, my daughter, my son, my pet cricket, Chooch, or any other children or pets that I might have or might want to have in the future, and their offspring, in aeternam.

MRI Images

The layout of MRIs is traditionally done in three different planes—sagittal, axial, and coronal. During medical training, doctors get a three-dimensional (3D) view of the body during the first year when we do gross anatomy. When the body is opened, a person gets the macroscopic view of how our organs are related to one another. MRIs allow us to see these organs (called *soft tissues* [74]) that make up the majority of our bodies without having to do any cutting. The older ways of looking at the inside of the body were two-dimensional (2D) pursuits, usually by passing high-energy waves through the body (transillumination, X-rays, and fluoroscopy). The images that were produced had a length and width. The only way to obtain a 3D understanding of what was going on in the body was to take a picture, rotate the patient, and then take another picture. Aside from being time consuming and expensive, it would require multiple doses of radiation that, except for certain situations, was not healthy.[75]

Eventually computed tomography came out and was able to provide rapid, low-dose 2D X-rays that, when given to a computer, could be compiled into a 3D image. Unfortunately, X-rays are not a useful modality to image soft tissues. MRIs, however, use magnetism, which is able to generate pictures with very good resolution. As computers continue to increase in processing speed, they are able to manipulate more data, faster. This allows for useful 3D image viewing on the host computer. Current personal computer processors are able to generate fairly good 3D images from the data they are given. As it stands currently, physicians and their patients still have to understand how to read 2D images and then use their inbred processors to manipulate the data and decide what to do about what was seen.

How MRI Images of the Brain Are Presented

The MRI machine's computer lays out images in three planes—sagittal, axial, and coronal. In figure 21, the image on the left is a T1 weighted, sagittal image of my brain. On the right is a picture of me. In the MRI, I am looking toward the left. The MRI is a longitudinal section through my head (the vertical line is where the cut is made through my head).

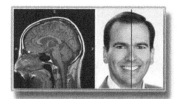

Figure 21. Sagittal brain MRI image. The picture next to the MRI is the orientation and location of the cut made through my head.

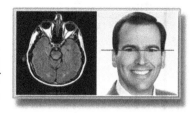

Figure 22. Axial brain MRI image. The picture next to the MRI is the orientation and location of the cut made through my head.

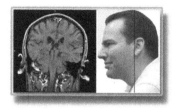

Figure 23. Coronal brain MRI image. The picture next to the MRI is the orientation and location of the cut made through my head.

The MRI in figure 22 is a T1 weighted, axial image. The cut through my head is at the level of my eyeballs. I'm lying on my back with my feet pointing out of the page toward you, so it is like my head was cut open at the level of the black line and you're looking up into my brain.[76]

The MRI in figure 23 is a T1 weighted, coronal image. I'm facing you. If you were to cut through my head at the point indicated by the black line and move my face out of the way, that's what you would see. You can tell that I received gadolinium for this study because the blood vessels are bright.

What You Are Looking At

In figure 24, I have labeled two images with numbers—a sagittal, T1 weighted MRI and an axial, T1 weighted MRI. By matching the numbers with the structures, you can learn what you're looking at when you see an MRI image. Each of the structures is described. Note that not all numbers appear on both MRIs since you cannot always see the same things on different views. Tables 6 through 8 name each labeled structure and give brief descriptions of their functions.

Table 6. List of structures and functions of the brain (1 of 3).

#	Structure	Function
1	frontal lobe	Guides behavior and social interactions, helps with initiative, helps in eye movement, contains the precentral gyrus which is where motor actions are born
2	temporal lobe	Deals mostly with memory, this is the part of the brain that is affected in Alzheimer's disease
3	parietal lobe	This area deals with spatial relationships, it contains the post central gyrus which is where almost all sensory input winds up
4	occipital lobe	Input from the eyes eventually winds up here. This is where things you see get interpreted and sent to other association areas that help to figure out how to deal with what was just seen
5	"head" of the corpus callosum	The corpus callosum is the place where most of the connections between the two hemispheres cross from one side to the other. It is grossly split up into the head (most anterior), body (middle) and tail (most posterior) parts
6	"body" of the corpus callosum	Middle of the corpus callosum
7	"tail" of the corpus callosum	Posterior part of the corpus callosum

Table 7. List of structures and functions of the brain (2 of 3).

#	Structure	Function
8	lateral ventricle	This is one of the largest spaces in the brain and it is filled with a fluid called the cerebrospinal fluid (CSF). This fluid travels around the entire CNS and contains proteins and white blood cells (among other things). Sometimes when trying to diagnose a disease affecting the CNS we doctors get a sample of CSF by inserting a needle into the spinal column in the area of the low back and removing a few cc's of fluid. The CSF is made by something called the choroid plexus which is also located in the lateral ventricles
9	midbrain	This region has to do with the control of eye movement, coordination and smooth movement (via the substantia nigra)
10	pons	This holds the nerves (the cranial nerves) that control many functions of the face and head. All input from the body and output to the body passes through here. This is VALUABLE REAL ESTATE in the CNS when it comes to how much trouble can come from even a tiny, tiny lesion
11	medulla	This is the last part of the brainstem which also contains cranial nerves which control the face, head and neck
12	cerebellum	This is the part of the CNS which is responsible for putting together all of the sensory input coming from the body - it processes the input from the inner ear along with muscles and tendons and then sends signals out to the muscles to produce coordinated movements

Table 8. List of structures and functions of the brain (3 of 3).

#	Structure	Function
13	cervical spinal cord	This is the start of the spinal cord proper and mostly contains axons that are covered in myelin.
14	nose	This is used as a receptive organ for the sense of smell. It is also used to hold up eyeglasses and is often admired if it looks like a button.
15	tongue	This is used to stick out at people who do not understand jokes about noses.
16	ear	Works in conjunction with nose to keep eyeglasses in place.
17	eye	Transmits impulses along optic nerve to occipital lobe.
18	optic nerves	These are the nerves that carry action potentials from the retina in the eye to the brain. The axons are susceptible to demyelination and this causes optic neuritis.

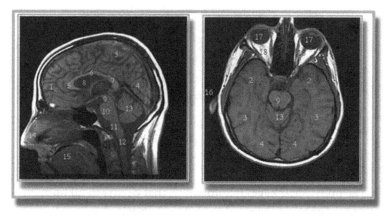

Figure 24. Labeled parts of the brain on sagittal and axial images.
1. Frontal lobe; 2. Temporal lobe; 3 Parietal lobe; 4. Occipital lobe; 5. Corpus callosum—"Genu"; 6. Corpus callosum—"Body"; 7. Corpus callosum—"Splenium"; 8. Lateral ventricle; 9. Midbrain; 10. Pons; 11. Medulla; 12. Cervical spinal cord; 13. Cerebellum; 14. Nose; 15. Tongue; 16. Earlobe; 17. Eyeball; 18. Optic nerve

MRI IS GREAT BUT NOT PERFECT—YET

There are many manipulations the MRI computer can do with the data that it gets from our bodies. It can differentiate many things like inflammation, blood, dead cells, and living cells. It can show where the brain is functioning and where it is not. It is a wonderful machine, but it's not perfect. Something I always try to teach my patients is that MS is a disease that's going on all the time in the central nervous system on a microscopic level. The human eye cannot see the demyelination that happens around each axon without using a microscope. It's important to remember when looking at an MRI that just because you don't see a lesion, it doesn't mean that there aren't thousands of microscopic lesions going on all throughout the white matter that you cannot see. A common term we use in MS neurology, when looking at an MRI of a person with MS, is "normal-appearing white matter" (NAWM).

This constant, microscopic demyelination can best be appreciated when you compare the MRIs of someone who has MS and who is not taking any disease-modifying therapy to slow down the disease process. MRI images seen in figure 25 are based on brain atrophy data in people who have MS but who did not start therapy. The loss of brain tissue occurred over seven years.

139

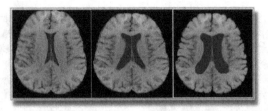

Figure 25. Atrophy.
Note how the brain on the left is "plump like a grape" and the brain
on the right is atrophied and "shrunken like a raisin."

This atrophy (shrinkage) is something that occurs in all humans. Note that this sort of change is normal in all people, but it usually takes over fifty years for this degree of atrophy to occur even when there is no degenerative disease process going on. With MS in the picture, this can happen for some people in well under a decade.

Summary

MRIs provide us with beautiful pictures of our brains (as well as many other parts of the body). They show us what things look like in detail. However, it is crucial, at this point, for us to remember that MS is a microscopic disease, and an MRI machine provides us with macroscopic images. Using this knowledge, we can put "lesions" into perspective. Just because we might not see a lesion in the white matter of our brains, it does not mean that demyelination is not going on. Demyelination goes on continuously, on a microscopic level. If we do see lesions, we can see if they are active by using gadolinium. If there is gadolinium enhancement, it means that a person's immune system is vigorously attacking their CNS myelin. If you see enhancing lesions on your MRI, it might mean that your MS is not under good control. Speak with your MS doctor/health-care professional, discuss what the enhancing lesions mean in your disease, and make a plan for what approach you will take to slow down your MS.

---

[73] http://www.quotationspage.com/search.php3?Search=&startsearch=Search&Author=escher&C=mgm&C=motivate&C=classic&C=coles&C=poorc&C=lindsly.

[74] This is in contrast to bones, teeth, and fingernails, which are the "hard tissues" in our bodies.

[75] C. R. Williams, "Radiation exposures from the use of shoe-fitting fluoroscopes," *New England Journal of Medicine* 241, no. 9 (September 1, 1949): 333–5.

[76] Please excuse the bottom of my feet.

Eleventh

What MRIs Look Like from the Other Side of the Desk

As was mentioned in the last chapter, for many people, viewing a picture of part of the body is a very personal thing. Some health-care professionals are sensitive to this issue. Others are not. The following is a conversation between a patient and a doctor while viewing the patient's brain MRI. Only the patient's half of the conversation is included in the text.

WHAT I HEARD THE DOCTOR SAY

So how did it look?
Yes, I remember learning to read when I was in first grade.
"House." "Car." "Pool."
I got older, and the words became more complex.
"Domain." "Freedom." "Natatorium."
Life became more complex.

Pictures? Well, yes.
I've seen them too.
In fact, I remember them from
before I was able to read.

I can describe pictures with the words
that you asked about before.
The simplicity of your questions—
it provokes some concern.

What's this that you present?
A picture. My brain?
No. I think I know what a brain looks like.
That is no brain.

What do you say? It's a cut?
Of what?
Again—my brain, you claim.
But I see no blood.

A slice?
Kind doctor, you propose that
this picture is a brain,
yet you speak of it as if it were a ham.

But whose brain?
Yes. As I said, I can read.
Yes. I can see the words.
I see your "slice" labeled with my name ...

But this cannot be.
I've seen a picture of a brain before.
It was smooth and regular with curves and lines.
It was a picture of a wondrous machine.

This picture you present appears angry.
It's irregular.
And spotty.
And hostile.

Lesions?
What do you mean lesions?
Lesion like a wound, you mean.
Then say wound.

By convention.
What convention?
This isn't a caucus!
It's my brain!

You're sorry?
That's it?
You lay a picture in front of me,
showing my brain full of your "lesions."

You show me, in cold black and white
in your self-deified fashion,
the thing that makes me, *me*
has been wounded!

That, Doctor, is the deepest of all lesions.
I could say that what you have done
is a gouge to my heart.
But that would only be to my heart!

A mere muscle.
A pump.
A thing that you medicals have already copied.
However poorly.

But with your picture and word,
you have assaulted me.

If this is my brain,
then it is the most special brain.
It is the brain that watched
and played ball with my father.

It is the brain that learned all
that was required of me in school and
then led me to the things
that I truly needed to know.

It is the brain with which
I met a beautiful woman,
and it led me to ask her
to become my beautiful wife.

It was the brain that watched
my mother pass
and then felt and witness
my father join her.

The brain that celebrated the birth of my daughter
and then my son!
The brain that now tries
to play ball with them!

The brain that holds
the dreams
of all
that could be.

Now you show me with your MRI "slices"
that you found holes in my brain.
These are not mere lesions in a brain that you have shown me.
They are terrorists punching holes in my life!

Doctor.

You have shown me more than you know.
You have shown me that while your knowledge
might be immense,
you wield it in a reckless manner.

Doctor.

Go back to your books and add some more.
Alanlects. Bible. Koran. Talmud. Tao Te Ching. Veda.
Start with a famous one and how Luke tells it.
Heal yourself before damning others with your diagnosis.

Doctor.

There is a fine line between caring and killing.
Mark this day.
This is the day you have not cared.
This is the day you have killed.

Twelfth

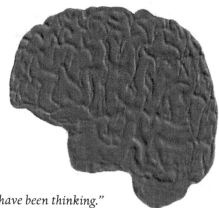

NEUROCOGNITIVE TESTING FROM A NEUROLOGICAL POINT OF VIEW

"Poirot," I said. "I have been thinking."
"An admirable exercise, my friend. Continue it."
—Agatha Christie, *Peril at End House*

While MRI scans are excellent ways to see the structure of the brain, neurocognitive testing is an excellent way to get an objective measure of the functioning of the brain. For our purposes, functioning of the brain is how the different areas of the brain, when working well together, are able to produce thoughts. The process of thinking, or cognition, includes being able to acquire information via our senses, remember information, compare old and new information, make conclusions from what we have learned, and much more.

AN EXAMPLE OF COMMON COGNITION

Here's an example of cognitive functioning that goes on in many people's lives. You're eating breakfast when your wife tells you that she has a meeting this afternoon and the kids need to be picked up from school. You ask what time they need to picked up, and your spouse says three o'clock. You think about your schedule for the day. You remember that you have a hair appointment at the same time. You say to yourself that you have to change the time of your appointment. You make a mental note to call and reschedule your appointment when you get to work. You know that the school is on the way home from the hair place, so if you can get an earlier appointment, you'll be able to pick up the kids after the haircut. You tell your wife, "No worries. I'll pick them up." You kiss her, finish your breakfast, and then leave for work.

When you get to work, you call your hair stylist and move the appointment up to 2:15 p.m. The day moves on. At two o'clock, you go for your appointment. You get your haircut. You look fantastic. You pay your bill. You pick up the kids. They comment on how great your hair looks. You return home. Life is good.

The spheres of cognition used in this example include attention (being able to focus on what your spouse is telling you), short-term memory (taking in new data), long-term memory (recalling known data), visual spatial (understanding the spatial relationship of items), executive functioning (making a decision about what to do with the data), verbal (communicating data through speech), and processing speed (doing all these things in a timely fashion).

AN EXAMPLE OF MS COGNITION

In the mind of the person with MS, the same situation commonly follows a slightly different course.

"Honey. I have a meeting today. Can you pick up the kids from school at three o'clock?"

"What?" you ask as your MS brain tries to focus on not pouring salt into your coffee like you've done every day since your beautiful wife bought new salt and sugar holders.

"Can you pick up the kids today for me?"

"Yeah. I guess."

"Thanks," she says, and turns toward the door.

"From where?" you ask.

"School."

"What time?"

"Three o'clock," she answers, with disappointment in her voice.

You notice that she's unhappy, and you try to cover up by saying, "Of course! I know they're at school, but I just thought maybe they had an after-school thing going on."

She has heard this before, so then she asks, "Do you want to put it in your PDA?"

"No," you reply. "I can remember the kids!"

She leaves, and you finish your breakfast, proud that you avoided the sugar/salt coffee conflict. As you get cleaned up, you notice your hair is long and remember that you have a haircut appointment today. You say to yourself that you can't miss that appointment. The day goes on, and the PDA alarm that you set when you made the haircut appointment goes off, saying you have a haircut appointment at three o'clock.

It's not until you're halfway through your haircut, when your stylist asks how your kids are doing, that you remember that you were supposed to pick them up today. You look at your watch and see that it's 3:27 p.m. You start to pull the hairdressing gown off as you get up and tell the hairdresser that you have to go. You rush out to your car and drive rapidly to the school to get the kids, but when you arrive, no one is there. You then call your wife, who says that she called her friend to pick them up when the school called her and said no one was there to pick up the kids. She goes on to say that she had called you first, but your phone had gone to message, so she called her friend.

In this example, we see deficits in attention (being distracted by the salt-sugar coffee confusion), immediate memory (not paying attention prevents normal memory tracks from being laid down), remote memory (forgetting about the hair appointment until seeing long hair in the mirror), and executive functioning (running out of the hair salon right away without thinking about the best way to find out what has happened to the kids). The fact that you are walking around with half a haircut and a hairdressing gown wrapped around your leg, while inconsequential in comparison to the welfare of your children, really compounds the pathos of the situation.

That is not normal functioning.

Quite often, people who have MS (and many others, as well) have deficits in these spheres of cognition.[77] The only way to tell if a brain is working properly is to do a functional test. We do functional testing all the time. When you first meet a person, you do your own personal cognitive testing. You introduce yourself to a stranger and then you find out who they are.

"Hi," you say.

"Hello," he or she says back. Okay. Now you know that he or she speaks English and he or she did not shun you even though you have a big mustard stain on your shirt.

"My name is Fred," you add.

"Oh my God," the person replies. "My frog's name was Fred, and he got run over by a Big Wheel when I was six years old, and I still haven't gotten over it yet. Would you like to come home and see my collection of lint?"

So the test yielded results. If you continue your testing, you might find that the frog story/lint thing was just a joke and you become best friends. Then again, the comment about him being a lint collector might trigger a memory about a string of lint-related bank robberies that you heard about on the news, and so you decide to excuse yourself so you can alert the LRCTF (Lint-Related Crime Task Force) that you might have a break in the case.

What I'm trying to point out is this:

A PERSON'S APPEARANCE DOES NOT INDICATE THE COGNITIVE STATUS OF THAT PERSON![78]

Likewise,

A PERSON'S APPEARANCE DOES NOT INDICATE HOW THAT PERSON IS FEELING![79]

And to take it one step further,

THE MRI OF A PERSON'S BRAIN INDICATES NEITHER THE COGNITIVE STATUS OF THAT PERSON NOR HOW THAT PERSON IS FEELING![80]

There are people with MS who are physical quadriplegics and are good lawyers, accountants, doctors, artists, and just about everything else. At the same time, there are people with MS who are triathletes, models, doctors, teachers, lawyers, electricians, and regular people who cannot remember what you just said to them! They cannot remember what they were just reading about in a newspaper article. They do not understand what's going on in the TV show they're watching because they forgot what happened in the last scene. They have kids who need to be picked up from school, but they know that no matter how many times they're told that they have to get the kids at two thirty, they'll forget it as soon as the next distraction enters their life! We MSers know that we should write things down and make a list—like everybody tells us to do—but when we do, we lose the damn list that we wrote everything on. And do you want to know why we can't find the damn list? We can't find the list because we have a stack of lists of stuff that we haven't finished because for every task we start, we think of five other things that need to get done. This unrelenting, disorganized, *underappreciated* world of attention deficit continues to balloon until we become mental quadriplegics![81]

This trouble with basic cognition has far-reaching effects. Sometimes a person with MS who has cognitive issues can no longer do his or her job well, if at all. This can lead to the MSer's coworkers thinking that they're slacking off at work. The MSer might appear to be joking around all the time when actually the laughing and kidding come from the fact that the MSer, who cannot concentrate and remember, is just trying to "get by" until the next sentence with the hope that they might be able to pick up from the context of the conversation what it was that they were supposed to be doing for the "big project" that's coming up. The same goes on at home when they get yelled at by a spouse about what a mess the whole house is because they started fourteen different projects and have finished none of them. Or when your children say that they know they told you that they had to have the money for the class trip in by yesterday and now they can't go because it's too late and that you do this all the time and that you don't love them and that's why Daddy left.

Is it hard to see why depression is so common in MS?

Here's a useful intervention, for patients and doctors alike.

COMPUTER-BASED NEUROCOGNITIVE TESTING

Computer-based neurocognitive testing has been developed. It has been proven to be a reliable and effective modality in the evaluation of cognition in people with MS.[82, 83] While the testing can be used to help diagnose and track many different diseases that cause trouble with thinking, I will address only MS in this chapter, since that's the only neurodegenerative disease that I have.

As of now.

That I know of.

In neurocognitive testing, there are areas of cognition that are more commonly affected in people with MS than in the general population. These include:

1. Attention
2. Short-term memory
3. Executive function (a.k.a. judgment)
4. Processing speed
5. Psychomotor processing

If a person cannot pay attention, he or she cannot lay down memory tracks. If a memory track cannot be laid down, then it's very hard to make decisions based on recently acquired data (executive function). Processing speed goes down because of the demyelination of the axons.[84] Psychomotor processing is the time it takes for the body to follow a motor command generated by the mind, such as finger tapping.

The beauty of computer-based neurocognitive testing is multifold. First, after a person with MS takes the test, she or he can see physical documentation of how their brain is functioning. When MSers see data showing that they have lower scores in attention, memory, judgment, and processing speed, when compared to age and educationally matched people without MS (as well as to themselves prior to MS), the effect that MS has had on their thinking becomes vividly clear.[85] After the doctor sees the results of the testing and puts together what was found on the neurocognitive screening questionnaires, the doctor can then discuss using various combinations of cognitive therapies and medications to help ameliorate whatever problems are found.

If a person has ADD and a medication is part of the treatment plan, their response to therapy can be both immediate and life changing. Having improved attention, leading to better memory and judgment, allows for a person to say to him or herself, "Wow, I can concentrate and remember again. Maybe I can do some things again like go back to work or manage a household—things I thought were lost and gone forever."

HERE'S THE LIBERATING PART FOR MSERS

Neurocognitive testing can also allow a person to show the test results to a spouse, friend, or child and say, "Hey, look. I have it here in black and white. I can't concentrate and remember things very well. By taking some medication and doing neurocognitive training exercises, there's a good chance I can start to think the way I did before I developed MS!" By having tangible evidence of their intangible cognitive functioning, MSers can feel empowered.

➤ When we see the results, we can say, "I knew I wasn't crazy! The changes in my thinking are caused by MS!"
➤ We don't feel all alone in our dysfunctional brains when others can see the results.
➤ We know there are therapies for ADD, so if we get on therapy, there is a good chance that we can start thinking like we used to.
➤ We can show the results to those around us who did not understand why our behaviors changed after we got MS.
➤ Additionally, we can say that, with therapies, we could possibly start to behave like we did before we got MS!

After starting and staying on therapy for MS-induced ADD, quite often we MSers start to realize some things:

• We don't talk nearly as much anymore.
• We don't interrupt people nearly as much anymore.
• We don't lose track of what we were saying nearly as much as we did.
• We don't forget nearly as many things anymore.
• We don't make *nearly* as many stupid comments anymore.
• We shut up and listen a lot more.

Computer-based neurocognitive testing is a reliable tool that can measure how our MS-ravaged brains function! Additionally, while others still can't feel what it's like to have MS, they're at least one step closer to understanding us.

HERE'S THE LIBERATING PART FOR DOCTORS

Computer-based neurocognitive testing is a useful tool for us doctors. We listen to our patients and hear the troubles that they have with their thinking. The dogma has been that depression is *very* common in MS. We are taught that we should be aware of it and start appropriate treatment for it. Yes, depression, along with anxiety and bipolar disease, is common in MS and can affect cognition. These should always be screened for, along with attention deficit hyperactivity disorder and substance abuse. However, we need to appreciate the fact that mood disorders can be both causes and effects of impaired cognition. Use of screening tools like those in the list that follows can rapidly provide objective evidence of dysfunction for particular cognitive spheres:

1. Computer-based neurocognitive testing
2. Patient screens for:
   a. attention deficit disorder
   b. hyperactivity
   c. depression
   d. anxiety
   e. bipolar disease

Therefore, after obtaining a pre-MS cognitive history of a patient from the patient (and/or from family and friends as appropriate), it can be combined with the psychological screens and the objective results of valid neurocognitive testing, allowing for initiation of indicated therapies, including neurocognitive training, medication, and/or emo-cognitive therapy.

It should be noted that while computer-based neurocognitive testing is a quick and reliable screening tool for cognitive functioning, as it stands right now, that's what it is—a screening tool. Screening tests should always be followed by complete neuropsychological evaluation by a trained neuropsychiatrist or neuropsychologist. Psychiatric and psychological therapies should be continued as indicated for the appropriate care of the patient. The brain/mind continuum is an incredibly complex creation that needs to be respected. Computer-based neurocognitive testing can quickly render sensitive and specific data to a neurologist that, when combined with neurological examination and evaluation, can lead to treatments that have meaningful impact in the lives of MSers and those around them.[86]

LOOKING AT THE ONES WHO LOVE US AND OURSELVES

We have people around us who love us. They put up with us. They take us to our appointments. They know that we say that we'll pay the bills like we always do, but they know that we've missed a few, so they check up on us. Some of our loved ones check to make sure the bills were paid, but they never tell us because they know that we were always the check writers and we would be upset if we knew that they couldn't depend on us anymore. They hear us make inappropriate comments in social situations and try to laugh it off, shaking their heads and making excuses. "It's a new medication that Jerry just started ..."

It's normal to think that we can control our behaviors on our own, but with MS, those control mechanisms have been disabled. As a last resort, we hide behind the usual phrases:

○ I was tired that day.
○ We were at your parents' house, and your mother and sisters always put me in a bad mood.
○ I don't like to take a medication if I don't need it.
○ My cousin took a medication like that and got worse.
○ I don't want to put any more chemicals in my body.
○ I only use all-natural remedies.

I used to think like that.

It wasn't until years after I was diagnosed with MS and I had started becoming a neurologist that I could look back on my life and start to see the changes that had gone on in me as a person:

I had always been a good student, but after getting MS, my grades took a precipitous drop and never fully recovered.

I had always been a conscientious student, but one specific day, when I had an exam scheduled, I specifically remember that I did not care that I was not ready for the test!

I had always tried to act like a gentleman, but there came a series of incidents where I was actively hurting a girl that I thought I loved.

I was saying mean things to people that I would have never, ever said before I got MS.

I was acting like a jerk around my family and friends.

I was acting like a jerk around everybody.

After I got married, there were times when I was not respecting the greatest person in my life, my wife.

Through all these years, I knew that somehow my thinking had changed. While going through my years of medical training, the pieces of the puzzle began to come together. Between what I learned from medical school, internship, residency, being married, watching my kids grow, being a computer geek, and everything else I have ever lived through, I came to one *huge* conclusion:

It's okay to ask for help.

I finally got on a disease-modifying therapy. I finally did neurocognitive testing, which revealed findings consistent with ADD. I realized that I should start taking medication for it. I was reluctant at first, but then I asked myself, "How would you treat a patient who had the same disease?" Thinking logically, I started taking medication.

Now I'm better at being a husband, a dad, a brother, a doctor, a friend, and just about everything else that I try to do, like writing a book.

THINKING OF OTHERS—THE ONES WHO GET SCARED

For some people, once they notice the emo-cognitive changes that have gone on in us MSers, they have a different reaction from those who put up with our behaviors. They say things like this:

- o You're such a baby.
- o You're so lazy.
- o You're so disorganized.
- o You don't take care of the kids.
- o You don't love me anymore.
- o You've changed.
- o I'm outta here.

We don't think we've changed because the change that goes on in us is insidious. If we tell them that we feel like garbage or our memory is shot, they belittle it:

"Look, we're all tired," Billie says. "You. You're always sitting there on the couch. You say you don't have the energy, but I saw you get up and go to that sale to buy that stuff you love to use. You had energy then. And you say you can't remember nothin'! We're all getting older. I couldn't find my cell phone at work the other

day, so I retraced my steps until I found it! But you. You forgot the
kids at the park and they could've been picked up by some crazy
person! I'm taking them to my mother's house. See ya later."

They don't realize how different it is in MS.

Yes, that's true.

But don't let that be an excuse!

We have a disease that causes changes in our thinking, but we have stuff that can help us out. After getting and staying on a disease-modifying therapy for MS, ask about what can be done to help out your thinking. If your doctor doesn't know, ask another doctor. And if that doctor doesn't know, ask another doctor or a nurse or a therapist or the National MS Society or look it up on Pubmed and don't stop until you find someone who can say, "I know what can be done. Let's make a plan about what we can do." Don't give up! There are people in medicine who can help us with our thinking who don't realize that they can. By sharing with them some of the concepts laid out in this book, you might spark new ideas that help others understand the mind.

SUMMARY

A person's appearance does not indicate the cognitive status of that person!

A person's appearance does not indicate how that person is feeling!

The MRI of a person's brain indicates neither the cognitive status of that person nor how that person is feeling!

Computer-based neurocognitive testing can be a quick and easy screen to show what areas of cognition have been affected in a person.

Finding out what areas of cognition have been affected can allow for appropriate and rapid institution of therapies to improve a person's quality of life and the lives of the people around him or her.

Evaluation by a trained and licensed neuropsychiatrist, neuropsychologist, or neurologist is necessary for complete emotional and psychocognitive evaluation and treatment.

---

[77] These deficiencies are very similar to those seen in attention deficit disorder, both adult and childhood types.

[78] Excuse me for shouting, but this is the most important idea in the book.

[79] This is the second most important idea in the book.

[80] This is not the third most important idea in the book. I just did not want to mess up the punctuational rhythm.

[81] I intentionally went from the third person to the first person in that paragraph to underscore the fact we can get lost in the middle of our thoughts—and it blows!

[82] A. Achiron, G. M. Doniger, Y. Harel, N. Appleboim-Gavish, M. Lavie, and E. S. Simon, "Prolonged response times characterize cognitive performance in multiple sclerosis," *European Journal of Neurology* 14 (2007): 1102–1108.

[83] M. R. Piras, I. Magnano, E. D. Canu, K. S. Paulus, W. M. Satta, A. Soddu, M. Conti, A. Achene, G. Solinas, and I. Aiello, "Longitudinal study of cognitive dysfunction in multiple sclerosis: neuropsychological, neuroradiological, and neurophysiological findings," *Journal of Neurology, Neurosurgery & Psychiatry* 74, no. 7 (July 2003): 878–85.

[84] As mentioned in chapter 1, the axons are the cables coming off of the nerve cell bodies, which are the computers in the brain. Since the cables are being stripped in MS, the transmission speed of a nerve decreases or is lost entirely. Having MS is like going from high-speed Internet access down to dial-up service.

[85] This is why I have my patients put down on their intake form what their GPA was in the last schooling they had before being diagnosed with MS.

[86] If evaluation is needed, here are some good places to start looking for a professional. For neuropsychiatry, the American Psychiatric Association's Healthy Minds website is www.healthyminds.org. For neuropsychology, the American Psychological Association's website is www.apa.org.

Thirteenth

Neurocognitive Testing from the Other Side of the Desk

Neurocognitive testing is useful in quantifying certain parts of what humans have decided to label as thinking. Attention, memory, judgment, visual spatial, and verbal are three-dimensional constructs of an other-dimensional entity called the mind. These things are useful ways to evaluate and help people exist in our three-dimensional world. However, just as the swollen MS brain is the lesion that everyone misses because they are looking so closely at the little white dots, the mind is the thing that is missed when we try to define it. I think Mr. Jobs's quote, which I used at the beginning of this book, was on the right track. Our hearts and intuition are the things that already "know." I believe that if we sometimes stop thinking and just let our minds be, we can more easily see ...

Imagined—Wished—Possible

The universe,
with its billions of light-years of space
and its infinitely incessant time
is everything
and at the same time
nothing.

Comprised of all and everything,
it renders the individual
infinitesimal;

impotent
to traverse its eternity.

Yet a person
holds the power of boundless travel
within their mind.

The expanse of the mind
where no one else can go
is an unfettered place.

There are no speed limits,
or dimensions
                              or rules.

Unless the mind decides to allow them.

It speaks with images
and fragments
and transformations
and compositions
that we don't see in our shared space.

Unless it allows it.

It traverses a hundred million, billion, *gajillion* light-years in a

blink.

And then it returns
even faster

at an extraordinarily subjunctive speed

to help others and
share ideas and
find intimacy and

be amazed

by each person

whose entire world
of space and time
ranges all the way from
here
     to
        here
           and from
              this instant
                  until the next
                      but whose mind too
                        holds a power
                            of boundless travel
                                through their own
                                      unique
                                          universe.

Fourteenth

The MS Therapies from a Neurological Point of View

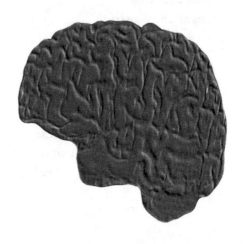

*Medications don't work in
people who don't take them.*
—C. Everett Koop, MD
Surgeon General of the
United States, 1982–1989

As described in the preceding chapters, when nerves are demyelinated, they cannot work properly, if at all. When nerve function is compromised, it can lead to disability, both cognitive and physical. In this chapter, we will explore the therapies that have been found safe and effective in slowing down the course of multiple sclerosis. Please note that everything written about the drugs for MS in this chapter are my personal interpretations of the FDA approved package inserts (PI) as of 2012. The medication or medications that are right for each of us can only be determined by us MSers working with our doctors. The intention of this chapter is for education only. The order in which the drugs are listed is chronological, according to the date they were first approved for use by the FDA in the United States.

When I started medical school in 1990, there was no specific therapy available to slow down MS. We had steroids, which could be used to treat a flare up, but over the long haul, steroid use had not been found to change the overall course of the disease.[87] By the time I graduated from medical school in 1994, three therapies had come out. Over the next eighteen years, six more drugs came onto the market to slow down our disease. Now, since we have a selection of medications to choose from, it's important for those of us who have MS in our lives to understand the differences between the medications. However, before we can talk about the medications, we need to know how the white blood cells (WBCs) that cause demyelination get into the central nervous system (CNS). It is with this knowledge that you and your doctor can start to find the medication that's right for you.

Table 9. Therapies available to slow down the course of multiple sclerosis.

Year	Generic name	Brand name	Mechanism of action	Decreases relapses by about...
1993	beta-interferon 1b	Betaseron®	Affects inflammatory response	1/3
1996	beta-interferon 1a	Avonex®	Affects inflammatory response	1/3
1997	glatiramer acetate	Copaxone®	Affects inflammatory response	1/3
2002	beta-interferon 1a	Rebif®	Affects inflammatory response	1/3
2004	natalizumab	Tysabri®	Directly affects WBCs	2/3
2008	beta-interferon 1b	Extavia®	Affects inflammatory response	1/3
2010	fingolimod	Gilenya®	Affects inflammatory response	1/2
2012	teriflunomide	Aubagio®	Directly affects WBCs	1/3
2013	dimethyl fumarate	Tecfidera®	Affects inflammatory response	1/2

THE JOURNEY OF THE WHITE BLOOD CELL

White blood cells are born in the bone marrow of the long bones in our bodies, like the femur (the thigh bone) and in the thymus gland, which is a gland located in front of the heart and behind the sternum (see figure 26). They are made from hematopoietic stem cells[88] and are lumped into two groups—B-cells and T-cells. Both bone marrow and the thymus gland have lymph capillaries in them that allow the newly made WBCs to enter the lymph system.

The lymph system is a passive fluid collection and distribution system in our bodies. It handles the fluid that is present in between the cells in our bodies (called *interstitial fluid*).[89] The WBCs move through the lymph system by forces that are exerted on them. These forces include: 1) contraction of muscles squeezing the lymph fluid back into the central part of your body so the fluid can be returned and redistributed via the circulatory system, and 2) gravity, which is constantly pulling the fluid down to your feet.

You can easily see the passive nature of the lymph system in your body. After standing or sitting at a desk all day while wearing socks or stockings, you might often notice an impression left by the elastic band. This happens because the extracellular fluid, which is being pulled down by gravity, has no force squeezing it back up into the main part of your body where it can be redistributed. The muscles in your legs, while sitting or standing, do not contract very much. This then allows the extracellular fluid to pool in your legs. Eventually, the lymphatic fluid gets squeezed from the lymph capillaries to the lymph vessels to the lymph nodes and then to the main lymph duct that empties into the blood stream. Many of the WBCs stay in the lymph system until called upon by other WBCs that are out scouting for trouble in other parts of the body. If you get bitten in the leg by a bug, WBCs stationed in the leg sound the alarm that your body has been invaded. These WBCs send out various chemical messengers called *chemokines*. Some of the chemokines send a message to blood vessel walls, telling them to put out receptors, called *vascular cell adhesion molecules* (VCAMs). These receptors can then catch (bind with) the WBCs that pass by in the blood. After a WBC and a VCAM grab onto each other, the VCAM can then do the following:

➢ pull the WBC out of the blood stream
➢ help it to squeeze out of the blood vessel by going in between the cells that make up the blood vessel wall
➢ let the WBC go, once inside the tissues, to help fight off the invaders.

This process is represented in figure 26. The numbers 1 through 4 represent each step that the WBC goes through to do its job.

1. WBCs are made in the bone marrow and thymus gland and then travel to the lymph system.
2. The WBC can only leave the lymph system after a molecule called *sphingosine-1-phosphate* (S1P) binds to the $S1P_1$ receptor. When this binding occurs, it allows the cell to become activated, bind to other cells, and then leave the lymph system to go into the circulatory system.[90]
3. They then can bind to a VCAM, which has appeared after the blood vessel wall got a help message from a WBC in the peripheral tissue, and leave the bloodstream.

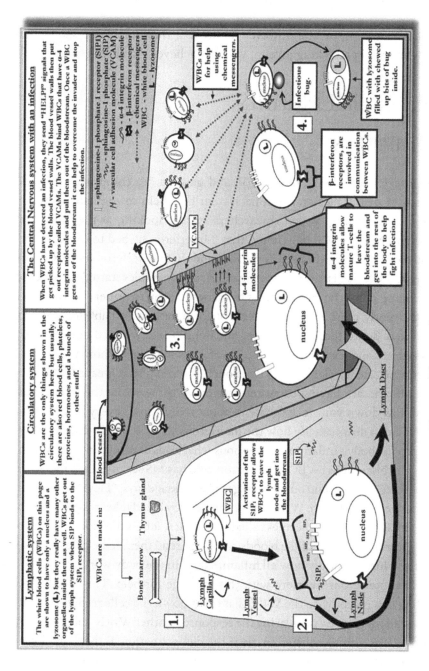

Figure 26. The normal immune system.

4.   Once in the peripheral tissue, immune cells can communicate with each other so they can get together and attack the invader/infection.

In the setting of MS, however (figure 27), the fourth step shows the immune system attacking myelin, which it believes is an invader.

THE PLATFORM THERAPIES

THE INTERFERONS

The interferons (alpha [α], beta [β], and gamma [γ]) comprise a class of molecules in the human immune system that help to regulate immune system functioning. When researchers started looking at the effects of the interferons on MS, they found that β-interferon helped to decrease the frequency of exacerbations. They also found that γ-interferon increased MS exacerbations. As discoveries were made, drug companies started the process of bringing β-interferon molecules to market for the treatment of MS.

Currently, there are four β-interferon formulations available for MS: two versions of β-interferon 1a (Avonex® and Rebif®) and two for β-interferon 1b (Betaseron® and Extavia®).[91] These interferons have been shown to reduce the relapse rate in relapsing MS by about 33 percent. That means that if you have MS and are having three relapses every three years, the interferons could slow down your relapse rate to about two relapses every three years.

No one knows exactly how the interferons work. It is believed that they dampen the body's inflammatory response that leads to demyelination. When the white blood cells (WBCs) in a person who has MS see myelin in the brain or spinal cord, they send out a message. The message says, "Hey! We have an invader here. Send more WBCs so we can destroy it and take it away!" When that gets sent out (by molecules called *chemokines*), it tells the blood vessels to divert some WBCs out of the bloodstream and send them to help destroy the myelin. This is basically how all inflammation in the body works.

The interferons interfere with this message for help. They do this by binding to a receptor on the WBC that turns down the cells response to the initial call for help. By decreasing the response to other WBCs' calls for help, fewer WBCs will be enlisted to cause the demyelination. If there are fewer cells showing up to do the dirty work, then the disease process in multiple sclerosis will go on more slowly.

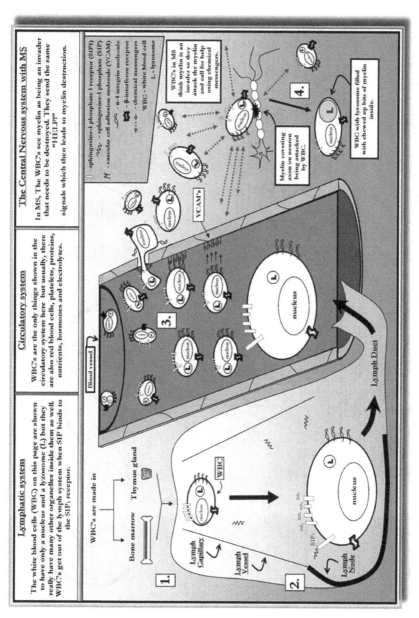

Figure 27. The immune system in MS.

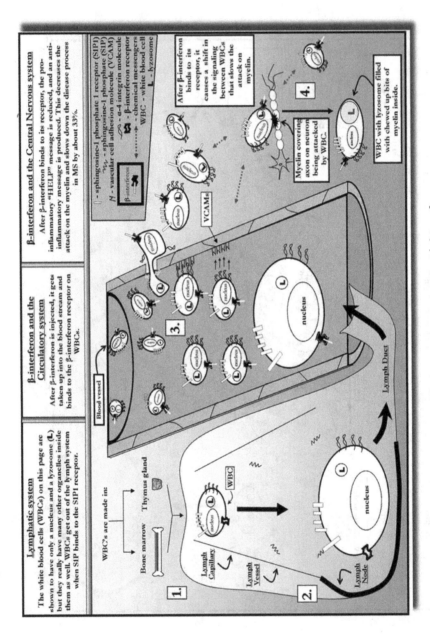

Figure 28. The immune system in MS with β-interferon.

While the difference in efficacy between the interferons is minimal, they do have differences, including the following:

1. Route of administration
2. Dosing frequency
3. How they are made
4. How likely they are to produce something called *neutralizing antibodies*

INTERFERON ROUTE OF ADMINISTRATION AND DOSING FREQUENCY

All four β-interferon medications are given by injection. The needle length for a subcutaneous shot is a little shorter because it goes down to the subcutaneous (SQ) space, and the intramuscular (IM) needle is a little longer because it has to get down to the muscle layer (see figure 29).

β-interferon 1a—IM is taken once per week. It does not matter what day of the week it is taken or what time of day it is taken. Headache, fever, chills, and malaise are some of the side effects seen with β-interferon 1a. Use of acetaminophen, ibuprofen, and good hydration can often help reduce the side effects of the medication. After you take the shot a few times, you will be able to figure out what works best for you. While β-interferon 1a—IM

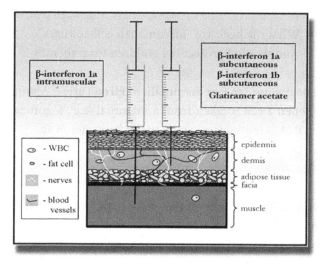

Figure 29. Cross-section through skin comparing intramuscular and subcutaneous injections. Glatiramer acetate is not a β-interferon but was included in this figure since it is given by subcutaneous injection.

is taken once per week, β-interferon 1a—SQ and β-interferon 1b—SQ are taken every other day or three times per week, respectively. The side effects can be similar to β-interferon 1a—IM and can be treated the same way. The main thing to remember about side effects is that side effects are different for everybody! Some people have no side effects from these medications. Some people have such bad side effects that they cannot stay on the medication. It is a spectrum in between. When I prescribe a medication, I tell people what the known side effects are with the medication. After that, I tell them to use the power of positive thinking and believe that they will be among the lucky ones who have no side effects. However, if they do experience side effects, I tell them to get in touch with me so we can work together to try to find ways to improve the situation at hand.

How the Interferons Are Made

β-interferon is a compound that *all* humans have in them normally. It helps to reduce the communication between WBCs. When those of us who have MS take extra β-interferon, it decreases cellular communication even more and thereby helps to slow down MS. Avonex® and Rebif® are β-interferon 1a. They are identical to the β-interferon that we humans naturally have in our bodies. Avonex® and Rebif® are made from things called *mammalian cell cultures*.

> What the heck are "mammalian cell cultures"
> and should I protect my children from them?

No. You do not need to fear mammalian cell cultures.[92] Mammalian cell cultures are when a cell is taken from a mammal (e.g., a guinea pig ovary cell) and the DNA is reprogrammed to make β-interferon 1a.
That's all the cells do.
Make β-interferon 1a.
24/7.
They swirl around in a big vat of nutrients and make β-interferon 1a.
No vacations. No TV.[93]
It is booooooooorrrrrrrrrinnnnnnnnnnng.
The cells try to keep it interesting though.

"Hey, Paul, what cha doin'?" one cell says to the other.

"Making β-interferon 1a. How 'bout you, Rich?" the other cell asks, just to be polite, knowing what the other cell is going to say.

"I'm making grain alcohol," Rich answers.

"What!" Paul screams.

"Just kidding. I'm making β-interferon 1a too."

The thing is that what Paul, Rich, and the other cells are doing is actually making an *exact* copy of the β-interferon that we humans have in our bodies. This way, when we MSers inject β-interferon 1a into our bodies, it will not look foreign to our immune systems.

THE NEUTRALIZING ANTIBODY ISSUE

If something is injected into a human body, it has a chance of causing the generation of antibodies. This is called *immunogenicity*. Several things go into immunogenicity. These include:

1. How similar the injected drug molecule is to other things in that body
2. How big the injected molecule is, and
3. where the molecule is injected into the body.

It is important that the β-interferon we inject look as much like the β-interferon that is already in our body as is possible. If the molecule is not similar, then our immune system is more prone to think that it's an invader. Also, since β-interferon is a comparatively large molecule, even if it's identical to the native β-interferon, our body might still want to get rid of it. Finally, if β-interferon is injected into a place where the immune system is ready to attack it, then antibody production rates could potentially be higher. The important thing is that if a medication has antibodies made against it and the antibody binds to a critical location on the medication, the medication might not be able to do its job as well. This type of antibody is called a *neutralizing antibody*.

The β-interferon 1a that is made from mammalian cell cultures is identical to the naturally occurring β-interferon that is present in all of us. This means that when a human immune system sees it, it doesn't spend too much time worrying about it. β-interferon 1b is made from bacterial cell cultures. Bacteria cannot do everything that a mammalian cell can do, and because of this, the molecule that bacteria make has a different structure from human β-interferon. Since the molecule looks different, it has a greater chance of having the human immune system view it as an invader. The immune system, therefore, is more prone to making neutralizing antibodies (NABs) against β-interferon 1b because it looks different.[94]

The location of the injection is also important. We have more WBCs stationed under the surface of the skin (called the subcutaneous space) because we humans are getting cuts on our skin all the time. We want to have a strong defense system ready to fight off bugs that are trying to get into our bodies right at the point of entry. So, if we inject a medication directly into the subcutaneous space, we're putting it into a hostile area.

Alternatively, we do not usually cut ourselves down to the muscle layer. Because of this, there are fewer WBCs stationed in the muscle layer. It can be viewed as a less hostile area. If we put a medication like β-interferon 1a (that looks like the β-interferon that we naturally have in us) into a less hostile area (like the intramuscular space), the chance that we will develop NABs to it should be lower.

The concern with NABs comes from the fact that if a person develops NABs to a therapy, the efficacy of that therapy could possibly be reduced. If the efficacy is reduced, the medication will not slow down MS as much as it could if NABs were not present. Additionally, if a person develops NABs to one therapy, those NABs have the chance of neutralizing the efficacy of the other interferons as well. Because of this, if your MS worsens rapidly while on a β-interferon and you are found to have NABs to β-interferon, a non-interferon therapy should be considered.

SHOULD I BE CHECKED FOR NABS?

That's a question you need to talk over with your doctor. When someone asks about checking for neutralizing antibodies, several things go into the answer. How is the patient doing on the therapy? Is their MS getting worse faster than what is expected for that person? Does he or she have new enhancing lesions on their MRI? If the person is getting worse quickly or has a bunch of new lesions seen on MRI, NABs could be the cause.

THE NONINTERFERON PLATFORM THERAPY

The other platform therapy that's currently available is glatiramer acetate. While the exact mechanism of action for glatiramer acetate (Copaxone®) is also not known, it is believed to work in a combination of ways. [95] Its structure looks a bit like myelin. Therefore, it can act like a decoy. If the immune system spends its time with the glatiramer acetate, then it will have less time to chew up the myelin in the CNS. It also might have some anti-inflammatory properties, which help to dampen the body's immune response when attacking the myelin in the CNS. Overall, glatiramer acetate slows down the MS disease process by about one-third (see table 9).

As far as neutralizing antibody production goes, glatiramer acetate has not been found to form neutralizing antibodies! It is felt that since the molecule is relatively small, it's less immunogenic—hence the body's immune system does not form antibodies against it. One of the challenges that glatiramer acetate users had to face was that they had to take a subcutaneous injection every day.[96] In 2014, the drug's dose and dosing were modified to allow for the medication to be given three times per week. It's crucial that injection sites are rotated to a new location for each injection. If they do not, a person taking multiple subcutaneous injections can develop something called *lipoatrophy*, where the fat layer under the skin breaks down. When this happens, it can cause some indentations in the skin. I've had some patients who have been on glatiramer acetate a long time (about eight years) and have not had this happen. I also have had some patients who religiously rotated their injection sites and still wound up with lipoatrophy. Hopefully the decrease in frequency of injections will help to reduce the occurrence of lipoatrophy.

THE SECOND-GENERATION THERAPIES

THE MONOCLONAL ANTIBODY

In 2004, a new generation of therapies for MS emerged with natalizumab (Tysabri®).[97] Natalizumab is a protein called a *monoclonal antibody* that was developed to decrease the number of white blood cells that cause MS from getting into the CNS. Here's how it works.

As was mentioned earlier, WBCs cause demyelination in MS. There are many types of WBCs, but the main one that causes demyelination is called a *helper T-cell* (also known as a Th or CD4 cell). There are protein molecules called *α4-integrins* on the surfaces of helper T-cells. When there is an infection or invader in the body and the immune system is needed, the blood vessels in that region put out molecules on the surfaces of the blood vessels called VCAMs.[98] The VCAMs bind the α4-integrin molecules on the helper T-cells that are floating in the blood. Once the T-cell binds to the VCAM, it can be pulled out of the bloodstream and go help to fight off the invader (or demyelinate a nerve). Natalizumab is a specially designed protein molecule that fits over the α4-integrin molecule on the WBC (figure 30). It is put into the bloodstream by an intravenous infusion, once every twenty-eight days. By covering up the α4-integrin molecule, the WBC can no longer bind with the VCAM molecule, be drawn out of the blood stream, and get into the CNS where the MS is going on. This leads to a slow down in disease activity in MS. In 2004, the thirteen-month interim results of two randomized, multicenter, double-blind, placebo-controlled, phase three studies involving more than 2,100 patients with MS comparing natalizumab with placebo looked good and the FDA decided to license natalizumab for use in people with relapsing forms of MS to reduce the frequency of relapses.[99, 100]

SIDE EFFECTS

The process described above is good to help slow down MS—it slows down the relapse rate by 67 percent. But how safe is it to reduce the number of T-cells in the CNS? In the AFFIRM trial, natalizumab was shown to be safe and efficacious in slowing down MS when compared with placebo. While the absolute number of infections was higher in the group that was on natalizumab when compared with the placebo group, the difference was not statistically significant. That means that the difference in the number of infections between the two groups might have been due to chance. People in the study developed urinary tract infections, lower respiratory tract infections, gastroenteritis, vaginitis, tooth infections, herpes, and tonsillitis during the study, but they were able to overcome the infections when they were treated with the appropriate medication (antibiotic, antiviral, or antifungal).

There was a second trial run (the SENTINEL trial), which compared natalizumab + β-interferon 1a with natalizumab + placebo to see if adding

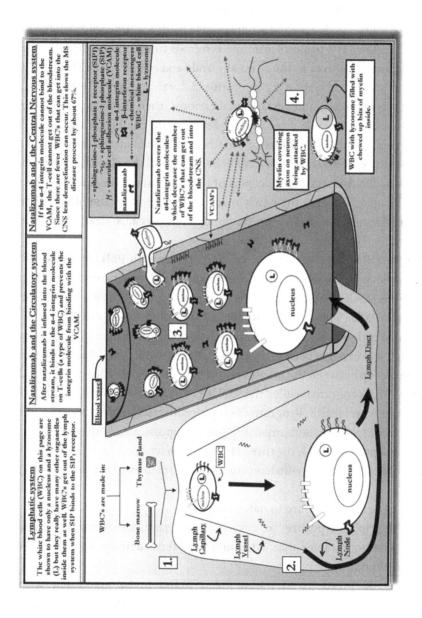

Figure 30. The immune system in MS with natalizumab.

β-interferon 1a could reduce the relapse rate even more. In this study, two cases of progressive multifocal leukoencephalopathy (PML) occurred. PML is a disease that is caused by the JC virus. The JC virus is a common virus. About 52 percent of people in the general population have this virus living in them. The virus causes a disease called *progressive multifocal leukoencephalopathy* (PML).[101] As long as a person's immune system is functioning normally, the virus stays quiet (it lives in the adrenal glands and lymph tissue.) However, if a person's immune system is compromised (by things like HIV infection, leukemia, lymphoma, and certain medications), then the virus can come out and cause trouble. It does this by getting into the blood stream and then getting into the CNS. Once in the CNS, it starts to attack the cells that make myelin (called *oligodendrocytes*). When it attacks the oligodendrocytes, it injects its DNA into the cell, copies of the virus are made, and then the cell bursts open allowing the newly made JC viruses to go and infect other oligodendrocytes. The virus can move rapidly and cause death or severe disability.

In the SENTINEL study, one of the patients with PML died and the other was severely disabled. After this happened, the makers of natalizumab (Biogen Idec) took natalizumab off the market since they did not want anyone else to get PML. They wanted to see if they could figure out why PML occurred in patients taking natalizumab. A thorough investigation was done, and then it was brought back to the market. It is now only available through a program set up between the manufacturer of natalizumab (Biogen Idec) and the FDA. This program is called the TOUCH (TYSABRI® Outreach: Unified Commitment to Health) Program. This program tries to minimize the risk that a patient taking natalizumab will get an opportunistic infection.[102]

As of September 2013, the three factors that have been found to increase the risk of PML in people who have used natalizumab include the following:

1. Length of exposure to natalizumab
2. Previous exposure to cytotoxic or immunosuppressive drugs (chemotherapies that can cause long-term damage to a person's immune system)
   a. Medications that have been found to be associated with developing PML while on natalizumab include drugs that suppress function or production of a normal immune system (e.g., mitoxantrone, azathioprine, methotrexate, cyclophosphamide, mycophenolate mofetil).[103]

3. History of JC virus infection
    a. The determination of whether a person had a history of JCV infection was determined by a sensitive, two-step test looking in the blood for antibodies to the JC virus.

In 2013, Biogen Idec developed a very sensitive test to determine if a person has the antibody to the JC virus in him or her (by having an antibody to a virus, it implies that the person has the virus in them). The problem with increasing the sensitivity of a test is that it becomes less specific. That means that anything that even remotely looks like an antibody to the JC virus will return a positive result. This means that a person who has a positive test might not actually have the JC virus in them (called a *false positive*). Biogen Idec now reports the results of this very sensitive test as an index. If a person's index number is less than 0.4, then it is believed that the person does not have the virus. The test is repeated every six months to evaluate if the person has picked up the virus since the last time they were tested. The incidence of PML in people who have taken natalizumab for less than twenty-four months and have not had prior treatment with immunosuppressants is less than 1 in 1000.

THE WBC SEQUESTRATOR

In 2010, fingolimod (Gilenya®)—was approved to help people with relapsing MS.[104] It was the first oral medication proven to slow down progression of and disability in MS. The goal of fingolimod, like natalizumab, is to decrease the amount of WBCs that get into the CNS and thereby decrease the amount of demyelination that goes on. However, its mechanism of action is different (see figure 31). After taking the fingolimod capsule:

1. The fingolimod gets absorbed into the blood stream.
2. It goes into the WBC.
3. The WBC goes into the lymph system.
4. The fingolimod gets changed (phosphorylated).
5. The changed molecule binds to a S1P receptor that is on the wall of the WBC.
6. After being bound, the receptor can no longer get the WBC out of the lymph system and back into the circulation.

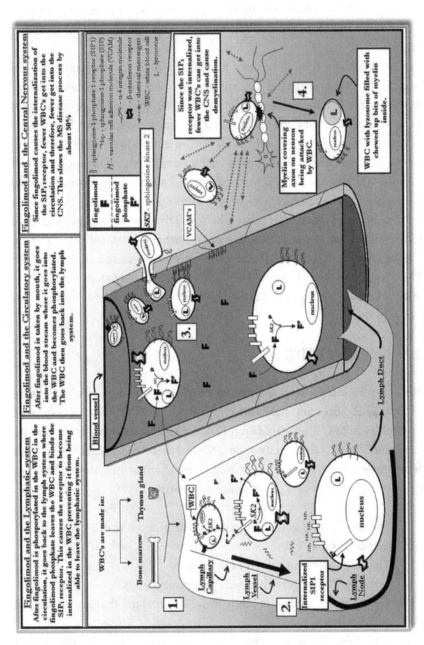

Figure 31. The immune system in MS with fingolimod.

Table 10. Studies and primary endpoints for natalizumab and fingolimod.

Medication	Study	Primary endpoints
natalizumab	A Randomized, Placebo-Controlled Trial of Natalizumab for Relapsing Multiple Sclerosis. Chris HP, O'Connor PW, Havrdova E, Hutchinson M, Kappos L, Miller DH, Phillips JT, Lublin FD, Giovannoni G, Waigt A, Toal M, Lynn F, Panzara MA, and Sandrock AW for the AFFIRM Investigators. N Engl J Med 2006; 354:899-910	Compared the annualized relapse rate and the rate of sustained progression of disability at two years, between natalizumab 300mg IV every 4 weeks vs. placebo. Natalizumab reduced the risk of sustained progression of disability by 42% and reduced the relapse rate by 67%.
fingolimod	A Placebo-Controlled Trial of Oral Fingolimod in Relapsing Multiple Sclerosis. Ludwig Kappos, MD, Ernst-Wilhelm Radue, M.D., Paul O'Connor, M.D., Chris Polman, M.D., Reinhard Hohlfeld, M.D., Peter Calabresi, M.D., Krzysztof Selmaj, M.D., Catherine Agoropoulou, Ph.D., Malgorzata Leyk, Ph.D., Lixin Zhang-Auberson, M.D., Ph.D., and Pascale Burtin, M.D., Ph.D. for the FREEDOMS Study Group. N Engl J Med 2010; 362:387-401	Compared the annualized relapse rate at two years between fingolimod 0.5mg and 1.25mg orally, everyday. The annualized relapse rate was decreased by 54% in the 0.5mg group and 60% in the 1.25mg group. The time to disability progression, which was a secondary endpoint in the study, was longer in both doses of fingolimod.

If the white blood cell cannot get out of the lymph system and into the blood, it cannot get into the CNS and cause demyelination. In the study that got it approved by the FDA, fingolimod decreased the relapse rate in MS by 54 perent.

Side Effects

Like natalizumab, fingolimod was found to have some side effects. The side effects are mostly due to the fact that the S1P family of receptors is found throughout the body. The receptors are found in smooth muscle, including the heart and lungs, and the macula of the eye (located on the retina). They are also crucial in fetal development, and since the number of WBCs in the blood stream is reduced by 20 to 30 percent, the risk of certain infections is a concern. Therefore, before therapy with fingolimod is started, there are certain precautions that need to be taken.

Cardiac Effects

It can cause the heart rate to slow down. Because of this, the first time a person takes the medication, he or she has to be under medical observation for six hours to make sure that his or her heart rate does not slow down too much. If you go off of fingolimod for more than two weeks, you have to be observed for six hours again when you restart the medication. If you take certain heart medications or have certain heart diseases, you should have an ECG done before getting the first dose.

Reasons why a person should not take fingolimod include:

1. Recent (within the last six months) occurrence of myocardial infarction, unstable angina, stroke, transient ischemic attack, decompensated heart failure requiring hospitalization, or Class III/IV heart failure
2. History or presence of Mobitz Type II second degree or third degree AV block or sick sinus syndrome, unless patient has a pacemaker
3. Baseline QTc interval ≥500 ms
4. Treatment with Class Ia or Class III anti-arrhythmic drugs

INFECTION RISK

Since fingolimod reduces the WBC count in the blood, the possibility of getting certain infections can be higher. It is recommended that if the person starting fingolimod has not had chickenpox or had the chickenpox vaccination, he or she should get the vaccination before going on the medication. This precaution is because there were two deaths in the 1.25 mg dose arm of the approval study (one case of disseminated primary herpes zoster and one herpes simplex encephalitis). It should be noted that these cases occurred only at the 1.25 mg dose. The dose that was approved for use by the FDA was 0.5 mg every day. There were no deaths in the 0.5 mg arm of the study. The main infections at the approved dose were bronchitis and, to a lesser extent, pneumonia.

MACULAR EDEMA

Part of the retina in our eyes is called the *macula*. This area is responsible for high acuity vision. Sometimes fluid and protein deposits can form under the macula and cause macular edema. Macular edema occurred in 0.4 percent of people in the 0.5 mg arm versus 0.1 percent in the placebo arm. People who have a history of diabetes mellitus or uveitis (inflammation of the uvea, which is the layer under the retina in the back of the eye) are at greater risk of developing macular edema and need to have an evaluation done by an ophthalmologist before starting therapy. Macular edema occurs more frequently in people with diabetes.[105] Fingolimod has not been tested in people with diabetes mellitus.

RESPIRATORY EFFECTS

Since sphingosine receptors are found on smooth muscle, there is a chance that it can affect breathing. Shortness of breath was reported in 5 percent of people on fingolimod 0.5 mg and in 4 percent of people on placebo.

HEPATIC EFFECTS

Like most of the MS medications, fingolimod is metabolized by the liver. In the study, 8 percent of people on fingolimod 0.5 mg had a threefold increase in liver enzymes versus 2 percent in people on placebo. As with other MS therapies, your doctor needs to follow your liver function tests on a regular basis.

FETAL RISK

The sphingosine receptors are also crucial in fetal development. Because of this, women of childbearing age who take fingolimod need to use effective contraception if they are sexually active.

TERIFLUNOMIDE— THE SECOND ORAL MEDICATION TO BE APPROVED FOR MS

In 2012, teriflunomide (Aubagio®) was approved by the FDA after it showed that the medication reduced the relapse rate by 31 percent in either 7 mg or 14 mg doses.[106] It is a pill, taken by mouth once a day. It is a medication that decreases the number of activated white blood cells in the CNS that can cause demyelination. For complete information on the drug, go to www.aubagio. com and then discuss with your doctor if the medication might be right for you.

DIMETHYL FUMARATE— THE THIRD ORAL MEDICATION TO BE APPROVED FOR MS

In 2013, the third oral medication, dimethyl fumarate (Tecfidera®) was approved by the FDA for treatment of relapsing MS.[107] Dimethyl fumarate, akin to the interferons, produces its effects on MS by decreasing the body's inflammatory response but in a more powerful way. Dimethyl fumarate increases a pathway in the body (the Nrf2 antioxidant response pathway), which is the main defense a cell has when it's attacked. In the DEFINE study, dimethyl fumarate, 240 mg, by mouth twice daily, reduced the annualized relapse rate in MS by 53 percent when compared to placebo. In the same trial, 240 mg was also given three times per day, and the annualized relapse rate reduction was 48 percent.[108]

SIDE EFFECTS

The side effect profile with Tecfidera includes a possible drop in the lymphocyte (a subtype of white blood cell) count. Your doctor needs to check your lymphocyte count before starting the medication and then continue to follow it while you are on the medication. In the DEFINE study, 40 percent of the people experienced some GI upset and flushing of the upper body (chest, head, and/or neck). To mitigate the symptoms, the drug is titrated up to full dose over the course of a month (or longer, sometimes) in hopes of ameliorating the incidence of side effects. Additionally, it is recommended that people make sure to eat a full meal before taking their medication. Several of my patients have reported that having a teaspoon of peanut butter with the capsule helped them tremendously with the side effects.[109]

PERSONAL NOTE ABOUT BEING ON β-INTERFERON 1A—INTRAMUSCULAR

My first disease-modifying therapy was β-interferon 1a—IM. Personally, I had headache and chills quite often when I first started taking β-interferon 1a—IM. I found that if I took it in the morning, I could take two 650 mg acetaminophen tablets an hour before the shot and two 200 mg ibuprofen tablets an hour after the shot. Then I would take two more acetaminophen four hours after the first dose and the same with the ibuprofen. Basically, I was taking two pills every two hours throughout the day of my injection. I did it because it kept the side effects away. I did that for nine years. Then, about two months before I went off β-interferon 1a—IM and started natalizumab, they came out with an eight-hour version of acetaminophen. I also realized that there was a longer-acting version of ibuprofen (called *naproxen*), which lasted about ten hours. I said to myself, *Great!* Now I could take my shot at night, since there were medications that lasted for at least eight hours that would let me sleep through the time when I had my worst side effects. So I switched my shot from morning to night. I took two eight-hour acetaminophen at 8:00 p.m., my shot at 9:00 p.m., and one naproxen tablet at 10:00 p.m. I was able to sleep through the night and most of the side effects as well! The next morning, sometimes I would wake up and feel a little headachy. If I did, I would take two more eight-hour acetaminophen.

I used to take my shot on Wednesday morning because Wednesday always seemed to be a crummy day. It was the day furthest away from the weekend, and there were no good shows on TV. As far as the areas on my body where I would inject, I rotated my sites between my thighs and my buttocks. If I injected in one of my thighs, I could give myself the injection.

If the injection for the week was in the buttocks, I would have to have my wife do the shot.

If I did not mention it before, my wife is a pediatrician who specializes in breastfeeding medicine. For almost everything we do together (except for a few special things[110]), we make sure to include the kids. So on Wednesday morning, if I was going to get my shot in the buttocks, I would lay bare-butt, facedown on my bed. Lauren would bring our kids in, and then they would start fighting. "I want to do the alcohol pad," my son would shout. "No," Abby would shout back. "You did it last time. You do the bandage!" "Okay," Vincent would answer, "but only if I get the remote control tonight." Abby would frown. "How about a great idea," she would say. "You can do the alcohol pad and get the remote control tonight as long as I get to do the alcohol pad for the next two weeks and you give me some of your Halloween candy." The negotiations could continue like this for hours. Abby once asked for her lawyer to be present.[111]

After one of the kids cleaned off the injection area, Lauren would give the injection, and then the other child would put on the bandage. I found that when I took my injection, it was better to push in the medication slowly (over about thirty seconds), which would allow it to seep in between the muscle fibers as opposed to pushing it in quickly. I felt that if I let it seep in, it would disturb the muscle tissue less, and hopefully less scar tissue would form. Scar tissue, by its nature, is less vascular, which could possibly lead to decreased absorption of the medication over time.

After Tysabri came out, I was happy to not have to take a shot anymore. And when the cure comes out, that means one thing—I'll be out of a job. It won't be all bad though. I'll finally be able to become a writer …

SUMMARY

There are multiple disease-modifying therapies currently available to slow down MS. If you have MS, make sure you get on one. If you have tried them all and they did not work, you can either find a study to get into or find out when the next drug is coming out. Stay in close contact with your MS doctor/health-care provider.

I want to reiterate that the summaries presented above are my interpretation of the data that were in the package inserts at the time when the summary for each particular drug was written. Data for medications are changing constantly. I wholeheartedly encourage you and your doctor review the most recent data for any drug that you might consider starting to help alter the course of your disease.

---

[87] There have been several studies done over the years that have attempted to evaluate the question of whether corticosteroid use can decrease long-term disability in MS (Miller 1961; BPSM 1995; Zivadinov 2001; Ciccone 2008). With resurgence in the use of ACTH and its decreased side effect profile, another study might be warranted.

[88] Hematopoiesis comes from two Greek word roots, *hema*—*blood* and *poiein*—*to make*. Pure stem cells can make *any* type of cell in our bodies. Hematopoietic stem cells have already differentiated into making *only* blood-related cells.

[89] Interstitial fluid is an *extracellular fluid*. It does not include the fluid that's inside of cells, blood vessels, the intestinal tract, or the central nervous system.

[90] C. Bode, M. H. Gräler, Molecular Cancer Research Centre (MKFZ), Charité University Medical School (CVK), Berlin, Germany, "Immune regulation by sphingosine 1-phosphate and its receptors," *Archivum Immunologiae Therapiae Experimentalis (Warsz)* 60, no. 1 (February 2002): 3–12, doi: 10.1007/s00005-011-0159-5. Epub 2011 Dec 8.

[91] *Avonex* is a registered trademark of Biogen Idec; *Rebif* is a registered trademark of EMD Serono, Inc.; *Betaseron* is a registered trademark of Bayer; *Extavia* is a registered trademark of Novartis Pharmaceuticals Corporation.

[92] However, "Mammalian Cell Culture" would be a great name for a PBS special about terrorist koalas. Voiceover: "Watch now as FuzzyWuzzy slowly soaks the eucalyptus leaf in a bowl of hemlock, wraps it in a package with several other leaves, and then offers it as a sign of peace to CuchieCoo, the leader of a rival koala pack. Unfortunately, after he takes the 'gift' back to share with his spouse, the outcome is inevitable."

[93] And you thought your job was boring.

[94] Here is a reference that sums up the incidence of neutralizing antibodies in interferons: C. Gneiss, P. Tripp, F. Reichartseder, R. Egg, R. Ehling, A. Lutterotti, M. Khalil et al., "Differing immunogenic potentials of interferon beta preparations in multiple sclerosis patients," *Multiple Sclerosis* 12, no. 6 (December 2006): 731–7.

[95] Copaxone is a registered trademark of Teva Neuroscience.

[96] This is something that our autoimmunological friends with type I diabetes mellitus also have to deal with when taking their insulin injections. They, however, usually have to take more than one shot per day.

[97] Tysabri is a registered trademark of Biogen Idec.

[98] VCAM stands for "vascular cell adhesion molecule," and ICAM stands for "intercellular adhesion molecule."

[99] A short tutorial. A clinical trial is the scientific process that medications and other treatments for humans need to go through in order to prove that the drug or treatment is both safe to use in humans and effective in doing what it claims to do. Trials usually have four phases. Phase I is testing the item in a small number of people to see what

dose is safe and identify side effects. Phase II is essentially the same with a larger number of people. Phase III is the critical stage where safety and efficacy are studied in a large number of people. Phase IV is for therapeutics that passed stage III and are now available for use in patients where further risk, safety, and usage information is acquired. You can find more complete information at http://ClinicalTrials.gov

[100] The final results of the AFFIRM were published here: C. H. Polman, P. W. O'Connor, E. Havrdova, M. Hutchinson, L. Kappos, D. H. Miller, J. T. Phillips et al., AFFIRM Investigators, "A randomized, placebo-controlled trial of natalizumab for relapsing multiple sclerosis," *New England Journal of Medicine* 354, no. 9 (March 2, 2006): 899–910.

[101] PML is where the JC virus infects oligodendrocytes (the cells that make myelin), makes copies itself, breaks open the oligo, and then infects more cells. The outcome can be fatal if left unchecked.

[102] An opportunistic infection is an infection that can be stopped by a normally functioning immune system but cannot be stopped if a person's immune system has been weakened by things like chemotherapies or HIV infection. Examples include PML, toxoplasmosis, and pneumocystis carinii pneumonia.

[103] Tysabri (natalizumab) Package insert, I61061-11 Revised 03/2011, Biogen Idec Inc., 14 Cambridge Center, Cambridge, MA 02142 USA.

[104] Gilenya is a registered trademark of Novartis Pharmaceuticals Corporation.

[105] F. E. Hirai et al., "Clinically significant macular edema and survival in type 1 and type 2 diabetes," *American Journal of Ophthalmology* 145: 700, 2008.

[106] Aubagio and Genzyme are registered trademarks of the Genzyme Corporation.

[107] Tecfidera is a registered trademark of Biogen Idec.

[108] R. Gold, L. Kappos, D. L. Arnold, A. Bar-Or, G. Giovannoni, K. Selmaj, C. Tornatore et al., DEFINE Study Investigators, "Placebo-controlled phase 3 study of oral BG-12 for relapsing multiple sclerosis," *New England Journal of Medicine* 367, no. 12 (September 20, 2012): 1098–1107.

[109] As of this writing, there has not been a well-designed, double-blind, placebo-controlled study comparing the efficacy of smooth versus chunky forms of peanut butter in ameliorating the flushing/GI upset symptoms from dimethyl fumarate. While research on this topic might be of gustatory significance, as far as medical science is concerned, many might consider it to be just plain ridiculous.

[110] Like when we play canasta.

[111] He got her a good deal. She wound up getting to do the alcohol pad for the next four weeks, two pieces of Halloween candy, and a first-round draft pick of any new stuffed animals that either party brought home in goody bags from birthday parties and/or Grandma's house. I told Vincent that he shouldn't have tried to represent himself. He didn't have the guile. He was five. He tried smiling, but cute only gets you so far in negotiations.

Fifteenth

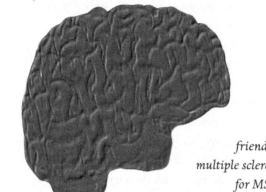

The MS Therapies from the Other Side of the Desk

*The following is a novella.
It is about Samantha, who is a
senior in college. She has a good
friend Matilda, a boyfriend Charlie, and
multiple sclerosis. This is a story about therapies
for MS that do not require a prescription.*

(N.B. Everyone and every place in this story is fictitious.)

MY LIFE WITH YOU

Sam opened the front door of her four-story walk-up with her book bag slung over her left shoulder. She looked up and down the street as she took a deep breath of the cool air. The streetlights were on, casting a glow on the clean, white sheet of snow that had fallen overnight. Not much had come down—maybe an inch or two. Sam decided it was pretty, validating her decision to take the longer, more scenic route to class. Moreover, she had just gotten a new pair of boots and was still breaking them in. The pair from last winter gave out after she went trekking across the Guadalupe Mountains with her boyfriend at the time. They had been good boots—rugged but cute and warm. Charlie had been rugged, cute, and warm as well, she thought, but she didn't know if he was the one. It was her last year at school, and her insides felt restless. She needed something. She didn't know if it was something or someone or somewhere. She just knew it had to be different.

As she took her first step into the snow, she had a flashback to a night in freshman year.

Sam had just finished a long night of studying at one of the campus libraries. Several times while studying, she had looked out the window and seen snow falling. She was excited because she had just gotten a brand-new used car from her parents. The idea that she would be able to get in her car, crank up the heat, and drive home without having her hands turn blue made her feel warm inside. After finishing her studies, she gathered her books, left the library, and walked to the parking lot. She slowly walked down the row where she was certain she had parked, but all she saw were sedans and SUVs. She brushed some snow off a few of the smaller cars, but none turned out to be her gray, two-door Toyota. A small knot of anxiety grew in her stomach. Moving more quickly, she walked to other rows and brushed off snow from more cars. Honda. Audi. Subaru. Chrysler. She found one Toyota, but it was red. She went back to the first row, thinking she had skipped her car. With increasing fervor, she wiped snow off of every car, regardless of size. Range Rover. Bronco. Isuzu Pup pickup truck. No gray, two-door Toyotas.

Standing in the darkness, with only the cold, hollow song of the wind around her, the knot in her stomach tightened. The car was stolen, she thought as she clutched her crossed arms to her stomach. Instinctually, she decided to call Charlie. After relating the situation and then waiting the longest ten minutes of her life, Charlie showed up in his car with a smile, a blanket, and a thermos of warm soup. She got in his car, and they slowly drove through the snow to the police station. Sam, shivering and almost in tears, cursed her carelessness for not having gotten a better antitheft device to protect her first major gift. Five minutes later, they rolled up to the station. Once inside and directed to the proper official, she was given some forms, which Charlie took and started to fill out. The officer got out some other papers, and Sam started to give her report. After several minutes of rapidly recounting her story and answering what seemed like an unending stream of questions, Sam suddenly stopped. The officer, followed by Charlie, looked up from their paperwork. Sam blushed as she remembered that she had parked her car behind a different campus library, where she had had lunch before going to the library where she had studied. She apologized effusively to the officer and then to Charlie. It wasn't until they had gotten back to her apartment that Charlie told her that her face had turned a shade of red best described as "cooked lobster." He helped her shake off her embarrassment by saying that it wasn't her fault and that the school really had way too many libraries, especially ones with parking lots.

Yes, she thought, as she made her way down the block, Charlie had been a comfort—and on more than one occasion. However, graduation was approaching. Things in her mind were changing. She was realizing that, for her, college was the end of childhood. What she had amassed over the last four years at college was not enough. She figured if she cut bait, reloaded, and cast again, she would have a better chance of finding what she was looking for. She decided to get rid of the boots, get rid of Charlie, and start her quest anew.

At the end of the block, Sam made a right onto Hawthorne Row. Before senior year began, she had decided to move off campus, wanting to start the "wean" off of college life. In high school, she had thought she wanted to be a math major in college, but after being asked to her third "What the Frak?" party, she decided to branch out. She took a creative writing class in second semester of freshman year, and after about ten or twelve milliseconds, she knew she had discovered her passion. Interestingly, that was where she had met Charlie. She started to wonder if she had fallen in love with writing because she fell in love with Charlie around the same time or if she had fallen in love with Charlie because she loved writing so much. Or was it just a coincidence? It didn't matter, she concluded. Writing was a constant, she thought, and she knew she loved it. Boys, from what she had seen in college, were inconstant. She wanted more.

There was no one out yet. The snow absorbed the sound of her footsteps. Sam started to think about what life after college might be like. She had applied to several graduate programs in journalism so she could continue to write, but she wasn't sure how her career would evolve. If she became a journalist, she would be writing about other people's lives. She didn't want that. She wanted to create something with the written word that *other* people would want to write about. She thought about some of her favorite writers. Hemingway. Carver. Plath. Fitzgerald. Then she thought about how they all had personal troubles. Alcoholism. Bipolar disease. Depression. Did their issues beget or limit their genius? Were their psychological schisms the necessary ingredient for their compositions or were they just emotional baggage that got in the way? Sam knew that she didn't really have to worry about it, one way or the other. She was far from a literary genius. However, she also knew that when she did hit her literary stride, she would have the "personal trouble" half of the equation all locked up with her multiple sclerosis. Thus far, she had some trouble with her walking but not much more than that. Her fear, however, was that her disability would define her life. That, in her mind, would be a damning epitaph.

She reached the roundabout and went right at the second spoke onto Campus Hill Road. She realized it was becoming lighter out when she noticed the streetlamps shut off. Two students were holding hands about thirty yards in front of her, walking up the big hill to campus. Their tracks, two sets of staggered footprints, were the only ones in the newly fallen snow. They produced a curving, needlepoint-like pattern. Sam stopped and sat on a bench to rest her weaker left leg before continuing up the hill. She turned and looked back at the sidewalk where she had walked. Unlike discrete, pretty, curving needlepoints, hers was a track of messed-up snow. She knew she didn't want to leave her limp as her signature. She pulled off her right mitten and reached into her left breast jacket pocket so she could listen to some music during the last ten minutes of her walk to breakfast. Upon taking out the phone, she saw a text message on the screen.

"R u coming home 4 spring break?" it read. It was from her younger brother, Jeremy. As far as brothers and sisters go, Sam and Jeremy had always been tight. Being a quick wit and four years her junior, he was able to keep pace with his sister on many things, both athletic and intellectual. On the things where he did not, or could not, matchup, she acted as his tutor and guidepost—especially after they lost their father. Theirs had been a happy family of four until Sam started her junior year of high school. That's when her dad started having stomach problems. It only took some blood tests, a CAT scan, and a needle-guided biopsy to discover that rapidly dividing cells in his pancreas were the culprits. Some say that cancer is a horrible disease, but her father viewed it as an opportunity. It gave him a chance to get his affairs in order and gain an awareness of the beauty of each of the moments he spent with his family. In turn, his family learned the importance of appreciating the moment. Done this way, those six months provided Sam, Jeremy, and their mother with more important memories than most people have in a lifetime. Between her father's planning, some community support, and her mother picking up a second job, Sam was able to leave for college a year to the day after her father had passed. By the time she departed, the bonds with her brother and mother had been made fast. She told Jeremy that he better continue his mental and physical workouts because after she left, all further communications were going to be linguistic smackdowns.

"Yes," Sam texted. "I need a break. I can't wait to see you and mom again!" After pressing send, she looked at the initial message. It was timed less than a minute ago. She checked her notification settings to confirm that Messages was set to vibrate. It was. She wondered why she hadn't felt the vibrations when the message came in. She pressed the Home button to get out of Settings and swiped down to Search. She tapped out "Big Yel," and the song auto-filled in the search bar. As the song came on and she put the phone back into the jacket pocket, she noticed that the left side of her chest felt weird. She compared how it felt with the right side. It felt different. Definitely different. She knew her MS was acting up again. Zipping up her jacket and sliding her mitten back on, she stood and faced the hill to get up to campus. Jodi Mitchell's voice came up as she started to walk.

> *"Don't it always seem to go*
> *That you don't know what you got till it's gone.*
> *They paved paradise*
> *And put up a parking lot."*

★ ★ ★

Maddy had just moved her vase to a safe place near the kiln at the studio when she realized it was almost time for the breakfast meeting with her advisor. She quickly picked up her scarves, threw them around her neck, and moved purposefully out the door. It was only after she had gotten halfway up the stairs that she remembered that she had rescheduled her academic advisor meeting for next week. She paused on the stairs in midstride, her left foot hovering over the next step. Looking down at her sandaled, uncommitted foot, she figured that there must have been a reason why she had forgotten that she had postponed the meeting. Moreover, there must have been a reason that she had felt compelled to leave. During her last session, her spiritual advisor had told her that she needed to listen to "this" more and "that" less. She knew on some level that her rushing out for a meeting that did not exist was definitely a "this," so she decided to continue up the stairs. Additionally, Maddy knew that when she heard the door to the studio lock behind her, her vase's spirit would be safe—along with the bag that contained her wallet, keys, and extra scarves.

"I need to let go of this world, so I can see it for what it is," she said aloud as she reached the ground level, anticipating her next "this" moment.

Opening the door, she saw the fresh snow coating the Arts courtyard. She placed her left foot on the snow and felt the cold ring around its edge. She closed her eyes, took a deep breath, and walked blindly. She started by taking long, slow steps, trying to absorb the cool energy. She figured the longer it took her to make each stride, the more energy could be absorbed to infuse her with pure, natural power. She thought how much healthier this was than drinking coffee. She was not sure if she was having a "this" moment or not. After having gone about five longs steps with her eyes closed, Maddy began to feel a sensation of cold coming up her body. She felt that it was a warning. She heard people walking around her. She decided that it would be wise to open her eyes before some frat boys tried to pone her. When she opened her eyes, Sam was standing in front of her.

"Sam!" she shouted. "You're my next 'this'!"

"Hi, Matilda," Sam answered, knowing that she could not possibly understand what Maddy was referring to.

"My advisor said that I had to enjoy 'this' more than 'that,' and since you appeared when I opened my eyes, you must be 'this'!"

"I'm honored," Sam replied dryly. "Ya wanna go to breakfast?"

"Sure," Maddy answered, with a big smile. They started to walk together toward one of the dining halls in silence. Sam took out her food card as they got to the building. She noticed that Maddy did not have her bag with her.

"Did you lock your bag in the studio again or did you finally decide that the universe redistributes all energy sources evenly among living things and you could save money by not wasting it on a meal plan this semester?"

"Locked in the studio. Can you spare ten bucks?" she asked. "I'll pay you back."

"Don't worry," Sam replied as she took out some money from her wallet. "It's on me."

"You can add it to my tab," Maddy replied, with a smile.

Sam turned and looked at her. "If I actually kept a record of all the things I've lent you," she said, "I'd go broke buying paper."

"That's horrible," Maddy exclaimed as her smile turned to a frown.

"Because I'd be broke?" Sam asked.

"Oh no," Maddy said, shaking her head.

"Because I wouldn't have any more money to lend you?" Sam offered.

"Samantha, it's not about the money," Maddy said righteously. "No. With a list that long, imagine how many trees you would have to kill!"

"Of course," Sam said as she pulled the heavy wooden door open for Maddy, "I forgot about the trees."

They walked through the dimly lit hallway that led to the dining area. Not many students were up yet, and there was no line at the cashier. Sam gave the cashier her card and a ten-dollar bill.

"This is for my friend. Give her the hot buffet. I'm not sure when she's going to get a chance to eat again," she said, smiling. Maddy had already gone in and picked up trays for them. After she put her food card away, Sam walked over to Maddy, took one of the trays, and followed her to the hot table. While Maddy loaded her tray, Sam got a bowl of oatmeal and a banana. Turning to walk toward the drink dispensers, Sam's bowl slid rapidly across the plastic tray. She stopped it just before it fell off. *Not this time*, she thought. Sam knew something goofy was going on with the way her right hand had been acting. It felt like sometimes it was there and sometimes it wasn't.

Meanwhile, Maddy was trying to balance a saucer that held a Danish on top of a cup of hot tea in her right hand while supporting a tray loaded with food using her left. Sam headed for a corner table by the window and sat with her back to the window. Maddy, with a surprising amount of grace for a full-figured gal carrying half her own body weight in food, slid into the opposite seat with her back to the room.

"How are things going with your MS?" Maddy asked in her squeaky, happy voice.

"I don't know," Sam began as she put a napkin in her lap. "My leg is still acting weird."

"Did you see your doctor?" Maddy asked.

"Yeah," Sam began as she started to cut up her banana into her oatmeal. "But she just told me that I had to get back on treatment with one of the drugs."

"They're just trying to turn you into a zombie with those drugs, you know," Maddy commented, shaking her head. "You gotta be careful about what you put in your body," she added as she positioned a knife in her right hand and a fork in her left, like a seasoned boxer putting on a pair of gloves.

"Why do you think they were trying to turn me into a zombie?" Sam asked, trying to find out if Maddy knew something she did not.

"You seemed so tired when you were on that first one," Maddy responded. "What was it called? Nefeterun?"

"It was an interferon," Sam clarified. "And yes, I felt tired, but now I'm thinking that the tiredness was nothing when compared with the trouble I'm having with walking," she said, staring at Maddy.

Maddy nodded, indicating that she understood. After a moment, she then opened her mouth and started swinging her jaw side to side.

"What's the matter with your jaw?" Sam asked.

"Nothing's wrong with my jaw," Maddy began, "but I just read a book that said people wind up absorbing only 5 percent of the energy of the food they eat because they don't chew it thoroughly." She pointed her knife at Sam. "That's a waste of natural resources." She turned her knife 90 degrees, pointing to the ceiling. "Now, I make sure that I chew my food very well. This way I can eat less often." She looked down, intensely surveying her plate as if she were tracking prey on the plains of the Kalahari.

Sam nodded as she listened to Maddy's reasoning and mixed her banana pieces into her oatmeal. She took a spoonful and enjoyed the warmth of the oatmeal mixing with the cool banana in her mouth. Picking up her glass and taking a sip of juice, she watched Maddy make the initial strike on her food. Using surgical precision and minimal effort, Maddy aligned, sliced, folded, and shoveled half a pancake covered with an egg-scrapple mixture into her gaping maw. She began chewing with her jaw, making long, circular undulations. After seven repetitions, she stopped.

"Look," Maddy began, talking through the food in her mouth. "It's obvious that medical people don't know how the body works." She then swallowed as her fork made its way back to her plate. "I've always told you that you neglect your chi and that, by neglecting it, it has become undernourished." Sam nodded and took another scoop of oatmeal. She didn't remember Maddy telling her anything about undernourished chi, but she was afraid to contradict Maddy as she ate. "You need help," Maddy continued. Sam watched Maddy's knife perform a finishing move on a pancake-wrapped sausage that her fork had assembled, unassisted, while she was talking. "I think you should see the doctor I see. He's down on Bates Street, and his prices are very reasonable."

"What do you see a doctor for?" Sam asked as she watched grease leak out the side of Maddy's mouth and drip off her chin.

"Remember that earache I had?" Maddy said, lowering her lips to her cup of tea as her hands continued to manipulate food on her plate. "Well, after I went to the infirmary like *you* told me to, they gave me some pills." Placing her lips to the teacup, she slurped some tea and then raised her head. "Do you know what happened when I took those pills?" Sam shook her head while Maddy took another slurp of tea.

"Well, I'll tell ya," Maddy said, somewhat indignantly. "I got diarrhea." Her hands reloaded her fork with scrapple and egg.

Sam nodded and then paused. "How long were you on the medication for?" she asked.

Maddy raised the food-laden fork to mouth height. "Until I got diarrhea!" she said, moving the fork into her mouth at the precise moment she finished the word "diarrhea."

"Of course," Sam replied. "I'm sorry for asking a ridiculous question."

"It's okay," Maddy reassured her.

"May I rephrase the question?" Sam asked.

Maddy made a "go on" motion with the knife in her right hand while her fork picked up a yolk-covered biscuit-half and hurled it into her mouth.

"How many days of medication did you take before the diarrhea began?"

"Two days," she garbled through the biscuit, holding up the pinky and ring fingers of her left hand so the message would be clear. Sam decided not to ask any more questions until her friend swallowed her food for fear that she might choke. It was apparent that over winter break Maddy had reached a Yoda-esque level of gluttony. She hoped the Force would be able to do the Heimlich maneuver on her if needed.

"How about the earache?" Sam asked.

"It was still there!" Maddy responded, before taking another slurp of tea.

"How long were you supposed to be on the medication for?" Sam asked.

"I don't know." Maddy shrugged. "I still have over half the bottle at home. I'm saving it for when I get constipated." She then grabbed her napkin between the pinky and palm of her right hand, which was holding her knife, and swiped it across her mouth. Sam held her breath as she watched the knife flash by Maddy's face. "Anyway, I went to this doctor on Bates Street after I saw his ad on the billboard down on the commons."

"What kind of doctor is he?"

"He's not a doctor in the traditional sense, but he's foreign and very much in touch with his chi."

"Where is he from?"

"I'm not sure. He appears Asian, but he might be Mexican." Sam felt like she was listening to a talk show about alternative medicine while watching a video of a lion disemboweling a wildebeest. "He has this machine you put your arms and legs into. After he turns it on, it draws the toxins out of your body and discards them."

"Which toxins?" Sam asked as she neared the end of her bowl of oatmeal. Maddy sopped up some more of the egg yolk on her plate with the other biscuit half.

"All of them," said Maddy's shiny, yellow mouth.

"Like what?"

"Well, I can't name them all. You know I'm more of a visual-spatial person. I know I saw mercury on the list along with lead and something that ended with a 'mum' sound."

"Chrysanthemum?" Sam asked.

"Yeah! That's it!"

"Chrysanthemum is a flower," Sam stated.

"Oh, yeah," Maddy conceded. "No, that wasn't it. But it was definitely a long word, and I knew I did not want it in *my* body." Sam finished her oatmeal and sipped some of her juice. She looked around the room and stopped when she got to the cashier. Her gaze rested on the back of a dark-haired guy dressed in chinos and a red pullover with a white turtleneck underneath. The sweater told her it was Charlie. The cashier handed his card back. After he put it in his wallet, he remained at the register. He was waiting for another person whose back she did not recognize. She turned back to Maddy, who had moved onto her next course—chopped fruits, assorted nuts, and Danish. Sam continued the conversation.

"What happens after you've been cleansed of the toxins?"

"Well," Maddy began, her right hand laying claim to a fistful of nuts. "After getting out of the machine, I sit on a mat. Then we go over my chakras."

"What? Like a massage?"

"No," Maddy replied as she started masticating the new chewier, harder foods. "It's more like guided meditation."

Sam knit her brow. "How so?" she asked.

"Well, he asks me questions to help guide me in meditation to help open my chakras."

"What are chakras?" Sam asked, half paying attention and half being aware of the rest of the room.

"They're points on your body, and each relates to different parts of who we are," Maddy began. "Each step requires deep meditation, and you need to open each chakra before going onto the next. The whole process can take a long time."

"How long?" Sam asked. She saw Charlie talking with his friend out of the corner of her eye.

"Years. But obviously I don't have enough money to see him for years, so we do a shortened version of it during the sessions, and I also try to do it on my own." Maddy finished off the dried fruit and nuts. "I have trouble with all of them, but the most trouble comes with crown. The doctor says that I need to live in 'this' more." Maddy pointed both index fingers downward as she said "this."

"Where do you usually live?" Sam asked.

"In 'that,'" Maddy replied, pointing her index fingers up and outward.

"What does that mean?" Sam asked.

"He means that I should deal more with the things I have control over at the current moment and not lose myself in the things that I can't control or might never happen. He calls them 'this' and 'that.'"

"Was that why you called me 'this' when I stopped you from getting hit by a bus before?"

"Yeah!" Maddy said, smiling and then looking concerned. "Wait. What bus?"

"Never mind," Sam replied as she noticed Charlie pointing in her direction. "Go on."

"So the goal is to open your chakras," Maddy continued as she picked up her Danish. "We need to get everything in balance."

"Who is 'we'?" Sam asked.

Maddy raised her eyebrows. "You. Me. Everyone. Your MS is probably related to your heart, brow, and crown chakras being closed."

"So if I get my chakras opened up, I'll be able stop my MS?" Sam asked.

"Maybe," Maddy answered between bites of the Danish. "Teacher Ng said he's had many people with brain tumors and seizures who got better."

"Teacher?" Sam questioned, knitting her brow. "I thought you said he was a doctor."

"Same thing—just less insurance crap to deal with," Maddy remarked.

"Ah." Sam nodded. She went back to noticing how Charlie and company had not even picked up a tray yet.

Maddy looked at her watch. "Oh dear," she said, urgently. "I would love to remain in the 'here and now' with you, but I have to catch Professor Urd before my free dance class. He wants to fail me because I didn't show up for the final at the end of last semester."

"What class was that?" Sam asked, thinking how Charlie usually liked to talk *after* getting his food.

"Set-building theory," Maddy replied. Sam turned suddenly, looking at Maddy.

"You took set theory?" Sam blurted.

"What?" Maddy exclaimed. "Are you nuts? Set theory is math. This was set-*building* theory. We had to come up with ideas for a set for my theatre group's spring production of *Obesity!—The Musical.*"

"Thank God," Sam said, sighing.

Maddy pushed back from the table and stood up holding onto the Danish. "Well, thank you for the food," Maddy said as she placed the remaining pastry in her mouth. "I'll let you know when the play is, and I'll text you Dr. Ng's phone number." She picked up her teacup, emptied it, and then replaced it. "Love ya, darling!" she quipped with a smile and a wink, turning and starting her quick waddle out of the dining room.

Sam turned her attention back to the table. She looked at a leftover fragment of biscuit sitting in a pool of syrup where the once proud mountain of food had stood. "If I knew she was bulking up for a play called *Obesity*, I don't know if I would have invited her to breakfast," she said under her breath as she started putting the napkins and silverware on the trays. While gathering the items, she sensed some people walking up to her table.

"Hey, Sam!" Charlie said brightly. Sam looked up and saw Charlie along the side of the table. "How are you doing?"

She noticed him reflexively lean into the table for a kiss but then stop. Sam thought about the agreement they had made when she brought up the idea that they might not want to see each other anymore on a girlfriend-boyfriend level since graduation was approaching. She had been somewhat surprised by Charlie's acquiescence.

"I'm doing pretty well," she said, smiling. "And you?"

"Not bad," Charlie replied, maintaining a happy tone. "I saw you eating with Madeline. Where did she go?"

"She had to go see a teacher about something," Sam said, allowing Charlie to redirect the conversation, which, after a pause, he did.

"I'd like you to meet a friend of mine. This is Kerry," he said as an attractive girl emerged from behind him, the top of her head slightly above the level of Charlie's left shoulder. "Kerry, this is Sam—the good friend I was telling you about."

Sam stood and put out her hand to the fair-skinned, hazel-eyed girl. She had a high forehead and blonde hair, fixed with a barrette in the back. She wore no makeup but had a pair of silver, drop earrings that led to an unadorned neckline. Her thick, dark blue sweater, not one of Charlie's, had large, white snowflakes on it. It loosely followed a healthy shape and hung slightly below the belt line of her jeans. She wore jeans that fit but did not hug her hips. The cuffs of her jeans covered the laces of her brown boots, which were shiny but had some scuffing.

"Nice to meet you," Sam said in an even tone.

"Nice to meet you as well," Kerry replied. Sam noticed a smile on the young girl's face, along with a hint of worry in her eyes. "Charlie has told me a lot about you." Sam looked at Charlie.

"I had to tell her how you were on your way to adding to the great tapestry of American authors." Sam nodded. "Kerry's taking that course you took with Professor Goofy Face—Letters about Literature or something?"

"Do you mean All About Alliteration in Literature with Dr. Geoffrey Faise?" Sam asked, turning to look at Kerry. "It was a fun course. Pretty easy. What are you majoring in?"

"I like writing," Kerri began, vigorously nodding her head. "Unfortunately, my dad wants me to get a degree in business."

Sam frowned. "That's a shame," she said.

"Well, it's so I can help out with the farm back home after graduation, managing the books and whatnot," she added, shrugging her shoulders.

"Ah," Sam replied, realizing that Kerry was more boots and jeans than jeans with boots. "What are you two doing now?" she asked.

"Well," Charlie began, "Kerry's mom was just diagnosed with MS. I was wondering if she could speak with you for a little bit."

"Sure," Sam said. "Anybody who has Goofy Face and MS in their life deserves as much help as possible." A smile crept over her face as she realized the different ways of interpreting what she had just said.

"Do you want to go downstairs for coffee and chat?" Charlie said.

Sam looked at Charlie. "Chat?" Sam asked, slightly taken aback. "Are you running a knitting club or did your grandmother leave you her trendy phrases book in her will?"

Charlie started to laugh.

"I'm sorry," he said. "Would you like to go and talk about current topics in an informal fashion?" he offered.

"Sure," Sam replied, looking at Kerry.

"That would be great," Kerry said, with some of the anxiety leaving her face.

"Super," Charlie said, smiling. "Besides, you know my grandmother, and she curses like a sailor." He turned to Kerry. "Give me your card, and I'll get vouchers from the cashier since we didn't eat anything." Kerry took her card out and handed it to Charlie. Their hands didn't touch. Sam noticed.

"Thanks," she said. As Charlie walked away, Kerry helped Sam finish gathering the plates and silverware onto the trays. They walked over to the garbage and tray-return belt together.

"Have you known Charlie for a long time?" Sam asked.

"Oh no," Kerry answered quickly. "Charlie and I just met this week in class."

"Oh," Sam said, with mild surprise in her voice. After placing the trays on the belt, they walked with Charlie out of the dining hall and into the dimly lit hallway.

★ ★ ★

"So what's the story with Kerry?" Sam initiated as she and Charlie found a table for three in the student-run coffeehouse. Kerry had gone to the restroom.

"None really," Charlie replied. "She's a nice girl I met in an econ class we have together." He put his bag down next to the seat facing the wall and then pulled out one of the other seats for Sam. "We sat next to each other and just started talking," he continued as Sam sat down, placing her bag under the table.

"She seems nice," Sam started. Charlie pulled the other seat out slightly before he sat down in his seat. "Have you gone out on a date yet?" she asked.

Charlie looked at Sam, mildly bemused. "With Kerry or with anyone?" he asked, drawing out the question.

"Either or," Sam said, nonchalantly.

Charlie sat back and looked up toward the corner of the room. He started mouthing random names, keeping track of the number with his fingers, first on his left hand and then on his right. "Do twins count as one or two dates?" he asked cautiously.

"If they were at the same time, one," Sam answered, coolly.

Charlie pulled one of his fingers back down. He counted the fingers and then looked at Sam.

"No," he answered as he interlaced his fingers and placed them, clasped, on the table. "How about you?"

"No dates," she replied, sounding neither happy nor sad.

"How's the MS going?" he asked in a similar fashion.

Sam's head and shoulders drooped slightly. "Crummy," she began. "My leg has been getting worse."

"Are you still taking medication?" Charlie said, leaning into the table slightly.

"Nah. It made me feel like crap." Sam saw Kerry wandering around looking for them. "Hey, Kerry!" Sam called out while waving her hand. Kerry turned and came over to the table. Charlie pushed the third seat out a little further.

"Would you like me to get the coffees?" Kerry asked while standing.

"Nonsense," Charlie said, rising from his chair. "I'll be the waiter for the day. What'll it be, ladies?"

"Small coffee with cream for me," Kerry said.

"Black for me," said Sam.

"What size?" Charlie asked as he started to back away from the table.

"If they have a hose that you can run over to the table and jam down my throat, it would be a start."

"One MegaGrossoCaffeineSlam coming up," he said, moving toward the coffee area with a bounce in his step. Watching him move sparked something inside of Sam as she turned to look at Kerry.

"Thanks for taking the time to speak with me," Kerry said, without pause. "Charlie has been talking about you all week. Ever since I met him on Monday, he's been like, 'I want you to meet Sam. She's great!'"

"When did you tell him about your mom being diagnosed with MS?" Sam asked.

"I think it was on Thursday in economics class," Kerry replied, after a moment.

"Health care was the topic?" Sam said, trying to make the connection.

"Nah," Kerry said. "Class was boring. It was about international econometrics or something. I was bored and started looking around. Charlie's book bag was on the floor, and the flap was open, and I saw he had a book about multiple sclerosis." Sam knit her eyebrows slightly. "I asked him about it after class, and he said he had a very good friend who had it."

"Did he say that I was the friend who had it?" Sam asked.

"I didn't know you were the one he was talking about until I met you upstairs."

Sam paused momentarily, putting together the sequence in her mind. She then looked back at Kerry. "Tell me about your mom," Sam said.

Kerry took a deep breath and began talking. "She was diagnosed just before Christmas, over break. When I got home at the beginning of December, she was having trouble seeing out of her right eye." Kerry's right eye squinted a little as she pointed to it. "She said it was painful, which I thought was weird because my mom *never* complains of pain. I knew something was up, and I was able to convince her to go see her doctor." Kerry paused, looking down at the sugar bowl on the table.

During the pause, Sam thought back to her trip to the doctor with her mother and brother. "Did you go with her?" Sam asked.

"Yeah," Kerry said. "We're pretty close. We went together, and the first doctor said he wanted to send her to a neurologist up at the university, but they didn't have anyone available to see her until February, so he sent her to a local neurologist."

"How did that go?" Sam asked, watching the corners of Kerry's eyes start to droop, ever so slightly.

"He was very nice," she said as if she were reporting the weather. "He did an examination and told us that it might be MS." Kerry's voice cracked a little, and her eyes reddened.

"Did he say it might be anything else?" Sam asked.

"Yeah, but they were all things I had never heard of before and had long names." She shrugged her shoulders and shook her head. "He sent her to get an MRI and some blood work."

"How was your mother feeling?"

"I think she was okay, but she's always been quiet and doesn't let on about her emotions much," she replied, folding her arms across her belly, holding her elbows. "I drove her to the tests."

"How were you feeling?" Sam asked. "That must have been a lot to throw on you."

"I don't really know. Things were moving along so quickly, I don't think I had time to think about it." Sam nodded. "So," Kerry continued, "we went for follow-up on Christmas Eve. He showed us the MRI of her brain and pointed out white spots …" Kerry's voice trailed off at the end of the sentence as she began to cry.

Sam took some napkins from the dispenser and gave them to Kerry. She took them without lifting her head. Several students at a table a few feet away had turned their heads to look at Kerry. Sam, casually repositioning herself, provided some privacy for her new friend. After a few moments, Kerry dried her eyes and blew her nose. "I'm sorry. I guess I've got so many emotions running around inside of me I don't know what to deal with first." She wadded up the napkins and wrapped them with a new one. "It hit us so fast," she continued, sounding like someone reporting what it feels like when a tornado hits. "It was eye pain. Doctor. MRI. Blam! MS. It came up out of nowhere!" Sam nodded knowingly. "I feel horrible coming back to school, leaving my mom and little brother to look out for each other."

"Is your dad around?" Sam asked, noticing Charlie paying for the coffee out of the corner of her eye.

"No," she replied, shaking her head. "He left home after Mom started acting differently."

Sam's eyes widened, her attention turning back to Kerry. "When did that start?" she asked.

Kerry looked up toward the ceiling, her eyes moving back and forth as she thought. "I guess about two years ago. He said my mother had changed— that she was acting like a baby." Kerry played with the ball of napkins in her hands. "I guess it was true. Her emotions were all over the place. She would go from laughing to crying to laughing again at the smallest things. She was acting weird." She stopped and looked at Sam. "That's weird, right?"

Sam's head started to nod slightly but then veered into a noncommittal shake and shoulder shrug. Kerry started listing her mother's abnormal behaviors while enumerating them with the fingers on her left hand.

"Along with the emotional stuff," Kerry iterated as she raised her thumb, "she became extremely disorganized and was always forgetting where she put things." Kerry's extended index finger made a gun shape pointed at Sam. Sam stared at Kerry's finger-gun as it rested on the table. "She would start ten different projects and complete none of them," Kerry continued. Sam watched Kerry's middle finger extend. "She was always complaining about how tired she was even though she was sleeping all the time." Kerry's unadorned ring finger stretched out. Sam became lost in her thoughts. "She also started making some inappropriate comments to people, which she never did before. She started to embarrass us in social situations! It was horrible!" Kerry finished with a loud voice and her open hand rising from the table. Sam continued to stare at the table, thinking about how hard it had been for her during her first year in college. She had noticed her own behavior change but had thought it was a normal part of development—a reaction to leaving home.

"My brother and I sometimes made fun of her as well because she had always done such a great job of being our mom," Kerry said, slumping in her chair as her hand came back down to the table. Her eyes reddened again. "We thought it would pass," she said as she took more napkins from the holder. "I thought she was going through menopause or something." She dabbed her eyes. "One time, she had started making dinner but then remembered that she had to get my brother at school." Kerry's voice sped up, growing more anxious. "She took off to get him, but she forgot that she left the stove on!" Kerry threw her hands up in despair.

Sam looked up and winced. "Oooh! Did anything bad happen?" she asked.

"Thankfully, no," Kerry said, meeting Sam's eyes.

"Thank God," Sam said.

"When she got back, there was smoke in the kitchen," Kerry explained. "She found the charred remains of a few bills that were lying on the counter, which must have caught fire because there was a big black V on the wall next to the stove."

"But nobody got hurt, right?" Sam asked.

"Yes, but no. There were no physical injuries, but my father couldn't take it anymore," Kerry replied. "That's when he left, saying that he was going to stay with his brother for a while. That was a year ago."

Sam nodded and then asked, "Have you seen him since?"

"Yeah," Kerry said, lifelessly. "He comes by every once in a while but never stays for long."

Sam watched Kerry sink into herself and decided to change the conversation's course. "Did your mom get steroids for her eye?" she asked.

"Well," Kerry started, "the doctor gave her something by an IV." She stared at the table. "I can't remember the name of it." She looked up at Sam. "I remember that it was a long word."

"Probably methylprednisolone," Sam replied, remembering her week in the hospital during winter break three years ago.

"Yes. That was it," Kerry said, smiling. "For five days. She gained some weight, but her eyesight was getting better by the time I left to come back to school."

"That's good," Sam chirped. "Did he mention that she needed to start a disease-modifying drug?"

"A what?" Kerry asked. Just then, Charlie, walking slowly, arrived at the table. He carried two cups in a cardboard tray and what appeared to be a small garbage pail with a lid, balanced in the other. He placed the cardboard tray on the edge of the table and Sam's coffee in the middle.

"Why did you put it so far away from me?"

"That thing is *so* heavy," he moaned. "If I put it too close to the edge, the whole table could go over." Sam stared at him as she pulled the MegaGrosso cup closer. Charlie gave Kerry her coffee and then took his from the holder. Sam looked at Charlie's cup, noticing the vast array of powders and foams in the cup. She looked at Kerry, motioning toward Charlie's cup. Kerry looked and then shrugged. Sam turned to Charlie.

"What's that?" Sam asked, pointing at Charlie's cup.

"That, my friend, is a Double-Whip ChocoFrap CinneCrumble with Maple Spice. It's their winter special," he replied, sounding like a car salesman. Sam lifted her cauldron of hot black coffee, took a slug, picked up a napkin, wiped her mouth, and looked to Charlie.

"If I might be so bold ..." she began.

"Please do," Charlie replied.

"Thank you," she said, taking a pregnant pause. "Exactly when and where *did* you lose your balls?"

Kerry choked on her coffee as a smile crept across Charlie's face.

"Well, while I appreciate your interest, I don't know if I can answer that directly," he began, standing straight and assuming a professorial demeanor. "While waiting in line, I had time to reflect upon the fleeting nature of life. Considering that the human life is but an infinitesimal blip on the timeline of the universe, I concluded that breaking habit and taking calculated risks would be a better way to spend my parcel of time." He looked back and forth at the two ladies sitting at the table before him. They nodded. "To that end, I have decided to become a dilettante, at least for the rest of my college career. New experiences are my goal. Each decision I make is another chance to achieve another goal. As of now, I have had enough black coffee. I need something different." Charlie motioned to his whipped, chocolate-smacked, cinnamon-coated, maple-punched drink and said, "*Quod erat demonstrandum.*"

Sam and Kerry gave a quiet, mini-applause as he sat down and rested his chin on his hands. "So what are you two gals chatting about?"

"Kerry was just telling me about her mom."

"Oh. How's she doing?"

"She responded to the steroids that she got, but now she has to decide which disease-modifying therapy to start." Sam turned back to Kerry. "Those are the medications that can slow down her disease."

"Why can't she just take the steroids when something comes up?" Charlie asked as he took a sip of his life-affirming drink. The foam left a mustache on his upper lip.

"You can't live off of steroids," Sam began. "They cause bone loss. They also make your body hold onto salt, and wherever salt goes, water follows." Sam motioned to Charlie to wipe his upper lip.

"I'm saving it for later," he replied, smiling. Sam handed him a napkin, which he accepted and used. "Some people," he chided, shaking his head.

Sam, ignoring Charlie, turned back to Kerry. "Because of that, you have to follow a low-salt diet or else you wind up gaining weight," Sam said.

Kerry cringed slightly. "Have you ever taken them?" she asked.

"I had 'em three years ago. They got me revved up, and I had to take a sleeping pill to fall asleep when I was on them."

"Did they make you sick?"

"No more than I did," Charlie chimed in. Sam stared at him. He quickly put his cup to his mouth and held it there until Sam turned back to Kerry.

"No. They gave me a whole bunch of energy, and my leg got better. They're good to handle an attack, but they don't change the overall course of the disease."

"The doctor gave us some binders about different medications," Kerry said, "but my mom didn't read them."

"Did you take a look at them?" Sam asked. Kerry shook her head. Sam remembered how overwhelmed she had felt when she was first diagnosed. "Did he spend any time telling you about the medications?"

"A bit, but not really," Kerry admitted, looking down at her coffee cup. "I like writing. I was never a science person."

"Me neither," Charlie said. "I think a lot of doctors forget that," he said, looking at Sam.

Sam nodded at Charlie and then looked at Kerry. "It's the doctor's responsibility to educate you and your mom about the medications," Sam said to Kerry. "If the doctor can't do it, he should have another medical professional around that you could speak with."

"He was busy but said that after reading the stuff he gave us, we could discuss them at follow-up," Kerry replied, encouragingly.

"That's good," Sam said. "So now you have to do your homework."

"But how do we know which one's going to be the best for my mother?" Kerry asked.

"It comes down to what your mother and her doctor decide to start with," Sam counseled. "Treating your mom's MS is a personal, daily activity. If one drug doesn't work, there are a whole bunch of other treatments to try."

"What do you mean 'your mom's MS'?" Kerry asked, with concern in her voice. "Isn't MS one disease?"

"Everybody with MS has demyelination in the brain and spinal cord," Sam started, "but how the disease affects each person's life is different. It's important that you and your mom and your brother stay close to each other and work with her doctor."

"It sounds confusing," Kerry stated, shifting in her seat with her hands around her coffee cup. "I'm nervous, and I don't even have the disease. I can only imagine how my mom feels."

Sam saw disquiet in Kerry's face. Sam decided to take another tack. "Here's another way to look at it," she said, leaning into the table. "There were no drugs available to slow down the course of MS until the early nineties. Now we have at least eight drugs available with many more coming," she said, becoming more animated as she spoke. "I like to think of it as a *dynamic* situation. People who were diagnosed with this disease before 1990 had nothing to look forward to like we have now," she continued, leaning in further. "It's up to us with MS to keep on top of our disease." Sam felt herself believing the words she was saying. "We need to do our research using reliable sources. We need to learn as much as we can about MS. And if we can't do it ourselves, we have to learn how to ask for help."

Kerry slowly nodded as Sam finished her address.

"And that goes for those of us who are around people with MS as well," Charlie added. Sam and Kerry both turned to Charlie, who looked only at Sam. Sam saw a wide-eyed, innocent look on Charlie's face. It reminded her of how he looked when she first met him. She turned back to Kerry.

"He's right," Sam stated. "And there are a lot of great resources out there. The first thing I would recommend for you *and* your mom *and* your brother *and* your scared father to do is go to the National Multiple Sclerosis Society website. They have almost everything there to help you and your family and your friends start to take control of the MS that's now in your lives."

After a moment of silence, Charlie turned to Sam. "You said *almost everything*. What's missing?"

Sam turned from Kerry and locked in on Charlie.

"A cure," she said.

Charlie held Sam's gaze. Sam began to feel his presence. Slowly scanning, she appreciated auburn eyes that were deeper and cheekbones more defined. In his silence, Charlie's quiet visage conveyed a comforting image to Sam. She then saw the corners of his mouth start to rise and turn into a smile.

"So, other than that Aceso," he asked, "it's a good site?"

"Yes," Sam replied, releasing his gaze. "It's an excellent site," she continued as her brain downshifted and came back to the table. "And thank you for the deification."

Kerry looked back and forth between Sam and Charlie. "Are we still talking about MS here?" she asked.

"I'm sorry," Charlie said. "It's an inside joke." He looked at Sam and back at Kerry. "Sam and I took a Greek mythology class together in sophomore year. Aceso was a daughter of Asclepius—the god of medicine."

"Aceso was the goddess of the healing process," Sam clarified. "She was the lesser known sister of Aphrodite."

"I still say she was *waaaaaay* hotter than her sister," Charlie insisted.

"They were really only half sisters," Sam said, looking at Kerry. "Aphrodite arose from the sea foam after Cronus cut off Uranus's genitals and threw them into the sea." Sam paused, thought for a second, and then pointed at Charlie. "Hey!" she exclaimed.

"No," Charlie said, cutting her off. "I already looked. They're not there." Sam shrugged and turned back to Kerry.

"The most important thing to remember is that the sooner a person gets started on a therapy, the better he or she does in the long run." Kerry nodded. She took a deep breath and let it out slowly.

"At least I've got a starting point now."

"What's that?" Sam asked.

"I'm going to call my mom and discuss what you just said with her. The way you put it makes it sound like the more involved we get, the better things will be."

Sam smiled. "That's right," she said. "The more involved you are, the better."

"My mom's doctor said the same thing," Kerry said. "We need to be proactive."

"That's great!" Sam said. "My first doc was so-so." She looked at Charlie.

"Maybe we—I mean—*you* could find a new one," Charlie suggested.

Sam's mind quickly processed everything she had learned over the past hour. Kerry and her family were entering into a new part of their lives. She knew they would do well as long as they stayed together. She realized that she needed to listen to herself and get back on a medication. She was starting to see Charlie in a new light.

"Sam?" said Kerry.

"I'm sorry," she replied as she looked back at Kerry. "I just made some connections in my head."

Kerry waved her hands. "Please don't apologize! You've been wonderful! I have to get to class now, but I want to thank you so much for your kindness and your help. Can I get your cell in case I need to ask any other questions?"

"Of course," Sam said, and gave her the number. "Call me so I have yours."

"My pleasure," replied Kerry, with a smile, picking up her bag and waving to Charlie. "See ya later." Sam and Charlie waved as Kerry disappeared into a thicket of students.

The coffeehouse was getting crowded. Charlie had started to gather up the coffee cups and napkins. Holding the sides of her vat of coffee, Sam sat back and looked at Charlie.

"Why do you have a book on MS?" Sam asked.

Charlie continued to busy himself bussing the table while answering. "Well, if you must know, given the sparse amount of time I have left on this planet," he began, "I've decided to read every book ever written." He placed all the items on one of the trays he had used to carry the coffees. "As it stands," he continued, turning to look at Sam, "I'm almost done with the Ms."

She took a long look at him before speaking. "It means a lot to me," she said.

"And you—you mean a lot to me," Charlie said, closing the loop.

And, for a moment, they sat, in the din of the coffee house, in the silence of their company.

"You wanna go to the Fishbowl and talk?" he asked.

"Unfortunately, I can't. I've got classes through the end of the day," she answered. "How about meeting there at about seven tonight?"

Charlie took out his phone and swiped until he got to his calendar. "I'm scheduled for an appendectomy then, but I guess I could let Emil take my place." He looked at Sam. "He's always wanted one."

"If tonight's no good, we could always meet sometime when we're in our mid- to late fifties," Sam offered. "Under the Biltmore clock, maybe?"

"Nah," Charlie quickly replied, dismissively. "I'm allergic to Biltmore clocks. I'll be there at seven."

"Good," Sam replied.

After gathering their bags and heading toward the exit together, they climbed the stairs single file, Charlie allowing Sam to pass in front. Sam noticed her left leg catch the edge of several of the stairs as she went up.

Charlie noticed what a cute butt Sam had.

At the door, Sam turned to look at Charlie. "I'm going to take the bus over to Sbroz Hall."

"Okay," Charlie said, looking toward the sky. "Stay safe. It looks like more snow's on the way."

"I'll see you later," she said, giving Charlie's hand a quick squeeze. He smiled, squeezed back, let go of her hand, and bounced happily down the hill.

Sam turned to go to the bus stop when she heard Bono's voice crawling out of her pocket. "... But I stiiiiiil ... haven't fooouuund ... what I'm looking foooorr ..." *It must be Kerry calling,* Sam thought. She took out her phone and saw the missed call on her screen. She added it to her contacts and then, for several seconds, stared at her phone. She went to her ringtone settings and tapped on a file named CS, reverting to her old ringtone. As she looked to see if the bus was coming, the ringtone played.

"All the promises we make
From the cradle to the grave
When all I want is you"

★ ★ ★

The Fishbowl was one of the less cerebrally intense study areas in what was the oldest library on campus. The library itself was situated at the top of a large and relatively steep hill. Located on the lower level of the library, almost half of the Fishbowl's curved perimeter consisted of windows overlooking the adjoining hill. Like its namesake, it had no ceiling, making it the place to see and be seen. Upon entering the library, a person could walk over to the Fishbowl and gaze down upon the undergraduates who were ardently being college students. Laptops were resting on tables, interspersed with some notebooks and pencils. Students were leaning over the shoulders of one another, obviously helping to explain advanced concepts learned in highbrow classes. It was the library scene in every promotional video for every college. Students in the Bowl were ready to go. Clothes, hairstyle, makeup, manicure, jewelry, accessories, behavior, volume, posture, height, speech, weight, smile, walk, look—all they needed was for someone to shout, "Action!"

Along the nonwindowed part of the Bowl ran a bank of personal computers interrupted by two doors that led to the restrooms. It was the least desirable location for being seen, and that's where Charlie sat. He had the National MS Society's website up on the PC in front of him while he was taking notes on his Mac. He still had his overcoat on even though he had been working in the Bowl for almost an hour. While he had made the twenty-minute walk from his apartment to the library in record time, the single-digit weather had left him with a deep chill, even with full winter gear on. He decided that the chill had lessened enough that he could lose the jacket. He saved the work on his Mac, placed it on the desk, and stood. As he began to take off his jacket, he saw Sam and Maddy descending the curved staircase. Sam wore a white turtleneck with jeans and had a burgundy sweater tied around her waist. She had purloined the sweater from Charlie two years prior, after he had gotten it as a Christmas gift. Her hair was pulled out in a pigtail through the back panel of the tan ball cap on her head. Maddy wore a paisley skirt, black stockings, and military boots along with a well-worn brown sweater that was draped in several scarves. A green, down parka was slung over her right shoulder, and her canvas messenger bag hung off her left. Charlie waved to them as they got to the bottom step on the stairs. They headed toward him.

"Hey ya, Chuck," Maddy started, using a Peppermint Patty inflection.

"Hey, ladies," Charlie replied. "Whassup?"

"Looking for the meaning of life," Sam replied in a tired voice. She put her book bag down on a chair near Charlie's. Maddy kept her bag over her shoulder.

"Either that," Maddy said, "or the answers to my upcoming test in Renaissance tapestry designers." Charlie nodded in acknowledgment. "Ya got that on your fancy light-and-noise machines?" she continued, waving her hand dismissively at the glowing screens behind Charlie.

"I might," he said, tilting his head to the side. "But that would be cheating, now, wouldn't it? And if *you* don't learn everything about Baldessari and Gossart, then who will teach the next generation about these great masters?"

"Aw, those crummy kids can look it up on those Internet things," Maddy said, getting grumpier by the moment. "I just need a pass to graduate so I can open my own pottery studio."

Sam turned to Maddy. "And become part of that fat-cat pottery lobby in DC?" she asked.

"Hey, leave me be!" Maddy rejoined. "I ain't no fat cat. I'm putting on weight for the show."

"Just kidding," Sam added quickly as she punched Maddy's robust upper arm.

"What show?" Charlie asked.

"*Obesity!—The Musical,*" Maddy announced.

"Is that like a remake of *Hair*, except shaved and heavier?" he said, stealing a glance at Sam.

"No," Maddy corrected indignantly. "It's an original, plus-sized piece. I'll let you guys know when the opening is so you can come," she said.

"Sounds good," Sam said. Charlie nodded.

"Great!" Maddy replied as she looked at her watch. "Oh, I gotta get going," she said, opening up her beleaguered satchel. "I have a dinner meeting with the rest of the cast, which I really can't miss." She started riffling through her bag, pulling out an assortment of sundries, scarves, and crumpled papers. "But first, I have to find my wallet."

"It's in your bag at the studio," Sam responded. "Remember? I had to buy you breakfast this morning."

"Of course!" Maddy exclaimed as she jammed the mess back into her bag and latched it shut. "How could I have forgotten?" she said, shaking her head back and forth. At a nearby table, some meticulously coiffed heads turned and glared at Maddy. Blissfully unaware of the volume of her voice, Maddy continued. "I have to get some money out of the bank machine."

"To pay me back?" Sam asked.

"Oh come now," Maddy said in a chastening tone. "Assuredly, you understand that by your donations, you are now considered a patroness of the arts. Your repayment will be the joy that you feel when you see the written word brought to life before your very eyes," she explained, sounding like the Good Witch of the South.

"Of course," Sam replied, turning to Charlie. "I'm a patroness who starved to death funding a play called *Obesity*."

Charlie shrugged as he looked at Sam. "Oh, the irony," Charlie said. "It's so thick ... you could ... I don't know ... choke on it?" Maddy frowned at Charlie.

"Please!" Maddy began in a theatrical voice, throwing the free end of one of her scarves around her neck. "My quest for money is not for compensation, but for further deglutition. The charge, for my fellow cast members and myself, is to dine, drink, and carouse ..." She drew in closer to Charlie. "All ..." she said, staring into his eyes and letting the word hang in the air before turning rapidly to Sam. "In the name of ..." she whispered intensely at Sam. Maddy then began a slow pull back from the duo. They watched as she raised her arms from her sides, lifting them as proud wings above her head while drawing a profound breath. At her apex, she stopped and then dramatically, bowed, exhaling the word "Obesity!" Charlie and Sam looked at her in silence. "I bid you ... farewell," Maddy concluded as she turned and began her exit. With an upright posture and taking grand strides, she approached a table of beautiful people near the stairs and paused. She surveyed the members of the table, stole a look at Sam and Charlie, and then turned back to the table. Grabbing a free end of another scarf, she drew it around her body, being sure to lightly drag it over the clique of committed, shag-cut scholarly scholars, and then slowly ascended from the Bowl.

"She's quite a character," Charlie said, still looking at the top of the stairs.

"She is special," Sam replied, turning to Charlie.

Charlie nodded and pulled out a seat for Sam. "How did the rest of your day go?" he asked.

"It was okay," she said, sitting in the chair next to Charlie. "I called my doctor. I mentioned my leg getting worse since I stopped the interferon." Sam looked at the table while she spoke. "She said I could come in to discuss what we should do." She paused for a moment and then looked at Charlie. "She'll probably want to give me steroids again."

"How did they work the last time?" Charlie asked, tilting his head to the side.

"Great. But I gained some weight and couldn't fall asleep."

"Did you let her know about your side effects?" Charlie asked.

Sam shrugged her shoulders and slumped in her seat. "No," she said. "I didn't want to bother her or sound needy." She moved the mouse to wake up the computer screen in front of her.

"But isn't treating your disease her job?" Charlie asked as he sat up in his chair.

"Yeah," Sam replied. "I guess." She shrugged again and stared at the graphics of the library's home page. There was an animation of a book dancing in front of a brain. After a few seconds in front of the book, the brain grew wings and then flew away.

"Well, how can she treat you if she doesn't know how you're feeling?" Charlie asked.

"I guess she can't," Sam admitted, still staring at the screen. After the brain flew away, the picture dissolved into text. *Let reading free your mind.*

"Okay," Charlie said as he opened a notebook. "So the first thing you can tell her when you see her is that you had some side effects the last time you got steroids." He wrote as he spoke. "Maybe there's something she can do about them."

"Actually," Sam said, looking at Charlie, "she told me that I had to stay away from foods that had salt in them, but I didn't really think it would make a difference." She turned back to the computer screen and watched the book dance in front of the brain again.

Charlie stopped writing and looked at Sam. "Didn't I bring you some soup when you were taking the steroids?"

"Yeah," Sam said nodding, turning back to Charlie. "That was very nice of you," she added with a smile.

"But soup's loaded with salt!" he exclaimed. "Why didn't you tell me you couldn't eat anything with salt in it?"

"I wasn't going to turn you away. What kind of jerk would that make me?" She turned away and noticed some pens lying on the table next to a computer.

"I wouldn't have thought you were a jerk if you explained to me how the steroids worked," Charlie said, looking at Sam. Sam leaned toward the table and picked up one of the pens. She looked at it and then clicked it several times.

"Well, it doesn't matter now," Charlie continued. "It's in the past, and we can't do anything about it except learn from it." He crossed out what he had written, turned the page of his notebook, and wrote *Disease-Modifying Therapy* at the top.

"So," he said in a spirited voice, "then you'll want to discuss what your next treatment's going to be, right?"

"Well, all I know is that I can't give myself anymore injections," Sam said, shaking her head and staring at the middle distance. The rate of her pen clicking increased slightly.

"Why?" Charlie asked, again tilting his head to one side.

Sam halted her clicking and stared at him. "Have you ever given yourself injections on a regular basis for two and half years, knowing that you were going to feel crummier before feeling only slightly better?"

"No," he acknowledged, shaking his head and looking slightly glum.

"Well, it's not fun," Sam said.

Charlie felt a little tightness in his stomach. "Is it painful?" he asked, trying to picture what it would feel like getting repeated injections.

Sam clicked the pen a few times. "Sometimes, but not usually," she answered. Her gaze dropped from Charlie's face and went to back to the pen. "I just don't want any more shots," she said to no one.

"Did it take a lot of time to give yourself the shot?" he asked.

"A bit," she answered. "But no more than brushing and flossing." She clicked the pen once, watching the tip appear and then disappear.

"Was it the size of the needle?"

"No," she said, clicking the pen in a couplet. *Click-click.*

"How about the frequency of the injections?" he asked. "You know, many diabetics have to do injections throughout the day," he said, hoping to lessen her pain by comparison.

Sam stared toward the floor. *Click-click, click-click.*

"I read that you can get skin breakdown too," he said, fishing for some way to make contact with Sam. "They mentioned on the website that you need to rotate your injection site to prevent skin breakdown."

Click-click, click-click, click-click.

"Did you get any skin breakdown? Did you rotate your injection sites? They also said sometimes people skip injections. Did you miss any injections?"

"No ... yes ... I don't know!" Sam said. "I don't want to have this damn disease anymore!" She squeezed the pen like she was trying to choke it. Charlie watched as the muscles in her hand and arm contracted and her arm shook. She slammed the pen down and lifted her left foot up onto her right knee. "Do you see this?" she asked, pointing at the worn toe of her shoe. "I just got these shoes for Christmas! The left one is shot already! It's not right!" she cried softly. "I'm twenty-two years old, and I walk like Quasi-freakin'-modo." She looked around the Bowl. "Why did *I* get it?" she asked. She turned and looked at some female cast members of the Fishbowl who were laughing. "Why the hell not them?" She turned back and looked at Charlie. "Why not you?"

His eyes widened for a moment but then softened as he realized that Sam was having a moment. Her eyes were reddened, but she wasn't crying. It was a face made of frustration and fear and uncertainty. Charlie had been diligently learning about the disease and wanted her to know that he cared and was trying to help. He had been going to programs for people who had MSers in their lives and had learned that emotions needed to be expressed. He had always been emotionally aware of himself. He was able to share his feelings relatively freely. He knew Sam to be more restrained; she wore her game face most of the time. She had told him that when she lost her dad, she learned that her mom and brother were all she had. *While at college, she must feel like she has no one*, he thought. When she had told him that she wanted to downshift their relationship from dating to friend status, he viewed it maturely. He wanted to give her the room to find herself, but he knew he didn't want to let her go. He continued to learn about MS via the Internet, reading books, and talking with people. More recently, he began to feel that there were some things that he couldn't understand and that he should just accept them for now and maybe someday …

"I'm sorry," Sam said as she lowered her leg to the floor and slumped back in her chair.

Charlie took in the apology and looked at his friend's young but tired face.

"It's just that there's so much going on right now," she said as she folded her arms and looked around the Bowl. More students had left. She turned back to Charlie. "Graduation is only four months away, and I still don't know what the hell I'm going to be doing next year," she said plaintively.

"Didn't you say that you had some interviews coming up for grad school?" he asked, hoping to lead the conversation to safer waters.

"Yeah. But I can't go into an interview like this," she said, motioning toward her shoe.

"You're right," he said, nodding. "I think my sweater looks much better when you're wearing it properly and not tied around your waist." Sam's expression didn't change. Charlie noted the response, modified his course slightly, and proceeded. "Ya know," he started, "if you get on some steroids and can't sleep, we can go late-night shopping for some new shoes."

Sam looked at Charlie. "Stores aren't open at night, brainiac," she said, with slightly less misery in her voice.

"Oh sure they are," Charlie said, making it sound like she had just doubted the existence of the sun. "There's a twenty-four-hour Shop-n-Eat-n-Go open out on Route 109 that has a *very* nice selection of flip-flops." He kept his eyes trained on Sam's face while she stared at him. "Of course, they're open toe, but they had a few with chunk heels, and I know I saw a really cute sling-back that I think would be perfect to wear to an interview. But I don't know if the color would be right for you." He paused and looked at Sam critically. "How do you feel about fluorescent mustard?"

"What?" she asked incredulously.

"Okay," Charlie said quickly. "How about a statelier peat moss?"

Sam shook her head. "Can't you see I'm trying to wallow here?" Sam lamented.

"Oh, I'm sorry," Charlie said. "Maybe you hadn't heard. They don't allow wallowing here. It was a rider on the 'Ban on Smoking in Public' bill."

Charlie caught a glimpse of the corners of Sam's mouth flicker. "No, I hadn't heard about it," she said.

"Yeah, they actually sent out a flier," Charlie stated. His brain saw the crack in Sam's negative space and wanted to drive a wedge in as quickly as possible. "As of some time in the recent past, there's only one sanctioned wallowing area on campus now."

"And where would that be?" Sam threw back.

"You know where the stables are, right?" Charlie began, looking askance at Sam.

"The stables?" Sam said, dropping her head and raising her eyebrows. "Really?"

"Yeah, you know, the ones past the Ag School," he said, pointing in a random direction.

"Okay, yes," she agreed. "I know the stables."

"Well, go a mile past there until you get to the barn where the cows are," Charlie continued, letting his imagination take over.

"So everybody who needs to wallow has to go where the smelly cows are?" Sam asked with disbelief.

"Oh, no, no, no," Charlie said, shrugging off the notion that the answer would be so quick and simple. "If people wallowed in self-pity around the cows, then the milk would go bad. There's an empty field about a mile past the cow barn. It's there that you can find the dedicated wallowing area, or the DWA for short," he finished, using air quotes for DWA while pronouncing the word "dwah."

"Heck, if I could walk that far," Sam reasoned, "I wouldn't need to wallow."

"I think that's why they put the smoking field another mile past the dwah," Charlie kept going. Sam laughed. "Hey, it's a serious situation," Charlie said, opening his eyes wide and waving a finger. "Every time exams begin, there's an exodus of stressed-out students, both smokers and wallowers, who go to the fields for respite." Charlie lowered his eyes. "Many don't make it," he said, remorsefully.

"You're telling me students are dying?" Sam asked.

"Oh no," Charlie corrected. "The smokers are so out of breath they can't even make it to the cow barn. Most just lie down and take a nap."

"They lie down in the fields that are loaded with cow poop?" Sam asked.

Charlie nodded vigorously.

"You can't really tell the difference with the smokers, but the nonsmoking wallowers really carry the odor with them," he said. "And that's not even the biggest problem. Since bodies are lying *everywhere*, the cows start tripping over the bodies and go down. Once they're down, their milk doesn't get pumped."

"Cows can stand up, you know," Sam tried to reason.

"Not the lazy ones," Charlie said, shaking his head like a defiant ten-year-old. "The lazy cows, which for your information are the majority of cows, stay down once they realize that they don't have to stand, and since they can't get their milk pumped, they start to swell ..."

"Swell?" Sam asked.

"Like a kid with a nut allergy getting a peanut-oil massage," Charlie said.

"What?" Sam asked.

"It's a common therapy for relief of muscle spasms," he assured her. "I can show you later, but let's finish with the cows first."

"Of course," she said. "The cows."

"So as the cows swell, the pressure increases until it reaches what's known as the Cow Tipping Point."

"Which is what?" Sam asked.

"The point at which the intra-udder pressure generates a bulk force that surpasses the elastic limits of the cow's internal elastic lamina, which leads to ...

"A lactic tsunami?" Sam offered.

"Holstein stream," Charlie rejoined, shaking his head back and forth.

"Dairy deluge," Sam added.

"Jersey jet, Guernsey glut—call it whatever name you feel softens the pain. It still spells tragedy," Charlie concluded.

The two sat in respectful silence for a moment until Sam looked up.

"What will the people put in their coffee?" she asked.

"What do you think?" Charlie replied soberly. Sam clasped her hands over her mouth.

"Oh, cheeses and crackers, no," Sam said with dread.

Charlie nodded, anticipating her answer.

"Nondairy creamer?" Sam weakly squealed.

"A dry, powdery, bovine-barren badland," Charlie replied dismally. A broad smile, framed in dimples, drew across Sam's face. Charlie took in the warmth of Sam's smile before they burst out laughing. Some well-coiffed Bowl amateurs at a nearby table turned to Sam and Charlie to demonstrate their chagrin by frowning. Charlie, still laughing, turned his head and looked at them. After surveying the three young faces, his expression turned from happy to that of a disappointed teacher.

"No," he began. "You didn't capture the moment properly." He turned to them full-face. "You turned too quickly. Plus, you're frowning way too much," he instructed. The newbies' faces went flat. Charlie turned back to face Sam and then demonstrated the movement. "It should be a slooooow head turn while simultaneously lowering your eyelids. Then … ever so slightly … you lower your brow for the kill shot." He executed the maneuver and then slowly turned back to Sam. "Freshmen," he said. Sam looked at the newbies, who turned back to their table and started to gather their things. She turned back to Charlie.

"Were we like that?" she asked.

"Of course we were," he replied. "Except ours was an independent production company. We didn't have the funding like they have in the big studios."

Sam smiled. "All right," she said as she sat up straight. "Let's forget about the cows for a minute. I have two things I need to share with you."

"Shoot," he said after scribbling something on the back of his notebook.

"I'm concerned that my leg might not get better after I take the steroids."

Charlie nodded. "But you won't know unless you try, right?"

"Yeah, but I'm still scared."

Charlie noted that her face was tightening up again. He reached over to his notebook and flipped through a few pages. "Things that help walking," he began reading. "Number one. Physical therapy for gait and safety training.

217

Number two. There's a drug out to help with walking. Number three. There are certain types of electric stimulators that can help if your foot is dragging. Number four. There are studies for different things that will hopefully help to cause nerve growth and/or regrowth." Charlie looked at Sam. "That last one is still down the road a bit," he finished.

"Where did you get that?" she asked, peaking at his notes.

"Went to a couple of websites. Spoke with a few people. Basic research."

Sam looked at him. "Didn't it take a lot of time?" she asked, looking at him quizzically.

"Not really," Charlie replied nonchalantly. "It's just another one of my classes."

"Which class?" Sam asked.

"It's an elective in the Arts School," he began. Sam looked puzzled. "It's a self-study thing I set up with this professor. Don't worry about it. For now, let's just get you some steroids, and we'll deal with whatever happens," he said, trying to turn the conversation back to Sam. "As far as how your leg does after getting a course of steroids, no one knows, right? So we just have to do what we can." She listened and nodded as Charlie spoke.

"What was the other thing?" he asked.

Sam paused for a moment, staring past Charlie, looking across the Bowl. She took a breath and then looked at him. "Will you come with me to my appointment?" she asked with some uncertainty in her voice.

"Of course," he replied.

"Thanks," she said. "It means a lot to me."

"No problem," he said, smiling. They looked at each other for a second before Charlie glanced at his watch. "Time. She has moved," he said, looking around the nearly vacant room and then back at Sam.

"Yeah," Sam said, surveying the empty tables. "I guess we should get moving."

Charlie began to gather his books and his Mac. "I've got a test tomorrow," he said. "Plus, I need to run some errands."

Sam nodded as she stood and threw her bag over her shoulder. They walked in tandem through the Bowl and up the stairs. The work-study attendant at the front desk smiled and whispered good night to Sam and Charlie. They waved good night to the young woman as they passed into the foyer. After zipping up their jackets, tying their hoods, and putting on their gloves, Charlie stepped ahead of Sam and pulled open the heavy wooden door. They stepped out into the cold night and descended the front steps in silence. Sam held the rail as she went down with Charlie on her right. At the bottom of the stairs, they stopped, turned to each other, and stood. A streetlamp cast a halo of light on the duo as they stood on the black pavement bordered by snow.

"Since we're both busy tomorrow," Sam said, with puffs of breath adorning her question, "can we meet for dinner?"

"Sure," Charlie replied. "After I get done with everything I have to do, dinner would be nice." He watched the puffs of his words intermingle with the clouds of Sam's breathing.

"What errands do you have to do?" she asked, knitting her brow.

"Well," he began, looking at the back of the notebook he had scribbled on earlier. "I have to pick up a raincoat ... an inflatable raft ... and some sympathy cards." He smiled and looked at back at Sam.

"You really care about those cows, don't you?" she asked, with growing bemusement.

Charlie took in the hint of a smile on Sam's face. He then shrugged and started slowly walking backward, in the direction of his apartment. "Just because you close your eyes," he said matter-of-factly, "it doesn't mean the problem goes away."

Sam nodded and smiled. "Dinner tomorrow, right?" she confirmed.

"Wouldn't miss it for the world," Charlie said, continuing in reverse. Sam's smile got bigger as she mouthed the word "Bye."

Charlie, feeling the moment, stopped.

He stood and saw the poised girl smiling, bathed in warm light in the cold night.

Closing his eyes, Charlie etched the image in his mind.

When he opened his eyes, Sam was still smiling. He smiled back at her, waved, and then turned to start his walk home. He jammed his hands into his jacket pockets as he turned over the situation in his mind. He knew that Sam had needed to break up with him so she could get her stuff together before graduation. However, from what had just transpired, it seemed like she needed him to be part of her life again. He didn't know if he was making too much of the encounter. Then he thought of how she had asked him. She had asked if he would "come with" her to the doctor's appointment. *She wasn't just asking for a ride,* he thought. *She wants me there to help out with something that will be affecting her life,* he reasoned.

A strong gust of arctic air knocked Charlie out of his head and almost into the bushes. He was starting to notice how much the temperature had dropped since he had arrived at the library. His glove-covered fingers were numb. He regretted not wearing his ski mittens. The skin on his face burned from the cold. As his path moved off the lighted main street and onto the side roads, all he could see were the clouds from his breath. The gusts had become a continuous wind. He had to lower his head and lean his upper body into the wind in order to cut through the bitter night.

Interestingly, the thing that he noticed most was that the chill, which had been inside him, was gone.

★ ★ ★

Friday night, Charlie was in his apartment getting ready for Sam's appointment in the morning. Earlier in the week, Sam had gotten the name of an MS doctor from a friend who had MS. The doctor was located in Waynesboro, which was a two-and-a-half hour drive from campus. Since Sam did not have a car anymore—she couldn't shift the manual transmission ever since her leg went bad—Charlie said he would take them in his front-wheel drive Honda. He and Sam had spent the past week gathering information about the latest therapies, getting copies of her records, filling out her intake form via the doctor's website, and talking about life. It was a peaceful time for both of them.

Charlie packed the question list that they had compiled along with some granola bars and sandwiches for the ride. He figured they could grab some coffee and have the snacks on the ride there and then have the sandwiches on the ride back. He checked the weather report and saw more snow was on the way. He called Sam and told her that they should push up their departure time by at least an hour to five in the morning. She groaned when he mentioned it but agreed that it was a good idea. After hanging up, Charlie showered, shaved, and laid out his clothes so he wouldn't have to get up until twenty minutes before pickup time. He had filled the gas tank when he had gotten the food that afternoon. Just before going to bed, he heard the door open.

"Steve?" he shouted down the stairs.

"Yo. Hey. How ya doin'?" came the voice. It was Steve.

"Fine," Charlie replied as he started down the stairs to the living room. Steve had been Charlie's roommate for all four years of college. Unlike Charlie, Steve had it all. He was brilliant. He could memorize anything on one pass and had gotten into medical school early decision. He was ripped like Rafael Nadal and was a four-year varsity athlete. He saw Steve's workout bag at the bottom of the stairs with a smaller, fluorescent pink workout bag on top.

Needless to say, he was not lonely.

When he got to the bottom of the stairs, Charlie stepped around the bags and looked toward the kitchen where he saw Steve and his friend searching for something in the fridge. The girl, who wore a fluorescent pink, braided-back headband around her blonde hair, had the face of a supermodel, except cuter. He walked to them through the living room.

"Hey, Steve," Charlie said, watching the couple wrestle an orange juice container out from the bottles of beer that were in the way. Steve stood up with the juice in one hand and his friend in the other. Steve wore gray thermal sweatpants and a navy blue Michigan shell while Pinky wore form-fitting, black thermal sweats. Her profile reminded Charlie of the engorged cow crisis he had discussed with Sam.

"Hey, Chuck," Steve said in his usual easygoing rhythm. "What's going on?"

"Not much," Charlie replied. "Just getting ready for bed." Steve looked at Charlie and then at Pinky, who looked at Charlie and then back at Steve.

"Hi," Charlie said, offering his hand. "I'm Steve's apartment mate, Charlie."

"Hi," she squeaked. "I'm Patty." She shook Charlie's hand while remaining affixed to Steve.

"Nice to meet you," Charlie answered, smiling. He looked at Steve. "Could I see you for a second?" he said, making a sign with his thumb toward the living room.

"Sure," Steve said. He turned to Patty. "Stay here for a minute," he said to her, handing her the orange juice. "I gotta go talk with Charlie." Patty nodded, released her hold on Steve, and took the juice. Charlie and Steve moved to the stairs.

"I'm going with Sam to a doctor's appointment in Waynesboro early tomorrow," Charlie explained in a hushed voice. "So if you could keep the noise down a bit, I would appreciate it mucho."

"Sure," Steve replied, and then knit his brow. "Why are you going to the doctor with Sam? Didn't the penicillin work?"

"Hah," Charlie answered flatly. "No. It's her MS. It's been acting up, and she wanted to see a new neurologist."

"Sorry to hear that," Steve said, shifting nervously. "She's not gonna die or anything, is she?"

"No," Charlie reassured Steve. "She's having an exacerbation, and she found a doctor, but his office is a couple of hours away." Steve nodded. "Plus, there's more snow on the way."

"No problem," Steve said, raising his hand. "I'll take ..." Steve turned and looked at Patty, who was reaching for something on top of the refrigerator.

"Patty," Charlie said. "Her name's Patty."

"I know, I know," Steve said, turning back to Charlie. "I was just distracted."

"Like whether or not you'll be able to keep up with her if she decides to bring up Plato's dialectic in conversation?" Charlie offered. Steve laughed.

"Don't worry," he reiterated. "I'll take Patty back to her place. She has a roommate."

"You know," Charlie started, "if I didn't know you so well, I might think ..."

"So might I," he said, smiling. "But we know dat ain't so. Right?"

"Of course," Charlie agreed.

"Have a safe trip," Steve said.

"Thanks," Charlie said as he turned his head toward the kitchen. "Good night, Patty. Nice to meet you."

"Nice to meet you too, Rollie," Patty said, waving.

"Close enough," Charlie said to Steve.

Steve laughed again and picked up his workout bag. "Patty," he said, "call Tara and let her know we're staying at your place."

Charlie turned and made his way up the stairs, thinking about Steve and Patty and lactic deluges and having everything. Then he thought about Sam and him and their conversation and what he wanted in life. He went into the bathroom, flicked on the light, and brushed his teeth. He considered himself lucky. He had already been accepted into several psychology graduate programs and was enjoying his reduced stress level. Additionally, he did not have any medical problems, or at least none that he knew of. He liked to jog and tried to stay in shape, but he wasn't an athlete like Steve.

After spitting, rinsing, and drying his mouth, Charlie flicked off the light and walked to his bedroom. He thought about the things that made him feel good. He liked reading and talking and listening, and of these, listening was his favorite. He liked to see how the people around him viewed the world.

He had had girlfriends, but none that stimulated him above the waistline until he met Sam. He turned off the lights and got into bed.

After he heard the front door shut, he listened to the silence grow.

He started to think about God and love and physics and faith.

They were all the same.

It's just that they appear differently to each of us, he thought as the darkness of the night changed softly into sleep.

★ ★ ★

Sam saw Charlie's car pull up in front of her apartment building. She checked her satchel to make sure the CDs that had her MRIs burned on them were there. She had checked the satchel the previous night and again that morning before leaving her apartment. After feeling the CDs and securely closing the bag, she checked her handbag for her wallet. Once certain that she had everything, she looked back to the car, where she saw the driver's side door open and Charlie get out. She opened the door of her apartment building and felt the biting wind hit her face. She took hold of the banister as she stepped carefully into the new snow. Two inches had come down since she had gone to bed. It continued to fall.

As she reached the bottom of the stairs, Charlie held the passenger door open for her. She gave him the satchel but held onto her handbag. Charlie took her hand and helped her over the edge of the curb, which was hidden by the snow. After sitting sideways on the seat, Sam clapped her feet together to dislodge the snow before turning to face forward in the car. Sam placed her handbag at her feet and then put her seat belt on. Charlie, after closing Sam's door, opened the back door and tossed her shoulder bag into the backseat. Charlie went around the car, sat in the driver's seat, repeated the shoe-snow dislodging process, and then buckled in.

Sam turned to Charlie. "Thanks again for doing this with me," she said in a sincere but tired voice.

"No pro-blame-o," Charlie said.

"Do you think we can get some coffee before getting on the open road?" she asked.

"My thought exactly," Charlie replied with a good amount of energy in his voice. "We'll hit the Coffee Hut before we get on the thruway," he said. "But first," he said, holding up a finger, "do you have your CDs?"

"Yes. Original and most recent."

"Cool." He turned on the CD player in the dashboard. The Ramones' "Blitzkreig Bop" started pounding through the car's speakers. "Let's rock!" he said.

Sam looked at him, with a smile. "You do realize that we're going to a doctor's appointment and not a football game," she said. "Right?"

"I'm sorry," Charlie answered. "I'm a little excited." His head continued to bob up and down. "It's just that I never went to a neurologist's office before."

"I got cha," Sam said, sensing Charlie's nervousness.

"How exactly is it different from a regular doctor?" he asked.

"You'll see," she replied. "The exam is kind of funky."

"Cool." Charlie slowly pulled the car away from the curb and headed up Brighton. The opening lyrics to the song started.

> *Hey. Ho. Let's go!*
> *Hey. Ho. Let's go!*
> *Hey. Ho. Let's go!*
> *Hey. Ho. Let's go!*

"I didn't know you liked the Ramones," Sam said.

Charlie turned down the volume. "Actually, it's my older brother's disc. I was talking with him a few nights ago. We talked for like two hours."

"What about?" Sam asked.

"College and life and stuff," he replied, somewhat nonchalantly. "He just got engaged."

"Wow!" Sam said excitedly and then added a slightly more subdued "Really" as she watched the snow hit the windshield. "Do you know her?"

"Yeah." He nodded. "She's nice. I just can't believe it's time for him to get married already."

"Do they love each other?" she asked.

"He said they do. He's a little uncertain about the financial end of things."

"Isn't he a cop?" Sam asked.

"Yep," Charlie confirmed as he started to brake the car for an upcoming stop sign.

"So what does she do?" Sam prodded.

"She does research in oncology, but she's also trying to get a law degree," he answered.

Sam nodded her head and started to think about how she could make money as a young writer. Charlie brought the car to a stop at the stop sign. Sam watched him look both ways even though no one was around. In fact, the only sign of life was some raccoon tracks around a group of overturned garbage pails. Charlie proceeded to make a right turn onto Hillside and start the descent into College Town. Sam noticed out of the corner of her eye that Charlie had stopped bouncing his head and was focused on the road. She could feel him ride the brakes all the way down the steep hill while maintaining a death grip on the steering wheel. She felt slightly nervous but did not want to make Charlie more nervous by looking at him. Once at the bottom, she saw him lean back and take on a slightly more relaxed pose, which relaxed her. As they sat at a stoplight, she felt a wave of dark energy come over her. Dark energy was the way she described the lethargy that entered her life after she developed MS. When it hit, she knew that her "normal" time was limited. Her eyelids were getting heavy. She noticed Charlie turn to look at her.

"We're almost at the Coffee Hut," he said, encouragingly. Sam turned to him, slowly lifting her head, which felt like it was supporting a loggerhead turtle. She nodded and then turned back to watch the steady stream of snow. After driving three more blocks, Charlie turned into the driveway of the all-night Coffee Hut and rolled down his window. "Two large, black coffees with milk and sugar on the side, please," he said to the pale, pimpled teen behind the screen. "Teenage Lobotomy" came over the speakers. Sam stared at the stereo.

"Sometimes I feel like I've been lobotomized by MS," she said, lifelessly.

"How so?" Charlie asked.

Sam shook her head and then shrugged. "I don't know," she said. After a few seconds, she turned to Charlie. "I don't have my punch anymore." Charlie looked at Sam without expression. "No ummph," she said, trying to explain what she felt. "I eat well. I do my exercises. I study." Her eyes lost focus on Charlie's face and settled somewhere between the two of them. "But when I sit down, I just have no drive to get up." She felt the weight of her eyelids. "The slugs and snails are passing me," she said.

"But you're much prettier than they are," Charlie said. Sam giggled slightly as she refocused on Charlie's face. "Plus," he continued, "you're not covered with nearly as much mucus as the average mollusk."

"Thanks for the positive thoughts," Sam said, feeling slightly more alive. "Unfortunately, that's exactly how I feel on the inside."

"You've been under a lot of stress though, right?" Charlie said. "That's got to be part of it."

"I guess, maybe."

The boy reappeared at the closed window and told Charlie the price of the coffees. Charlie counted out the money and handed it to him. In what appeared to be a well-practiced series of moves, the teen slid the window open, took the money, handed over the coffees, with milk and sugar on the side, retracted his arms, and slid the window closed.

"Thanks," Charlie said to the snow-filled wind before rolling up his window.

Sam picked up the conversation again. "I've been under stress before," she said. "Like when I was in high school trying to get into college. But back then, stress *gave* me drive. I thrived on it. Now," she paused, looking for her words, "MS just kind of blunts everything. My brain feels thick." She saw the confused look on Charlie's face as he started to arrange the coffees on the island between their seats. Keeping her head turned to look at Charlie was making her feel queasy. She faced front again, looking out the windshield. The snow continued steadily. Charlie had put the coffees in the holders and laid out the sugar and milk packets. "I think I'm going to nap a little before having my coffee," she said as she pulled the handle under the bucket seat, slid it back, and then put her seat back down. She adjusted her parka and seat belt before stuffing her hands in her pockets and closing her eyes.

"It feels like my head wants to bust open," she concluded as the sound of her voice was replaced by the rhythmic whisper of her breathing.

After arranging the coffees and preparing his own, Charlie looked at Sam in her cocoon. He had heard what she said and stored the information for processing later. He edged out of the Coffee Hut and onto the snow-covered street. Accelerating slowly, he made his way to the entrance ramp for I-86. There was no one on the road. He could tell that the plows had already started working since the highway had less than an inch of snow on it. He settled his body and mind into a cruising speed of forty-five miles per hour and then took a sip of his coffee. He decided to switch the music to something compatible with sleep so Sam could get some rest. Without looking, he counted through the CDs in the holder on the driver's side door. He selected the third one and put it in his lap. He then ejected The Ramones CD and put it in the first position in the door. He then took the CD off his lap and slid it into the player. He skipped to track three, put both his hands back on the wheel, and watched the road through the snow.

An electric sensation crawled up the back of his neck as the first chords of the song started. Sam had given him the Train CD when they first started going out freshman year. He briefly looked at Sam's soft face as she slept. He turned back to the road.

Now that she's back in the atmosphere,
with drops of Jupiter in her hair.
She acts like summer and walks like rain,
reminds me that there's time to change.

He had no idea what was going to happen after college was over. No one knew what role MS would play. He knew he loved Sam. His brother was getting married. That was forever. Or at least it was supposed to be. *You need to be ready to get married*, he thought. *You need to know that life isn't easy. You need to know that everybody has crap in their lives and the ones that make it are the ones who deal with the crap together. Communication. Understanding. Change. Acceptance. Growth.* He knew the definitions of the words, but he was concerned that he didn't know what they meant when they were shared exclusively between two people. He imagined that it was a beautiful thing when done properly. As the song played, he prayed that he would be able to learn.

And tell me,
did Venus blow your mind?
Was it everything you wanted to find?
And did you miss me while you were looking for yourself out there?

★ ★ ★

The doctor's office was a few miles off the highway in a town that had come up after a local university expanded and joined forces with the local health provider conglomerate. The snow had slowed slightly but was still coming down. Sam chewed on the granola bar that she had begun after waking from her nap. She had decided to skip her coffee because her stomach was acidy and churning a bit. An anxious feeling had been in her gut ever since she made the appointment earlier that week. Many of the doctors she had in her life had not left a positive mark in her memory. Most of her medical memories were associated with her father being diagnosed with cancer and then with her being diagnosed with MS. She knew that the doctors were not bad doctors, but none ever made her feel good. She knew that she needed to have a doctor to care for her MS. However, she also knew that if she felt uncomfortable with her doctor, it would offset, at least to some degree, any positive medical treatment she would receive. Her acid-producing concern was that this doctor was going to be just like the rest.

She looked at Charlie, who was looking back and forth between the GPS and the road.

"How much further is it?" she asked.

"It's supposed to be right around here," he answered, looking to the left. Sam looked out the windshield toward the right.

"There it is!" she said, pointing at a modern but quaint, freestanding building.

Charlie turned to look where Sam was pointing. "Ah," he said, slowing the car and moving to the right lane.

"It's small," Sam said.

"It's not like the university medical office buildings," Charlie added, glimpsing at Sam.

"I don't want a university," she said. "I want a person."

Charlie pulled into the parking lot behind the building and parked close to the entrance. Two other cars were there. One was covered in snow, and one just had a light coating. The parking lot had just been plowed.

Charlie looked around and saw a plow clearing the lot in the shopping center across the street.

"He'll be busy today," Charlie said. Sam didn't respond. She had her head buried in her satchel and was making sure she had all her stuff ready.

"MRI CDs. Intake form. Insurance card. Question list," she said. She looked at Charlie. "It's all here." Charlie nodded while keeping lips tightly closed. She stared at him for a second and saw the tension in his face.

"Are you nervous?" Sam asked.

"Me?" he said. "Nervous?" His hands started shaking while holding the steering wheel. She looked at his hands.

"You're doing that intentionally, right?" Sam said.

"Doing what?" he said as his shaking progressed into a flail. He reached for his coffee cup. "I'm just a little cold," he reassured her while clumsily bringing the cup up to his face. He held the oscillating cup about six inches in front of his face while his pursed lips comically attempted to take a sip. Sam smiled as his lips eventually docked with the coffee cup. He kept his lips pressed against the cup to dampen the shaking in his hand.

"I'm a little nervous too," she said, looking at Charlie. Charlie took the coffee cup down from his lips, put it back in the coffee holder, and then rested a hand on top of Sam's.

"It's a good type of nervous though, right?" he said. "Like before giving a speech or playing a sport. It's the nervous energy that pushes you on the field to get the job done."

"Yeah," Sam said, looking down at Charlie's hand resting on hers.

"Unfortunately," Charlie said, "some people don't have that last little push inside of them, and they run away."

"That's why it's good to be on a team," Sam said, placing her other hand on top of Charlie's.

"Because teammates cover each other's backs," he concluded. Charlie then lightly placed his left hand on top of Sam's, looked into her eyes, and quietly said, "Let's rock." They pumped their hands, smiled at each other, and got out of the car.

After walking into the building and stomping the snow off their feet, they stood in front of a window. The secretary looked up, saw the duo, and then buzzed them in. Charlie pulled the door open, and Sam walked into the office. On the far wall, there was a TV showing the local news. Sam looked around the office, noticing the wood trim that lined the room. It was a lightly stained oak with simple millwork. Behind a similarly stained wood desk, the receptionist, a blonde, middle-aged woman, sat.

"Hi," Sam began as she walked toward the desk. "I'm Sam Richmond. I have a nine o'clock appointment with Dr. Callcut."

"Yes, we've been expecting you," the woman said, with a smile. "My name's Margaret."

"We're not late, are we?" Charlie asked, looking at his watch.

"Oh no, no, no," the woman reassured Charlie. "It's just that with the snow, we do get cancellations from people who have to travel a good distance. Did you have any trouble in the snow?"

"No," Charlie said. "Just went slow and steady. That plow guy I saw outside is going to have a busy day today."

"Yes. That's my son, Scott. He loves using his truck to plow and pull people out of ditches when they get stuck." The receptionist turned back to Sam.

"Were you able to go to the website for the forms?" Margaret asked.

"Yep," Sam said, nodding as she reached into her bag.

"Great," Margaret replied. "I'll take them. And I'll also need your insurance card and drug plan card if you have one." Sam got the papers out and handed them over. "You can have a seat while I get your chart ready."

Sam turned back to Charlie, and they took their seats.

"Looks normal," Charlie noted as he looked around. "I like the hanging wall fountain."

"Where?" Sam asked. He pointed down a hallway that they had passed when they entered. After seeing the structure hanging on the wall, she walked to it slowly, stopping about a foot away. Charlie followed and stopped behind her, off to the side. The water hugged the surface of the granite slab so tightly that the rock had the appearance of a fluid, made of microundulations. She looked down at the catch basin that was covered with many small rocks. The little pools of water around the rocks, along with the sound of the water falling into the basin told Sam that it was indeed water, but her mind still questioned it. Raising her hand, she stuck out a finger and touched the falling water. The water tracked along her finger until she removed it. She wiped off her finger on her jeans while continuing to watch the water. Different colored LED lights were stationed at the top of the fountain, slowly fading in and out, making the water glisten like a liquid chameleon. The variable but constant sound of the water dropping into the catch basin gave her a peaceful feeling inside.

After a minute or so, Charlie moved up alongside Sam.

"It's quite calming," he said.

"Uh-huh," Sam said, stepping back from the fountain. She looked up at Charlie. "It also has prompted me to go to the restroom," she said. She walked back to the waiting room and saw the door to the handicapped-accessible bathroom. Upon entering, the cavernous spaces between the sink, the commode, and the walls were what took her attention. Blue-gray slate patterned tiles filled in the floor between the white pedestal sink to her right and the white elongated commode to her left. Both had matching brushed nickel hardware. A black, plastic garbage can sat under the paper towel dispenser. There were black-and-white photographs of nature scenes on the gossamer blue walls. The smell was clean, not barren and sterile like a hospital.

Sitting down, she looked around. She thought that she would dress such a big bathroom with some other softer items like flowers or wicker baskets. Then again, it was a doctor's office. It had a purpose to serve. She started wondering if she was going to have to get a big bathroom like this one for her house when she got older. She assumed it was bigger so it could fit people with wheelchairs. The first doctor she had seen after diagnosis had told her, in a reassuring voice, that 35 percent of people with MS were still ambulatory after thirty years. She realized that that meant 65 percent of people with MS were *not* ambulatory after thirty years. Then she thought about the woman she had met who had MS for over thirty years and she still jogged almost every day. She knew MS was different in everybody. She wondered how it would be different for her. After finishing up, she washed her hands and went back out into the waiting room. Charlie and the doctor were talking and laughing. They turned to face Sam as she approached.

"Hi," the smiling doctor began in a baritone voice. "John Callcut," he continued, offering his hand as he walked toward Sam. Sam put out her hand, and they shook. She liked his firm but warm handshake.

"Hi. I'm Sam Richmond," she said as she took in the doctor. He wore his hair parted on the left and was clean-shaven. His blue oxford shirt was crisp but looked comfortable with the collar open. The brown belt was cinched around a narrow waist and held up khaki, pleated chinos, which ended at dark brown, casual dress shoes.

"I was speaking with your friend here," the doctor said, motioning toward Charlie. The doctor had about an inch on Charlie height-wise, but Charlie's chest was broader. Dr. Callcut looked at Sam. "He says you're a writer."

"That's what I would like to be," she replied, smiling.

"Excellent," Dr. Callcut commented, broadening his smile. "Why don't you pick up your things and come on into the office?"

Sam nodded quickly and stepped over to the chair where she had left her bag.

"Can I come?" Charlie asked, looking at the doctor.

"It's up to Sam," Dr. Callcut said, turning from Charlie to Sam.

"Yeah," Sam replied. "He's been looking forward to this."

Sam and Charlie followed the doctor back to his office. The oak theme continued down the hall and into the combined office-exam room. Dr. Callcut stood by the door, allowing the couple to pass before him as they entered. Sam surveyed the assortment of wood-tone items that comprised the décor. A pair of mahogany bookcases lined the wall on her left; the first contained a Bose radio flanked by several autographed baseballs while the second had large textbooks. The long wall was covered in a mélange of photos and drawings carrying mostly a baseball theme. Closer to the doctor's desk, there was a wooden sign entitled "Physician's Prayer" along with prints of some water scenes. Above them all was a carved wooden plaque. The doctor's desk was at the end of the long wall, tucked in the corner with a bare wall behind it. An exam table, a sink, and a plant occupied the remaining wall.

"I guess you're a baseball fan," Sam said as she surveyed the wall.

"Aw, heck no," Dr. Callcut began. "Curling's my sport. These pictures were here when I moved in." Sam and Charlie simultaneously turned and looked at the doctor, who began to smile.

"That's a joke," he said. "Please, feel free to laugh," the doctor encouraged. Sam and Charlie smiled. "Really. Even if it's not funny, please laugh. It's the only thing that keeps me going." Sam looked at Charlie and laughed quietly. Charlie smiled.

"As it stands, I do like baseball," the doctor added. "The baseball pictures bring back good memories from growing up and the time I spent with my dad. The other pictures bring back good memories of some of the good people I've met in my life."

Sam looked up at the carved wooden plaque on the wall next to the doctor's desk. "What's the carving say?" she asked.

"It's Latin for *seize the day*," Charlie chimed in. "Right?"

"Precisely," Dr. Callcut confirmed.

"Oh," Sam said. "Where did you get it?"

"Actually, I made it," Dr. Callcut said, smiling as he walked past Sam and Charlie and stood behind his desk. He looked at the plaque. "I lost my son when he was young," he said gently.

"Oh," Sam said. "I'm so sorry."

"No worries," Dr. Callcut reassured her as he glanced back and forth between the young couple. "Now I have him looking over my shoulder, making sure that I take advantage of the time that I have with the people in my life. Like you," he said. He put out his hands toward the chairs in front of his desk. "Have a seat."

Charlie pulled a seat out for Sam and then himself. Dr. Callcut sat in his chair and started clicking on his computer. After a moment, he looked back at Sam.

"So, I see that you're looking to get on another therapy. It says you were on an interferon for almost three years. How were you doing on it?"

"Physically, everything was still working, but I felt like garbage. I had headaches the day of my shot and felt wiped out the next day. I felt like I was living but not having a life."

Dr. Callcut nodded. "How has it been since you stopped it?" he asked.

"Good. I mean it felt good not having to take my injections and not getting the side effects, but now my leg is dragging."

"She's going through shoes pretty quickly," Charlie added. The doctor nodded and smiled.

"I see you checked off that you're having some trouble with urination."

Charlie looked at Sam and then leaned in toward her. "You never mentioned that to me," he whispered.

"Yeah," she replied casually. "Sometimes when I get home, I suddenly feel like I have to go to the bathroom, and I lose control before I get there."

"Did that start after stopping your medication?" the doctor asked.

"Yeah," Sam replied while nodding her head.

"Did you tell your other doctor about it?"

"Yeah," Sam said lifelessly. "But she just said that I needed to get back on the interferon."

"Did you let her know how you felt while you were on it?"

"Yeah, but she didn't listen. She just kept on saying, 'Get back on medication.'"

"Did she ever offer you anything else?"

"She said there was a daily injection, but when I looked it up, I saw pictures of people's legs that did not look very pretty. I didn't want that."

"That's understandable," the doctor said, typing on his computer and nodding. When he was done, he paused for several seconds while looking at the computer screen. Then he pushed the keyboard away and looked at Sam.

"What do you like to do?" he asked. Sam put a questioning look on her face. "I mean, aside from the writing, what do you like to do for fun? Do you have any hobbies?" he asked.

Sam paused, looked at Charlie, and then looked back at the doctor before answering. "I used to like to ski," she answered. "And jog," she added quickly. Dr. Callcut nodded his head vigorously.

"And hike," Charlie added.

"Oh," the doctor responded brightly, looking at Charlie. He turned back to Sam. "Where do you hike?"

"Mostly here in upstate," she answered.

"We took a cross-country trip last summer and did some hiking in the Southwest," Charlie said.

"But I can't do those things now," she said resignedly, looking at Charlie.

"For now," Charlie responded. He turned to look at the doctor. "We, I mean, *she* was wondering if she could get a course of steroids to help her leg." Dr. Callcut smiled at Charlie.

"Well," Dr. Callcut said, looking at Sam, "we have to do whatever we can to get you back on the trails, right?" Sam nodded in agreement.

"Yes!" Charlie said enthusiastically as he pumped his arm.

"Charlie," Sam reprimanded. "This is a doctor's office. Not a football game."

"Do you like football?" Dr. Callcut asked, raising his eyebrows.

"Yeah, but this is a doctor's office," she replied.

"Are you saying that a visit to the neurologist can't be as exciting as a football game?" he asked in an incredulous tone. Sam was unsure of how to answer him. Charlie was smiling.

"Well, none of the other doctor visits that I've gone to were exciting," she said, making air quotes around "exciting."

The doctor then sat up straight and assumed a righteous tone. "If you think I'm boring because many neurologists are boring, that's profiling, and I think we all know that that's illegal." A wry smile drew over Dr. Callcut's face. Sam didn't know what to do aside from laugh, so she did. She looked at Charlie, who had his lips drawn tight.

"I hope he doesn't bring action against you," Charlie muttered, loud enough for all to hear.

"I would never do such a thing," Dr. Callcut said. "Unless, of course, insurance reimbursements continue to go down and they close the soup kitchen down at the city hall annex." He looked directly at Charlie. "The wife and I still have to eat, you know." Charlie nodded in agreement. The doctor turned back to Sam. "So, if that doesn't happen, you're safe."

"Good," she said as she stopped giggling. "Actually, I wanted to learn more about the other medications that are available."

"Great!" he said, smiling. "We have a bunch of them now. We have an infusion you take every four weeks, and there are at least three oral medications available." Dr. Callcut spoke slowly and looked at both Sam and Charlie. "By the way, if you have any questions about what I tell you, feel free to stop me. I'll also give you some information that you can take home to review at your leisure, and we can discuss any other questions you have at follow-up."

"We also brought some questions to ask."

"Excellent! I love questions," the doctor said. "And I love trying to answer them even more." He looked directly at Sam and then said, quietly, "Actually, my wife thinks I like the sound of my own voice." Sam smiled.

"And I also brought my MRIs," she added.

"Wonderful! How about we do the exam first and then look at your MRIs, and then we can start making some plans on how to make the MS in your life better and answer your questions at the same time?"

"Sounds good," she said.

"Should I leave?" Charlie asked.

Dr. Callcut looked at Sam. "Do you want him to leave?" he asked.

"No," she said, and then turned to Charlie. "Charlie, I want you here."

"Okay," Charlie answered, with a smile.

The doctor then turned to Charlie. "Do you want to leave?" Dr. Callcut asked.

"No," Charlie said, shaking his head.

"Okay. The resolution that Charlie will stay for the exam passes by a unanimous vote of three to zero," Dr. Callcut announced, and using a little orange rubber mallet as a gavel, he hit his desk. Sam got on the exam table as Dr. Callcut got his blood pressure cuff. Sam sat erect on the table and was slightly anxious.

"So, you want to be a writer. Who's your favorite author?" he asked as he wrapped the cuff around her arm. Sam wasn't ready for the non-MS question.

"Um. Steinbeck, I guess."

Dr. Callcut smiled. He put his stethoscope in his ears. "You sound uncertain. You can get back to me on it. No rush. Does Charlie know?" He started to inflate the cuff.

"I don't know," he answered.

"Did you two just meet?"

"No. We started going out three and a half years ago," Sam said.

Dr. Callcut started to let the air out of the cuff and got the reading. Then he turned to Charlie. "So who do you think her favorite author is?" he asked.

"She mentions Gertrude Stein quite a bit."

Dr. Callcut looked at Sam.

"Stein's not my favorite author," Sam said, shaking her head at Charlie.

Dr. Callcut cringed. "Ohhhh, I'm so sorry," he started to say in Trebekian fashion. "The correct answer was Steinbeck. We were looking for Steinbeck." He pretended to take off a pair of glasses and act like an old man. "Young man," he began, "I was throwing you a bone. She said Steinbeck not fifteen seconds ago."

"But she didn't sound sure."

"Doesn't matter. She's a woman. She mentions Steinbeck. You go with

Steinbeck. Until she changes her mind." Charlie laughed. "Do you have any sisters?"

"No. Just a brother."

Dr. Callcut shook his head knowingly. "I don't pretend to have any great knowledge about women, but after growing up with three sisters, my mom, and a grandmother, I learned one thing."

"Which was what?" Charlie asked.

"That the only true wisdom is in knowing that you know nothing."

"Socrates said that," Sam said.

"Yes! And who was Socrates's wife?" Dr. Callcut said. Sam and Charlie shook their heads. "Her name was Xanthippe, and from what I hear, she was the mother of all nagging wives." He paused and turned toward the door. "I'm blessed my wife doesn't nag me, of course," he continued loudly. "Just in case she's listening," he said quietly to Sam.

"You think he came up with that saying because of the way his wife treated him?" she asked.

"I don't know for certain, but from the stories I've read, I don't think Socrates was that upset about having to drink hemlock," he quipped as he wrote down Sam's blood pressure.

"Ya know," she began, "you're different from the other doctors I've met."

"What do you mean? I've got a diploma. I can show it to you," he said as he began to riffle through some papers.

"No. I trust that you're a doctor. But you're different."

"Because I can make you laugh?"

"Partly."

"Because you feel at ease?"

"Uh-huh."

"Because you were able to forget about your leg and MS for five minutes while sitting in the exam room of a neurologist?"

Sam looked at Charlie. They smiled, and then Sam turned back to the doctor. His face had assumed a milder emotion. Dr. Callcut looked at Sam. "Medical school and residency training taught me medicine. But it was my mom and my son who taught me how to be a doctor." Sam watched his gaze shift downward as he picked up the ophthalmoscope from the tray table. "When I was a kid, my mother would explain how my body worked and how it healed itself and how sometimes we needed a doctor to help it heal." Dr. Callcut looked back at Sam and pointed the ophthalmoscope at the carving. "My son was only three when he got hit by a car. He taught me that life goes by fast and that you have to enjoy each and every thing that you have, every moment that you have it." He shined the light at his hand and then into Sam's eyes.

"A lot of people worry about things that they have no control over," Dr. Callcut said, shrugging his shoulders. "They start to worry about the what-ifs. What if I go blind? What if I go into a wheelchair? That's wasted time. Look and think about your life," he said, looking at Sam. "If and when unfortunate things come up, ask for help, make a plan, and then do something about it. Other than that, go live life! That's when the good things happen. Open your mouth please and say ahhh." Sam followed the doctor's directions as he pointed the light into the back of her throat.

"Sometimes, when people have a problem," he continued, "they don't realize that they need help. If they're lucky, they have friends who help them realize it. If I look at my wife and see she's not happy, I want to know why so I can help carry the load until the next good point." Sam listened to the doctor as the spots in her vision faded.

"It's the same with my patients," the doctor continued as he switched the ophthalmoscope to an otoscope and started to look in Sam's ears. "They come to me when they need help. We talk and try to figure out ways to help treat their problem." Sam glanced at Charlie, who was listening to the doctor while staring at the floor. "Yes, medicine often falls short. There isn't always a cure, but that doesn't mean you can't help. That's when you have to be human." Dr. Callcut looked at Sam. "You've got your whole life ahead of you." Sam smiled. "We've got a lot of stuff that can help you lead your life they way you want to even though MS showed up." He motioned to Charlie with the otoscope before putting it down while continuing to look at Sam. "I think that guy might be able to help you." Sam knit her brow and tilted her head.

"How?" she asked.

"When we were talking before," Dr. Callcut continued, "he mentioned that the two of you spent the past week getting ready for the office visit today even though he was busy buying supplies for ... what was it again?"

"The Lactipocalypse," Charlie said.

"The Lactipocalypse—whatever that is. And even though he doesn't know who your favorite author is, he said his top priority was to get you here today despite the snowstorm." Just then, the doctor's phone rang. He turned, looked at Charlie, and said, "Uh-oh. The wife."

While he went over to the desk to answer the phone, Sam looked at Charlie and mouthed *thank you.*

Charlie mouthed back *you're welcome.*

Dr. Callcut hung up the phone and looked at Sam and Charlie.

"We better slap some bacon on a biscuit and get moving," Dr. Callcut said. "The state just declared a snow emergency."

★ ★ ★

"So," Charlie said as he looked across the dinner table in the motel restaurant at Sam. "Dr. Callcut said that he could get you your IV steroids by Monday. That gives us thirty-six hours to be snowbound refugees." Sam was staring at the snow outside the window. The snow was still falling as it had all day long, and it seemed to have intensified. The highway was closed soon after the snow emergency was declared. A jukebox was playing Jason Mraz. "The Remedy" was there, quietly, in the background.

"What are you going to get for dessert?" he asked while he looked at the menu. Sam turned her head from the window to look at Charlie. Charlie looked up.

"I love you," she said. Charlie held a questioning look on his face for a moment before he looked back down at his menu.

"I missed that," he said. "Is that one of the ice-cream flavors?" There was no response. He looked back up at Sam.

"I know I've been in a different place for the past seven months. My world has been in a fog. I needed to step back and get some perspective on my situation. You respected that. For that, I love you." Charlie put down his menu, listened, and kept his mouth shut.

"You kept me on your radar, making sure I didn't circle the drain. For that, I love you," Sam said.

Charlie remained motionless.

"You have shown kindness, dedication, and thoughtfulness that I have never seen in another man. And for that, I love you."

Charlie felt warmth in his heart as he let her words linger.

She went on. "Now, I have a question for you."

"What's that?"

"What's the title of your self-study course?"

He looked at the dark hair that framed Sam's face and fell to her shoulders. The pure skin of her cheeks had a blush across them that gave her a porcelain-doll quality. When he looked at her eyes, they told him that she was back.

"Friendship 402," he said.

Sam nodded. "May I have a follow-up?"

"Please do," Charlie said. He saw the playful Phoenix start to rise from her lashes.

"Who was your advisor?" she asked.

"It's complicated," he said, somewhat dismissively.

"Uh-huh," Sam replied.

"It's a rotating faculty thing," he said, stalling as he made a rotating motion with his hand.

"Oh?" she said, cocking her head to the side. "Are you getting good grades?"

"I'm taking it pass/fail," he explained.

"How do you think you're doing?" she asked.

"I feel good about it, but I'm waiting to get the final word," he said, nodding. "You know how these things are."

Sam looked back out the window. The snow was blowing horizontally. She turned back to Charlie. "I think I know one of your teachers," she offered.

"Well, it is a small school."

"Yes it is," she agreed. "I think I can solidify a pass for you."

"Great!" Charlie uttered, smiling.

"I just need you to do one thing."

"What's that?" he asked.

"You have to go up to her and tell her that you'll take her back," Sam said.

Charlie looked out the window with a worried look on his face.

"What's wrong?" she asked, raising a suspicious eyebrow.

"The snow!" he cried out in a hushed voice. "How can I get to her through the snow?"

"Really?" Sam pushed.

"Wait. I know how I can do it." Charlie pulled out his cell phone.

"She doesn't accept texts."

"What about e-mails?"

Sam shook her head. Charlie sighed. Then he motioned to the waitress. She nodded and went into the kitchen. Sam looked back. A song by Yaz drifted through the room.

"What are you doing?" she asked.

"I'm doing what I've wanted to do for the last few months." The waitress came back out carrying a large paper bag as Alison Moyet's voice softened the background. The waitress approached the table and handed the bag to Sam. It was heavy. Charlie's eyes were focused on her face as she opened the bag.

… All I needed was the love you gave …

The smile that blossomed on her face could have melted all the snow in upstate as she took out a new pair of hiking boots. "I figured since neither of us knows what we're going to be doing after college, we're going to have a lot of searching to do. With these boots, hopefully you and I can search around the country, together, for the thing—or things—we were meant to do. At least for a while. Or, you know, until the money runs out."

… Only you.

Sam held the boots in her lap with both hands. She smelled the leather and thought back to when they went up the Guadalupe Mountains. She remembered looking out over the desert during the day and being able to see the shadows of the clouds on the ground. After they had pitched camp, they were both amazed to see the enormous, red moon rise from the horizon. She looked at Charlie.

"Do you remember lying on the ground and watching the shooting stars?" she asked. He slowly, almost imperceptibly, started nodding his head.

"They kept coming and coming and coming," he replied, with a gentle smile growing across his face.

"They never stopped," she whispered as she held her gift. It was then, looking deeply at Charlie, she saw the constant man sitting across from her. And while the music played softly, Sam began to wonder, in a very happy way, what if …

Sixteenth

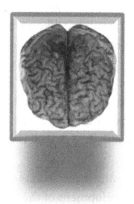

THE MS ICE FROM BOTH SIDES OF THE DESK

Oh Lord, please don't let me be misunderstood.
—The Animals, "Don't Let Me Be Misunderstood"

This chapter is different from the others. This is the chapter where patient and doctor are going to be speaking as one. What I will offer are insights learned from leading a bipartite and sometimes schizophrenic life. My learning about MS can be broken down into four parts:

1. Having learned about the brain before I got MS
2. Continuing to learn about the brain after getting MS
3. Discovering how the MS that had affected my brain had affected my mind
4. Discovering how I got my pre-MS mind back

Having gone through these stages, I have made some connections that can hopefully help all of us who have MS in our lives.

A. For non-MSers, I will lay out what I believe to be the microscopic, physical changes in the MS brain that lead to the cognitive and behavioral changes in MSers. By understanding the microscopic, physical changes that cannot be seen, hopefully you will be able to get an understanding of why we MSers act the way we do.

B. For us MSers, we know how we feel. Something's not right. We don't feel like who we were before we got MS. Sometimes we can see exactly how our minds are not working (like not being able to concentrate), but sometimes we don't even realize that we're not acting like the people who we once were. The part of our brain that can look at ourselves and govern our actions is all—to borrow a word from my friends in the hood—*fakakta*. But once we take a look at and understand the cause of the problem, we become empowered. We then can work with our doctors and other health-care providers to try to get our minds back.

This chapter is divided into three sections. Part I begins with a more in-depth discussion about development of the central nervous system. This includes where myelin comes from, what it does, and how myelination progresses through the nervous system, allowing us to become fully functioning people. Following that, we will explore things that prevent nerves from working properly, including demyelination and, as will be shown, elevated intracerebral (within the brain) pressure. In part II, we will put the concepts described in part I together to come to a new understanding of what's going on in the heads of many MSers. In part III, we'll try to formulate a logical process, involving both patient and health-care provider, to ameliorate the lives of those of us affected by MS.

PART I

DEVELOPMENT AND FUNCTIONING OF THE NERVOUS SYSTEM

FORMATION OF THE CENTRAL NERVOUS SYSTEM

After conception, when the egg and sperm have met, exchanged personal information, and decided to go ahead and make a new life, new cells are made according to the combined DNA blueprints. At this stage of the game, the cells that are created can become anything. They are said to be pluripotential. As they continue to grow and multiply, a disc is formed. From the ventral (front) side of the disc, most of the body is made. From the dorsal (back) side of the disc, something called the *neural plate* forms. The nervous system is made from the neural plate.[112]

Without putting too fine a point on it, the cells on the edges of the neural plate multiply, forming ridges on the neural plate. The ridges eventually fold together and make a tube that is to become the spinal cord and brain. The remnants of the hollow part of the neural tube can sometimes still be seen in the spinal cord of an adult on MRI. One of the critical steps for nervous system development is closure of the ends of the tube. The end that goes on to form the brain (called the *anterior neuropore*) closes about twenty-four days after conception. The end that goes on to form the tail of the spinal cord (called the *posterior neuropore*) closes around day twenty-eight. Once the tube is closed, development of the nervous system can really take off. The nerves start to grow and take their appropriate positions. The brain starts folding and making connections. Among the final things that go into making a complete nervous system is the coating of most nerves with myelin.

MYELINATION

Myelination—the wrapping of axons with myelin made by oligodendrocytes—begins during the third trimester of pregnancy and is not complete until a person is in their third decade of life.[113] The first area of the nervous system that needs to be myelinated in order to sustain life the moment the baby comes out of the womb is the cervical spinal cord (located in the neck). Some of the nerves in this region are what allow a baby to breathe, cry out for Mommy when hungry, and suck on a nipple for food.

Many of the nerves that control voluntary movement of body parts get myelinated over the ten years after birth. As a baby develops, it starts to hold its head steady and can coo. Soon, it makes noises and can track things that it sees. After a few more months, the baby can grab and hold things. Babies then start to babble and make "mumum" sounds. As the motor nerves continue to myelinate, they sit up, crawl, and can pull themselves up to stand. After a year, they can walk, and by two, they are going up steps. With the gross motor system well underway, myelination in the language and fine motor centers starts to take off. Sentences start to form, and circles can be copied. Another year passes, and they can ask an endless stream of questions and go to the potty on their own. At one point, they realize that there are others around who look just like them who like to draw and skip and hop too! They are then ready to go to school. This is when the most special part of the human brain—the frontal lobes—starts to get hooked up.

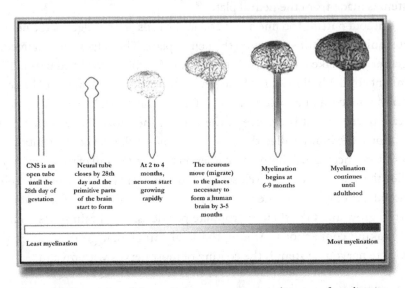

Figure 32. Formation of the central nervous system and timing of myelination.

THE FINAL, BIG CONNECTION—THE FRONTAL LOBES

The frontal lobes are what make each of us unique. It is the part that defines who we are. The occipital lobe gets input from the eyes and sees, but the frontal lobe decides what to do with what was seen. The temporal lobes store our memories as well as manage the comprehension and production of language. However, the final approval of what we say is controlled by our frontal lobes. The parietal lobes can come up with the spatial relationships between our bodies and the surrounding world, but it is our frontal lobes that decide if we are going to do anything to change that relationship. It is only after the pathways that are going to, coming from, and within the frontal lobes are myelinated that we can consider ourselves to be neuroanatomically complete. Our frontal lobes are in charge of our emotional control, judgment, planning, social propriety, concentration, attention, cognitive flexibility, verbal expression, and initiative. The frontal lobes are among the last parts of our brains to be myelinated. They start to do their jobs around age fourteen, which is when we humans start to

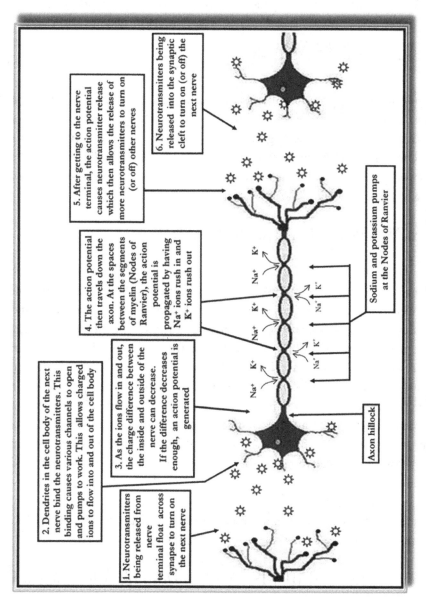

Figure 33. How an action potential is propagated along a nerve.

understand the consequences of our actions. They continue to myelinate into our late teens and can be reformatted after that through our education, jobs, and neurocognitive training. If everything goes according to plan, we develop into well-functioning individuals in the wonderful world around us.

FUNCTIONING OF NERVES

While all of the nerves in the central nervous system were made during the months after conception, they could not start working properly until they were myelinated. At the beginning of this book, nerve functioning was touched upon using the analogy of a computer network. The idea of the network still applies, but now we need to talk about the fundamentals of how a nerve actually works.

RESTING, THRESHOLD, AND ACTION POTENTIALS

We will start the lesson at the end of the nerve, which is called the *axon terminal*. In order to get a message to the next nerve, the axon terminal has to release neurotransmitters into the space between the axon terminal and the dendrites of the next nerve. This space is called the *synapse*. Once they get across the synapse, they bind to receptors on the dendrites. This binding can cause channels to open and let ions (like sodium, potassium, and calcium) move into or out of the cell. The binding can also cause pumps, which use energy, to move ions into and out of the nerve cell. Normally, the charge inside of a nerve cell (called the *resting potential*) is about -70 millivolts (mV). The charge outside of the nerve cell is zero. If more positive ions, like sodium (Na), flow into the cell than out, the charge difference between the inside and outside of the nerve will decrease (meaning that the inside charge of -70 mV can become more positive (e.g., -60 mV)). If the difference decreases enough, and the inside charge gets to be about -55 mV (called the *threshold potential*), something called an *action potential* (AP) is generated.

HOW AN ACTION POTENTIAL IS CONDUCTED DOWN THE AXON OF A NERVE

After being ignited where the nerve cell body and axon meet (called the *axon hillock*), the AP starts going down the axon. As the AP continues with a charge of -55 mV down the axon, potassium ions (K^+) are pumped out because the nerve cell wants to restore the normal resting potential of -70 mV. However, if the AP is going to make it all the way down the axon to stimulate the next nerve, then it needs to be bolstered along the way by having more positive ions come into the nerve to keep the charge around -55 mV.

This regeneration of the AP happens at each of the gaps between the bundles of myelin that wrap the axon.

These gaps are called the *Nodes of Ranvier*.[114] It is at these nodes that sodium ions (Na^+) can rush in to keep the cell depolarized (less negative) so the AP can continue. However, since the nerve cell wants to get back to its resting potential (which is more negative), there are also pumps that start pumping out positively charged potassium (K+) ions. At each Node of Ranvier, the sodium channels win out over the potassium pumps, thus allowing the AP to be regenerated just enough so that it can get to the next Node of Ranvier. The jumping of the current from one node to the next, all the way down the axon to the nerve terminal, is called *saltatory conduction*.

NEUROTRANSMITTER AND RECEPTOR SIDEBAR

Neurotransmitter = a key
Receptor = a lock that can initiate changes inside a cell

A neurotransmitter is only a key. Like most keys, if you put it into the wrong keyhole, the lock does not open. If you put it into the proper keyhole, the lock opens, and then whatever the lock is attached to can do its job. If it is a lock to get into your home, you can go inside and do all of your home activities. If it is to the ignition lock on your car, the engine will start, and you can drive to the beach. If it is to a lock on a safety deposit box, it will allow you to get your valuables out. Likewise, a neurotransmitter (key) fits into a specific receptor (lock). Acetylcholine unlocks acetylcholine receptors. Dopamine unlocks dopamine receptors. Serotonin unlocks serotonin receptors. These different receptors induce changes in the different cells that they are located on. This "lock and key" model for neurotransmitters and receptors is simple, but it becomes more complex when we appreciate that there are "receptor families."

Each receptor is part of a family of receptors. The acetylcholine receptor family is made of nicotinic and muscarinic subfamilies. And those subfamilies have their own subfamilies. Just like each member in a family, they might look similar, but their functions can be very different. The differences are linked to what type of cell they are part of and how they work. There are acetylcholine receptors of both subfamilies scattered throughout the body. Some are on nerves, some are on glands, and some are on muscle. They are almost everywhere. When acetylcholine binds to a nicotinic receptor on a nerve, the receptor changes shape and opens a channel that allows sodium to rush in and potassium to rush out of the neuron. If enough acetylcholine binds to enough nicotinic receptors, then the action potential can be started. The acetylcholine receptor, however, has just two subfamilies. Dopamine has at least five receptor types in its family. Serotonin has at least seven. New receptor subtypes are being discovered on a regular basis.

The next thing to appreciate is that the receptors for certain neurotransmitters in the CNS are specific to certain pathways (tracts). Dopamine is involved in at least four different pathways in the CNS. These pathways, for the most part, control movement, reward, and initiative. The dopamine receptors in each of these pathways differ from each other.[115, 116] The dopamine that gets released in these pathways, in combination with other neurotransmitters that bind to their unique receptors, generates desires, feelings, thoughts, and actions that are unique to the individual.

Grossly, our brains look similar. However, with the hundreds of billions of microscopic connections between neurons in our brains, each brain functions differently. They are constructed according to each person's unique DNA and are constantly changing in response to our interior and exterior environments. With the enormous range in these variables, every brain is unique. In the world of neurobehavior, doctors try their best at using pharmacotherapies to help a person attain the emo-cognitive functioning that they want. However, their attempts are based upon interpretations of data about drugs from population-based studies. Since a person is not a population, any one individual might or might not benefit from a specific intervention. If they do, hurray! If not, continued, open discourse between patient and doctor is necessary to get the best possible outcome.

HOW TO MAKE A NERVE NOT WORK

DEMYELINATION

In this book, we have been talking about the demyelination that goes on in MS. If the axon is stripped of myelin, then the charge difference between the inside and the outside of the nerve cell cannot be created and/or maintained. If there is no charge difference, saltatory conduction cannot occur. When conduction cannot occur in a nerve, messages from and to the brain cannot be relayed properly. This leads to many of the troubles that MSers face.

Aside from demyelination, there are other things that commonly affect nerve functioning in humans. These include things like medications, drugs, alcohol[117], temperature, and pressure. For our purposes, we will talk about only two of these—temperature and pressure.

TEMPERATURE

As far as temperature goes, the conduction of an impulse along a neuron can be interrupted when its temperature gets outside of a narrow range. This can happen with temperatures that are too high or too low.[118, 119] When nerve conduction is impaired, the speed with which we think and move slows down. The difference between demyelination and temperature (and pressure, as will be explained in the next section) is twofold. With demyelination, a focal lesion is produced that affects a select group of nerves, which causes a specific deficit (like weakness in your left leg or not being able to see out of your right eye). However, the effect of a change in temperature is global. It affects the whole brain, leading to a slight worsening of everything. Many people without MS know how lethargic they become on a hot, hazy, humid summer day.[120] Your whole body seems to be cloaked in a heavy coat that you cannot shake off. The only way you can start to feel better is by going into a place where you can cool down your entire body, like a pool or an air-conditioned room. If you put an MSer into a hot environment, you can see both global deficits *and* old, focal deficits reemerge. In the world of MS, this common symptom is called *heat intolerance*.[121]

Additionally, since nerve dysfunction also occurs with temperatures below the normal range, cold intolerance can also reveal a worsening of focal deficits in an MSer when she gets too cold. This past winter, I was shoveling snow when the temperature was four degrees. After shoveling for about forty minutes, I tried to make a joke with my neighbor from across the street who had just come outside to shovel his sidewalk. As I started to shout over the wind, I noticed that my speech was slurred. My speech didn't return to normal until after I had gone back inside and warmed up. The nice thing about temperature-induced deficits is that they resolve when the temperature is normalized.

PRESSURE

Akin to temperature, nerves can only work within a narrow pressure range.[122] Elevated intracerebral pressure can cause nerve dysfunction leading to troubles with many things, including cognition, gait disturbance, and urinary control. These symptoms are well documented in a neurological condition known as *normal pressure hydrocephalus* (NPH).[123] Normally, the fluid that surrounds the brain and spinal cord (a.k.a. cerebrospinal fluid or CSF for short) gets made by the choroid plexus in the lateral ventricles (see chapter 8, figure 20). The CSF then flows out of the lateral ventricles through the third ventricle, goes around the brain and the spinal cord, and then returns to the brain to be reabsorbed by the arachnoid granulations. In NPH, the CSF cannot flow out of the ventricles as quickly as it's being made. This leads to elevated pressure within the lateral ventricles. The elevated intraventricular pressure leads to an enlargement of the lateral ventricles, which can be seen on CAT scans of the head, and produces the classic presenting symptoms of NPH—wacky, wobbly, and wet. These patients start behaving inappropriately (wacky), are unstable when they walk (wobbly), and have urinary incontinence (wet).[124] A common treatment for this syndrome is to put in a bypass (called a shunt), which allows the CSF to be diverted from the ventricles directly into the abdomen, thus reducing the pressure in the head. By reducing the intraventricular pressure to a normal level, the patient's symptoms abate.

How then, we can ask, is the elevated pressure effect in NPH related to MS? Let's think about the process of MS. For some reason, the immune system has started to view the myelin in the CNS as an invader. The immune system starts to mount a response. Any immune response in the body is mediated by inflammation. For example, if you go jogging and twist your ankle, one of the first things you notice, aside from the pain, is that your ankle swells. The bones, tendons, and muscles in your ankle are surrounded by skin that can stretch. That's good because the immune system wants to get as many repair cells to the damaged area as possible along with a good supply of oxygen, glucose, and water.[125] The immune system starts taking away the damaged bits and starts rebuilding and repairing the original structure of your ankle. While swollen, you can't run on it very well (if at all) since you've lost the normal range of motion around the ankle joint and it hurts when you stand on it. When you touch it, the sensation feels different from the other, not-swollen ankle. Your ankle stays swollen for several days, but then, as the healing starts to wind down, the swelling slowly subsides. After about a week, you're back to your old self, and you can walk and run as usual.

In many ways, the inflammatory attack in the CNS of MSers is like a twisted ankle. The main difference between a twisted ankle and an MS brain is that the brain is trapped in a rigid box (called the skull) that is noncompliant (meaning that it cannot stretch like the skin around a twisted ankle).

Because of the continuous, low-lying, microscopic, inflammatory[126], demyelinating disease that is going on in the CNS of MSers, there is a constant, elevated interstitial pressure (pressure within the brain tissue) that has nowhere to go and winds up pushing upon the adjacent, compressible, jellylike nerves in the brain, brain stem, and spinal cord, which causes a significant number of them to not work properly.

Much like NPH, many of us with MS have trouble with thinking, walking, and urinary control. Of course, we have focal lesions of demyelination and nerve cell loss that can cause these troubles as well. However, the elevated pressure in the CNS worsens nerve functioning *globally* and affects areas in the CNS that control these and other systems. Unlike NPH, where the elevated pressure is in the ventricles and can be reduced by placing a shunt, the interstitial pressure in MS has hundreds of billions of microscopic areas of elevated pressure within the brain tissue that cannot be easily reduced by using a macroscopic shunt. Happily though, we do have medications that work on a microscopic level that can do just that.

THE KEY POINTS TO REMEMBER ARE:

1. MS causes a constant, covert, elevated pressure in interstitial spaces (the spaces between the nerve cells) of the CNS.[127]
2. This elevated intracerebral pressure comes from the WBCs that are demyelinating nerves and the inflammatory fluid that accompanies them in the CNS.

3. Elevated pressure can cause global, as opposed to focal, deficits since it affects the entire CNS.

4. The constant, elevated pressure in the CNS of people with MS causes changes in behavior and cognition that cannot be appreciated just by looking at the MSer. This is the invisible MS. It is potentially reversible with therapies that reduce the elevated interstitial pressure.

5. The constant, elevated pressure in the CNS of people with MS also causes a variable worsening of the visible, physical problems caused by focal demyelination and nerve cell loss.

PART II

A NEW IDEA OF WHAT IS GOING ON IN THE MINDS OF MSERS

UNDERSTANDING MS SYMPTOMS

If a person can accept the idea that elevated interstitial pressure causes a global lesion that worsens nerve functioning, then it becomes a lot easier to understand what has been described, until now, as the "hidden MS." Symptoms associated with the hidden MS are hidden because they are products of something no one can see—the mind. Our frontal lobes integrate the data that other parts of the brain collect. They get input from almost everywhere else in the brain and then make the decision about what action to take based on the information received. One of the responsibilities of frontal lobe processing is to govern behavior. If a percentage of the nerves in the frontal lobes have stopped working, because of the effects of pressure, temperature, and/or demyelination, then the processor cannot produce the behaviors the way it did before. The symptoms include troubles with:

1. Initiative
2. Concentration
3. Emotional control
4. Coital activity
5. Urinary control
6. BEhavior that is socially appropriate

These symptoms have been the bane of my time with MS, which has been the majority of my life. I call them the MS ICE CUBE or The MS ICE for short.

1. INITIATIVE

"MS FATIGUE" IS ACTUALLY A LOSS OF INITIATIVE

Quite often, when people see us MSers, they'll say that we appear to be tired. When asked, we MSers might say that we're profoundly exhausted. The observer might then say to him or herself, "That's weird. I know I saw him lying in bed for eighteen hours. How could he be exhausted?" This has been dubbed by many neurologists as the *MS fatigue*. But it is not fatigue. True fatigue comes from buildup of lactic acid in muscles after exercise and almost always resolves after sixty minutes of rest.[128] Even on a good day, we MSers look and feel like pieces of wet lasagna. We try to explain that it's not just tiredness. It's something more. And it's not just the physical weakness caused by MS lesions. It feels like we've been coated in tar, both mentally and physically, while our legs have been set in concrete and then coated in lead while a fifty-pound bag of uncooked pizza dough is draped upon our shoulders and a 310-pound loggerhead sea turtle takes up residence on our heads. We have no "get up and go." No pep. No punch.[129]

In fact, one might even say that it looks like we
MSers do not have any initiative …

"NO! YOU CAN'T SAY THAT! TO SAY THAT SOMEONE DOES NOT HAVE INITIATIVE IS A PEJORATIVE TERM IN OUR SOCIETY!"

Why is it pejorative? Because when it's said that a person has no initiative, it implies that he or she is lazy. To say a person has no initiative makes it sound as if the person could do whatever he or she wanted to do, but he or she just doesn't want to do it. Those around the MSer know that the MSer was not lazy before he got MS. They know that before the MSer got MS, he had a happy family, had a good business, acted gentlemanly, and enjoyed life. After getting MS, the MSer says that he feels like he doesn't have the energy to do his job anymore. He has no punch. He feels like he just doesn't want to do anything anymore. So he goes to see his doctor and says that he has no energy anymore. "Ah," the doctor says. "Fatigue is a big problem with MS." Then the doctor tries to give the MSer helpful hints on ways to avoid the MS fatigue. "Stay cool. Don't overdo it. Eat a healthful diet. Get exercise. Take your medication. I'll see you in six months."

Observers who are close to the MSer might start to think that the MSer is depressed. "Who wouldn't be depressed having a disease like MS?" they ask. "Maybe I'll speak with them." So they speak with the MSer, who might say, "No. I'm happy. I just have this overwhelming sense of lethargy and heaviness that never goes away." So the MSer goes back to the doctor, who listens to the patient. "The lethargy and fatigue just won't go away," the patient says. Then the doctor thinks and thinks. He or she then says that sleep disturbance in multiple sclerosis is well documented.[130, 131] The doctor might order a sleep study or recommend medications like amantadine and modafinil, which might work. The patient might come back and say that the medication is working all right, but he or she still can't get off the couch. Their children have to bring him or her their food. The doctor might start to think more about depression and how common depression is in almost all chronic diseases. So the MSer starts a medication for depression and feels a little better, but at follow-up, he or she still has many of the same feelings. The patient and the caregiver and the doctor look at each other and say it must be another part of the disease that is not well understood. It must be the *MS fatigue*.

Noooooooooooooooooooooo!

Let's go back to initiative. As defined, initiative is the ability of a person to start something. The "something" can be anything—an act, a program, a movement. As noted previously, the parts of the brain that control initiative, drive, and motivation are located in the frontal cortex (specifically, the orbitofrontal cortex[132, 133]). The amount of brain tissue that is involved is enormous.[134, 135] In the world of medicine, it has been shown repeatedly that if the frontal lobes are damaged, initiative can be greatly affected. It is known that in surgeries where lesions are made that interrupt the communication between the frontal lobes and the limbic system, people can lose their initiative.[136, 137] Almost any trauma to the frontal lobes may produce some loss of initiative.[138]

> In the setting of MS, the trauma is the constant, elevated
> pressure in the interstitial spaces (the spaces between
> the nerve cells) within the brain tissue.

We do know that natalizumab, fingolimod, and dimethyl fumarate, as noted in the therapy chapter, have mechanisms that greatly reduce the number of WBCs that get into the interstitial spaces in the brain and spinal cord. Many people who start natalizumab report having an improvement in the quality of their life as determined by the SF-36.[139,140] A decrease in brain volume after using the disease-modifying therapies has been well documented by radiologists who review MRIs in MS patients who start these medications. The reduction in calculated brain volume has been termed pseudoatrophy.[141]

CONCLUSION

MSers have a loss of initiative secondary to the elevated pressure within our brains.

2. CONCENTRATION

ATTENTION

The frontal lobes are also responsible for attention and concentration. As mentioned above, the frontal lobes don't really get hooked up and work until the early teen years. This can be seen clearly in children. If you put a child in front of the TV to watch the news, he or she will get bored and start playing with the remote. If you put on the music show that has songs about ice cream and a band that wears bright colors, the child will pay attention and sing along. After the frontal lobes are hooked up, a young person can start to pay attention even to things that might not interest him or her.

Some kids who do not myelinate as quickly as the rest of the children quite often have trouble paying attention. They may or may not be diagnosed with attention deficit disorder (either with or without hyperactivity), but if they are treated with medications that prevent the breakdown of the neurotransmitters that are responsible for attention and concentration (dopamine and norepinephrine), then there can be a rapid change in how they do in learning, both socially and academically.[142, 143] The nice thing about childhood ADD is that there's a good chance that once a child's brain has myelinated enough, commonly by the age of fourteen, they can come off of their medication. In MS, connections with and within the frontal lobes are either paralyzed by the swelling caused by MS or from being demyelinated. These factors variably reduce brain functioning to a childlike state. In short, MS cognitive dysfunction is, quite often, attention deficit disorder.

CONCENTRATION

In addition to the loss of the ability to pay attention, the swollen MS brain also has trouble with working memory and concentration.[144, 145] MSers quite often forget what they were talking about after they get distracted by the slightest of interruptions like a truck driving by or a light turning on or a mosquito flying by or a car honking or when a fire truck comes racing down the street. One time when I was a teenager, I was watching TV when I started to smell some smoke. I just figured the neighbors had built a fire in their fireplace, and while it did smell a little different from a normal fire, I didn't make too much out of it until I heard and saw the fire truck come racing down the street, and when the siren sound didn't fade away, I thought to myself, *That's weird. It didn't fade away. Then that must mean the fire truck stopped right here on my block. Oh my God! That smoky smell!* I ran down out of my house and saw the fire truck parked at the end of the block. It turns out that the house on the corner had gone up in flames! A kind lady lived there. I found out later that a space heater had ignited some drapes. What a shame. I should really replace the batteries in the smoke alarm when I get home ...

What was I writing about again ...?

So our swollen brains, when trying to pay attention, are distracted because the pathways that let us concentrate are paralyzed. Another way to think about it is that concentration is a filter that blocks out all of the things that you do not want to pay attention to. It's like going into an electronics store to buy a new TV. All the screens are on, and the volumes are all at the same level. You can't learn anything from any of the shows that are on because the surrounding images and sounds are getting in the way. Concentration allows us to see what we want to see and not be bothered by the background noise.

CONCLUSION

People with MS very often have findings consistent with attention deficit disorder.

3. EMOTIONAL LABILITY

Emotional lability (a.k.a. pseudobulbar affect) is when a person's emotions go from being happy to sad and back to happy from moment to moment. Control over emotions is mediated by connections between the frontal lobes and the left ventromedial prefrontal cortex.[146] Since little kids do not have their frontal lobes hooked up yet, they demonstrate this on a regular basis. For example, if they talk with each other and decide that they want to go to the amusement park, they get excited at the idea. When they're told that they cannot go to the amusement park (because Daddy doesn't have any money to pay for it), they start crying. They don't cry because Dad doesn't have any money. They cry because they cannot go to the amusement park right now and have fun! If, however, the quick-thinking dad asks the child if he or she wants to go and get some ice cream, the child immediately becomes happy again because he or she can have something else that's good right now! This is called emotional lability. Many of us MSers have labile emotions. We feel like babies sometimes when we start crying over little things. Then when others look at us and ask, "Why are you crying?" we say, "I don't know," and really feel foolish. The loss of emotional control from frontal lobe dysfunction often makes many of us MSers feel abnormal. We know we're not behaving the way we used to. If we don't understand why we're acting differently, we become insecure and turn in on ourselves. If no one can tell us why we're acting this way, we can feel abandoned—not only by others but by our own brain.

We MSers should realize that our change in behavior is coming from frontal lobe dysfunction caused by the swelling in our brains. We need to remember that we are still the same people we always were, but now we need some help to take back our minds.

We doctors have to realize that we cannot diagnose and treat what we do not understand. When it comes to treating the mind, we have to understand that we cannot understand what's going on in the mind of another. Once we accept that, then we can learn. We need to listen and then be open to using treatments that many of us are afraid to use.

And going back to us MSers, we have to understand that we cannot understand what's going on in the minds of our caregivers and health-care providers unless we listen to what they say.

CONCLUSION

Both MSers and doctors have to understand that we cannot understand what's going on in the mind of the other and that we have to listen so that we can learn.

4. COITAL ACTIVITY

As will be seen in the chapter on sex, the human sexual response cycle is a five-stage process. The stages are desire, arousal, plateau, orgasm, and resolution. The main rule guiding the cycle is that these stages must occur in sequence. If the sexual encounter is between two people, then both partners need to first pass through the desire stage before things can go any further. For the MSer, there are a few things that can get in the way of getting the sexual cycle going. First, let's define desire. Desire is a strong wish in wanting something to happen. In some ways, it can be thought of as "sexual initiative." If the MSer has trouble with initiative when the non-MSer has desire, we're already a strike down in the count. If the stimulus presented to us by our partner is strong enough, then maybe the decreased sexual initiative can be overcome and the cycle can start. However, if the stimulus is not as enticing, then the MSer might not be able to get to the desire phase. The partner might take the MSer's lassitude as sexual laziness. "Why do I have to be the one to turn you on?" he or she might ask. Or if he or she doesn't say anything, he or she might start to think to him or herself that their partner doesn't find him or her appealing anymore and that the spark is gone.

The other way that the sexual cycle can get a flat is when the MSer has desire but their partner does not. In this case, the MSer can start to act like the child who cannot go to the amusement park right now. He or she can become impatient and force the sexual encounter, which turns their partner further away.

CONCLUSION

Sexual dysfunction in MS quite often is not something that can be fixed with a drug for erectile dysfunction or vaginal lubrication. Sexual functioning starts with desire, which comes from the mind. If we think of desire as sexual initiative, we need to treat sexual initiative first in order for the sexual cycle to start.

5. URINARY CONTROL

Urination, on a basic level, is simple. Either you are urinating or you are holding it in. On a neurological level, however, it's one of the most convoluted systems we humans have. It's a reflex action that for most animals goes on without thinking. The urinary bladder fills with urine. Once it's stretched out enough, the reflex takes over. The muscles that hold the urine in (called *sphincters*) relax, and the muscle that squeezes it out (the detrusor muscle) contracts.

The complex part started when life moved out of the sea and onto land and waste material couldn't just float away. It got even more complex when we humans, with our great thinking brains, started to come up with "socially appropriate behavior."[147] Control over the urinary reflexes rests in the frontal lobes of our brains. As has been demonstrated multiple times so far in this book, the frontal lobes of us MSers sometimes function as well as a quadriplegic, blind dog performing cardiac bypass surgery on stage at CBGBs while singing backup for the undiscovered and greatly underappreciated band Habenular Nuclei.[148] In other words, the global dysfunction caused by the elevated intracerebral pressure leads to reduced control over urination. This is similar to the effects caused by normal pressure hydrocephalus.

CONCLUSION

Urinary control can be handled through drugs targeted at improving cortical functioning as well as using the standard medications that directly decrease bladder detrusor contraction or increase urethral sphincter contraction.

6. BEHAVIOR

The frontal lobes also control the way we behave in public and interact with others. Everybody has thoughts about others that they don't say because it's not socially appropriate. Incompletely myelinated kids don't understand that they should not ask Mrs. Floggerbottom why she has a moustache since only men are supposed to have moustaches. The frontal lobes act as gatekeepers, and since children don't have their frontal lobes hooked up yet, they make comments that are not socially appropriate.[149, 150] While everyone occasionally says things that they "didn't mean to say," we MSers, as a group, are above average in this category. If you ask anyone who has lived or worked closely with an MSer, he or she would probably agree with the statement that the MSer in their life has made comments that were not socially appropriate more often than most other adults.

CONCLUSION

People with MS don't want to say mean or stupid things! The problem is that we have lost our gatekeepers because of the swelling in our brains, so please don't write us off as a lost cause. There are interventions that can help!

So far in this chapter, I have presented the idea that some of the biggest issues that we MSers have to deal with are not visible. They are products of the swollen brain, which creates our minds. I have come to refer to it as the MS ICE. You can also call it the MS ICE CUBE to include coitus, urination, and behavior. I often trim it down to the MS ICE because it is easier to remember.

MS ICE SUMMARY

1. White blood cells are constantly getting into the brain to demyelinate nerves.
2. Nerves work in a narrow pressure range.
3. Since the brain is housed in a skull that has a fixed volume, the pressure goes up.
4. The elevated pressure causes loss of functioning in a percentage of nerves throughout the rain.

5. This general loss of nerve functioning produces diffuse, reversible frontal lobe dysfunction, which takes away our initiative, our ability to concentrate, and our emotional control.[151]

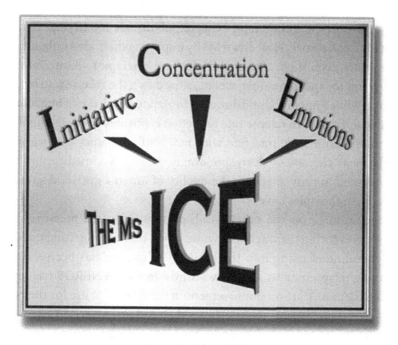

Figure 34. The MS ICE.
The MS ICE is a triad of frequent, often reversible frontal lobe deficits caused by the elevated interstitial pressure in the CNS of people who have MS.

PART III

HOW WE CAN MELT THE MS ICE

Global improvements (i.e., improvements of the MS ICE CUBE deficits) can come by reducing the elevated intracerebral pressure in MS. The medications that can do this include the disease-modifying therapies, IV steroids, and ACTH. As far as improving focal lesions where there has been nerve cell loss after demyelination, we will discuss medications that increase neurotransmitter release and improve conduction from the surviving nerves in those pathways.

The Global Lesion

The Disease-Modifying Therapies and Beyond

As described in the MS therapies chapter, all disease-modifying therapies, except for natalizumab, slow down MS by impairing the body's inflammatory response to myelin. In short, the platform therapies (β-interferon 1a, β-interferon 1b, and glatiramer acetate) slow down the relapse rate by about one-third while fingolimod and dimethyl fumarate slow it down by about one-half. The difference in relapse rate reduction is possibly because fingolimod and dimethyl fumarate interfere with more inflammatory pathways than the platform therapies. Correspondingly, these two medications have demonstrated improvements in the quality of life to a greater degree than the platform therapies have. [152, 153]

Natalizumab, on the other hand, prevents elevated pressure in the brain by preventing the offending white blood cells from getting out of the blood stream and going into the brain. Natalizumab has been shown to reduce the relapse rate by about two-thirds. In the TYNERGY trial, it was shown to demonstrate an improvement in the quality of life for the people who were taking Tysabri to slow down their MS.[154] This trial looked at the quality of life of MSers before and after being on natalizumab. In it, they asked the participants how they viewed their general, physical, and mental health and how any troubles with these areas prevented them from doing their usual activities. It also asked questions about sleepiness, cognitive functions, walking speed, and depression. The study concluded that starting natalizumab improved the quality of life for MSers. The authors of the study suggested that improvements in "MS fatigue" (which I believe is better defined as a loss of initiative) could possibly be due to the fact that certain cytokines (interleukins, tumor necrosis factor, and interferon-γ) break down the blood-brain barrier and allow white blood cells to get into the brain. They mention that these cytokines have been related to "fatigue-like" symptoms in animals.

Let's Take It One Step Further

While I concur with the TYNERGY investigators' reasoning, I believe that the culprit is not the cytokines but rather the pressure. The global dysfunction that causes the MS ICE is caused by the volume of white blood cells, other inflammatory cells, and fluid that's stuffed into the fixed intracranial volume, which raises the pressure. I feel that this is a subtle but important point. The point is important because it shows that the mechanism of action of natalizumab is an extremely important avenue for development of therapies for MS. Elevated pressure is a separate cause of dysfunction in MS. Our troubles do not come from demyelination alone. While inflammatory elements have an association with loss of initiative, the reduction in the intracranial contents is the thing that gives many of us MSers our minds back. The "pseudoatrophy" seen on the MRIs of MSers treated with natalizumab reflects the exclusion of white blood cells from the cortex. The "swollen ankle" brain of the MSer resolves, and we MSers can cognitively "run" again.[155]

A Personal Note on Tennis and Neurology

I want to insert an important experience that shows how the elevated pressure can directly affect focal lesions. Growing up, I played tennis quite often. I wasn't great, but I could hold my own. After I had my first exacerbation, which affected my balance, especially when I changed direction or turned my head quickly, I tried to go and play tennis with my girlfriend (who, eventually, became my wife). When I tried to serve, I would get dizzy just raising my head as I tossed the ball. If I tried to swing at the ball and it went in the service box, I was so off balance after bringing my head back down I couldn't fix my gaze on the ball or anything else for that matter. I would swing wildly at the ball when she would serve to me, and I would miss it by several feet. We continued to try to play for about twenty minutes, but it had started to become embarrassing. I looked like I was drunk and felt like an idiot.

Move ahead almost twenty years. After having been on natalizumab for six months and noticing that my balance seemed better, along with my coordination and concentration, I decided to see how I would do on a tennis court. After playing with my wife for two minutes, not only could I play tennis again but I was playing better than I had when I last played as a nineteen-year-old.

While I have always been humble in the gifts that I've been provided, that was a defining moment in my life. Something that I had always liked to do had been taken away from me. I felt down about it, but I decided to focus on the things that I could do. I stayed on top of the therapies that came out for MS. Eventually natalizumab came on the scene. I tried it, not expecting anything. The day I got tennis back, I felt like I had been given a gift. Since then, I have developed a specific viewpoint about the good things in life that has served me well:

I expect nothing, but I hope for everything.

This episode also taught me an important neurological lesson. While I had thought that tennis was gone forever because demyelinated nerves don't stay alive for twenty years, my balance came back after starting a medication that decreased my intracranial pressure. Interestingly, the lesion that caused my balance problems was located in a region where the top of the spinal cord meets up with the cerebellum, just below where the cerebral cortex starts. This told me that the effects that elevated pressure have on the cortex also apply to the other elements in the CNS, like the cerebellum and the spinal cord.

Additionally, when I play tennis with my wife, I play well for about thirty to forty minutes. Then, after getting heated up, I notice that I start to get off balance again. This tells me that I have lost nerves that control my balance and coordination because after the heat causes nerve dropout, I don't have any backup like I did before getting MS. When that happens, my wife and I take a break, drink some cool water, and then carry on.

So, if we accept the concept that lowering intracranial pressure has the potential for improving the lives of MSers, how else can we selectively prevent white blood cells from getting into the CNS? Natalizumab covers up the α-4 integrin molecule on the white blood cell so it cannot bind to the VCAM receptors on the blood vessel walls. What about selectively blocking the VCAM receptors and letting the WBCs continue to do their jobs in the rest of the body? This could possibly prevent infections caused by organisms (like viruses and bacteriae) that live in our bodies. Natalizumab is a monoclonal antibody. Maybe instead of using a monoclonal antibody, there might be a role for nanobots in producing this blockade.

Along with reducing the ingress of WBCs into the brain, how else can we reduce the pressure in the brains of MSers? Could shunt placement, which is used for normal pressure hydrocephalous, work? How about coming up with a way to reduce the production of CSF to decrease the amount of stuff contained in the skull? Can the volume of the skull be increased by attaching a negative pressure bladder housed in the abdomen to the subdural space?

I put the charge to all who read this book; you, by sitting around and by brainstorming with yourself and/or others, could come up with the next way to help the hundreds of thousands of people in the United States and the millions of people around the world who have MS. Remember, the only bad idea in brainstorming is the one that's not shared with others.

STEROIDS

When we have an exacerbation in MS, we use steroids, like methylprednisolone or dexamethasone intravenously, to shut down our immune systems. These steroids are known to be potent inhibitors of inflammation.[156, 157, 158] I know many MSers feel much more alive—thinking more clearly and having more initiative—while on steroids. Before I made my discoveries about the effects of brain swelling on initiative and cognition, I thought that the cause of the boost I felt came from the increase in blood glucose levels that IV steroids produce. However, I remember that the sensation I had while on steroids was more controlled than what one might feel after eating twenty-five candy bars in a row.[159] Unfortunately, high-dose, IV steroids have *many* side effects, including sodium retention, potassium loss, elevated blood sugar levels, bone loss, thinning of the subcutaneous fat, psychosis, gastroesophageal reflux disease, and ulcers, to name a few. Because of the myriad problems they can cause, frequent or chronic use of steroids can lead to problems that outweigh the benefits.

Another medication that can produce very good decreased brain-swelling effects is adrenocorticotrophic hormone (ACTH). It's a hormone made in the anterior pituitary gland. One of its actions is to produce an anti-inflamed state in our bodies. After ACTH is released into the blood stream, it binds to receptors on the adrenal glands, which then release melanocortins. The melanocortins then circulate through the body, binding to and activating melanocortin receptors, which are found on every cell in our bodies, including neurons. By producing an anti-inflamed state around each receptor, it can reduce swelling throughout our bodies. It also appears that ACTH only slightly increases production of the body's steroids (cortisol, corticosterone, and aldosterone) in comparison with IV steroids. The trade name for the medication is ACTHar Gel®.[160] ACTHar Gel® is indicated for use in the treatment of MS exacerbations. One of its biggest benefits is that it does not cause the deleterious effect of bone loss (osteonecrosis) to the same degree that comes with chronic steroid use.[161] Further research in its use, along with investigation of another hormone, proopiomelanocortin (POMC),[162] should be continued as a possible way of helping to give us MSers our frontal lobes back.

THE OTHER GLOBAL LESION—TEMPERATURE

As mentioned above, temperature is another main cause of global dysfunction. If we get too warm or too cold, we get nerve drop out. There are now myriad types of external cooling devices for MSers that can be used to keep core body temperature down. In medicine and surgery, cooling body temperature is commonly used in the setting of cardiac arrest and cardiac surgery. Some of the appliances are external, but some are internal. Shouldn't we be able to create an implantable device that could lower the temperature of the blood that's about to enter the brain by several degrees? It could be located close to a vessel that delivers blood to the brain, like the carotid or vertebral arteries. It should be a device that can either cool or warm blood, depending upon the surrounding temperature. I know it's possible; someone just has to make it. I would make it myself, but I'm busy writing this book right now. Plus, the Olympics just finished, and ever since the Norwegian men's curling team got knocked out in the quarterfinals by Great Britain, I have been ensconced in a state of great woe. I have to believe it had something to do with their *Partridge Family*'s bus-patterned trousers that caused a *Buksekrise*, which led to their fall.

PERSONAL NOTE ABOUT NATALIZUMAB AND WRITING

Other changes that I experienced after I started natalizumab reflected the difference in the anti-inflammatory effect of β-interferon 1a—IM and natalizumab. Among the changes that I experienced was that my initiative had come back. While I was on β-interferon 1a—IM, if my son wanted to play catch after I got home from work, I would usually refer him to my wife to play with him in the front yard. After starting natalizumab, I was able to change my clothes and go play with him. Eventually, I initiated having my son practice his pitching to me when I got home from work. If I was physically exhausted at the end of the day at work, I could lie down for twenty minutes, let my body recharge, and then I could get up and play. Around the house, I started to initiate doing the laundry one to two times per week. While watching TV, I no longer felt I had to lie down. I would sit up like a non-MSer. I also initiated doing homework with my daughter while my wife worked with our son.

The most vibrant example of the restitution of my initiative and concentration, however, is completion of this book. It's a defining example of restored initiative and concentration. In 2001, I started to write a book that was the precursor of this book. I started writing it on Wednesday, April 9, 2001. The first installment was called "MS BOOK 4/24" and had seven pages. Each time I wrote more in the book, I would usually save the file under a new name using the same format—MS BOOK 6/20, MS BOOK 6/25, MS BOOK 6/28, and so on. Between April 9, 2001 and March 24, 2002, there are seventeen different instances like this, yielding a grand total of thirty-three pages. There was little organization and nothing that could be considered a complete chapter. I had been on β-interferon 1a—intramuscular for five years.

The first two hundred pages of this book were completed between March 5, 2010, and October 5, 2010. I had been on natalizumab for four years.[163] This is not to say that β-interferon 1a—IM had not made me feel better than when I was on nothing. It did. But natalizumab caused a greater decrease in the swelling in my brain and gave me back a lot of my frontal lobe, limbic, hypothalamic, and basal ganglionic functioning. I had my initiative again, as reflected in how quickly I wrote the two hundred pages. I could concentrate and complete chapter after chapter. I (as well as my family and my patients) also noticed that I was less scatterbrained when doing tasks and had better emotional control. My emotions would not go from laughing to crying just from seeing an especially touching dog food commercial anymore.[164] Also, I didn't need the air-conditioner on from February until November anymore. In fact, I am no longer the first person in my house to turn on the air-conditioner when the weather becomes warm.

Focal Global Lesions

While treatment of the swollen MS brain has the potential to improve a great part of the MS ICE deficits, the restoration is rarely complete due to factors such as neuronal cell death and lack of response to medication. While, currently, we cannot regrow nerves for specific cognitive pathways, we can maximize the functioning of the nerves that have not been lost. As mentioned in the above personal note about being on natalizumab, I regained quite a bit of my ability to concentrate, and I accomplished a lot. However, I was still far from who I had been. Having programmed computers since 1981, I have been trying to incorporate their use in medicine without replacing the role of the human caregiver. While going through my training in neurology, I did rotations in neurobehavior where I saw neurocognitive testing performed. Among my first thoughts was that if the testing were done via computer, the results could be much more reliable than when done by another person. Plus, many other tests could be done by using a machine that had tremendous processing speed and could analyze data across multiple matrices. At the same time, I saw the importance of speaking with a patient (preferably face-to-face) as the critical piece in caring for another person. This then led me to learn more about FDA-approved computer neurocognitive testing, which opened a whole world of improvements for both me and my patients.

Concentration, Attention, and ADD in MS

In September 2010, I instituted computer-based neurocognitive testing at my office. MSers, more often than not, demonstrate cognitive challenges in attention, memory, processing speed, and executive functioning/judgment.[165] This is the cognitive profile of a person who has attention deficit disorder. Methylphenidate, which is commonly used in people with ADD, has been shown to improve attention in multiple sclerosis patients.[166] I took the MS battery of tests, which included evaluation of attention, memory, processing speed, executive functioning, and psychomotor (finger tapping) skills. The results showed that my deficits were greatest in attention and memory.[167] I did my research and decided to try dextroamphetamine/amphetamine (Adderall®), which decreases the reuptake and increases the release of two neurotransmitters, dopamine and norepinephrine. These are the neurotransmitters, via frontostriatal pathways, that have a major influence on attention and concentration.[168] I did this in concert with my neurologist and primary care doctor.

Pharmacology /Tolerance/Addiction/Abuse Sidebar

As we begin this part of the book, we need to come to a common understanding of the medical definitions for tolerance and addiction. When you take a medication, your body adapts to the medication by increasing the enzymes needed to break down (metabolize) the medication. Because of this, the dose of the drug often has to be increased in order to get the same effect that it originally produced. This is called *physiological tolerance*, and it is to be expected. The amount that the drug can be increased by is determined by several factors, including, but not limited to, side effects, toxicity, cost, patient history, clinical vigilance, and the doctor's knowledge of the medication.

Physiological Tolerance

An example of physiological tolerance is coffee. Coffee causes some people to function better at their jobs. By modulating the release of various neurotransmitters, it causes certain blood vessels to constrict and produces an elevation in blood pressure. If you start drinking coffee every day, your body says, "Okay, since caffeine is coming in every day at ten o'clock, I'm going to make sure to dilate blood vessels at ten o'clock every day so that we can still have a good blood supply to the brain while drinking the coffee." Because of this, regardless of whether or not you drink your coffee, the body is going to dilate blood vessels at ten o'clock every day because it has learned that you take your caffeine drug at ten o'clock every day. So, if one day, you do not take your daily dose of caffeine, your body is going to dilate the blood vessels anyway, because it had been reprogrammed to think that caffeine was coming every day at ten o'clock. When that happens, you wind up getting a caffeine withdrawal headache! Additionally, if you're a daily coffee drinker, your body has increased the enzymes to break down the caffeine and get it out of your system. So after drinking coffee for several days, you might need more cups of coffee throughout the day to give you the same effect that you had when you first started drinking it. This means that you have developed a physiological tolerance it.

Withdrawal symptoms depend upon how much and for how long you have been putting a drug into your body. If you're using something every day, you might notice more withdrawal symptoms than if you were taking the medication only a few days per week. To avoid withdrawal symptoms, a person needs to be tapered off of a medication (decreasing the dose over a certain period of time), based upon how long the drug lasts in your body. How long a drug lasts in your body depends upon the half-life of the drug.

The half-life ($t_{1/2}$) of a drug is the time it takes for your body to remove one-half of the drug from your body. A drug is considered to be out of your body 3.3 half-lives after you last took the medication. For example, if the half-life of a medication is two hours, it will be out of your body after 6.6 hours ($2 \times 3.3 = 6.6$). Short-acting drugs, having a shorter half-life, generally have less withdrawal than extended-release versions.

ADDICTION

Addiction is different. It's when a person continues to do something despite the fact that it's harmful to him or herself or others. Addiction, like many diseases, is a combination of genes and the environment.[169, 170, 171] It depends on the personality of the individual and his surrounding influences. One person can have a sugar-free, cholesterol-free cookie every day, and that's fine. If, one day, it turns out that he doesn't have any money to buy the cookie and he can say, "Oh well. No cookie for me today," that person is not addicted to the cookie. However, if he doesn't have the money to buy the cookie, and he feels that he needs the cookie so much that he has to rob a store to get the cookie, then that's an addiction. He is hurting others and, subsequently, himself.

If a person feels better or happier while taking a medication, that's not an addiction. If the person asks the doctor to increase the dose of the medication to get a better effect, that's not an addiction either. If the doctor says that it's unsafe to raise the dose or continue the medication for whatever reason (liver dysfunction, cardiac toxicity, etc.) and the patient decides to start "borrowing" some medication from a friend, then that's an addiction. If he decides to start buying the medication from a dealer on the streets, then that's an addiction. If he goes to another doctor and asks for the medication without telling the new doctor that the last doctor did not want the person to get the medication anymore because it was hurting him, that's also an addiction. The person is hurting himself and others.

DRUG ABUSE

Drug abuse is when a drug's use interferes with a person's responsibilities, health, social interactions, and/or conduct in society (legal issues), but the person's symptoms have not met the criteria of drug addiction. Anything a person puts in his body that causes a pleasurable sensation has the potential for abuse. Things that are more pleasurable are more likely to be abused.

Because of the genetic predisposition for addiction, I always review a patient's family history to see if there's a history of addiction in the family or if the patient has ever had trouble with addiction himself. At the same time, my staff and I routinely monitor requests for medications that have abuse potential that come in before the next refill is due. Pharmacists are required to contact the prescribing physician if they find that a patient has gotten the same or similar medications from another physician as well as when a person tries to refill a prescription too soon. Insurance companies send letters to doctors about a patient when they get billed from different pharmacies for the same medication that's being prescribed by more than one physician.

SO, IN SUMMARY ...

Tolerance is a normal physiological response that a person gets to a substance, which often requires an increase in dose to get the desired effect.

Addiction is a behavior that is governed by genes, the environment, and the coping mechanisms of a person that causes harm to the person and/or to others.

Drug abuse is when a drug's use interferes with certain spheres of a person's life, but their symptoms have not met the criteria of drug addiction.

Starting dextroamphetamine/amphetamine allowed me not only to increase my attention and memory but it gave me an insight into the treatment of ADD.[172] I remember learning in medical school about attention deficit disorder with hyperactivity. They showed us movies of children with this condition. The kids were put at their desks with their books and told what to do. Within seconds, they were up and running around. They couldn't finish any of their schoolwork. Then the professor told us that ADD was treated by using "stimulants" (methylphenidate, dextroamphetamine/amphetamine).

I remember thinking to myself, *How the heck can a stimulant calm down a child who's zipping around like a mosquito with sneakers?* The problem is that the medications that increase norepinephrine and dopamine levels have the pejorative appellation, "stimulant." Methamphetamine is known as "speed" on the streets, and when not given by a licensed medical professional, it can lead to disastrous results. People are fearful about becoming addicted to a medication that has amphetamine in it. It certainly is a potential drug of abuse, but as was defined above, addiction is governed by genes and the environment. A person who does not have the genes or the environment to produce an addictive behavior is at lower risk for developing an addiction. Of course, all patients on any medication need to have follow-up with their prescribing physician or caregiver.[173]

Personal Note about Being on Dextroamphetamine/Amphetamine

After I took dextroamphetamine/amphetamine (10 mg)[174] the first time, I felt how it worked. It didn't fire me up and make me jittery like coffee did. It seemed to quiet down the world around the thing that I wanted to concentrate on. It let me look at something and think about it without being distracted by things that were going on around me. I could perceive and process information in sequence before moving onto the next thing. Distractions, while they were still there, were now being ignored by my brain. The pathway of reading to remembering to integrating was no longer interrupted by the sounds and lights and voices of the immediate surrounding world. For me, it was a pathway that I never knew existed until after it was taken away from me by MS and then given back by using amphetamine/methamphetamine. I felt like I was eighteen years old again. I could sit and write and do research and write and go eat and write and go to the restroom and then go back to writing again, all without getting lost in distractions.

After being on it for four days, I noticed that I was not getting the same response I had on day one. I then titrated the dose up. Eventually, I noticed that I felt best around 20 mg. I also noticed that some days when I had a full complement of patients, I could use the extended-release version, and I was able to concentrate better on everyone, from the first patient to the last. I also noticed that on days when I was just attending a few hours of lectures, I could take the short-acting form of the medication so I could concentrate, thus allowing me to learn. On days when I was just watching a baseball game, I didn't have to take it at all. I didn't have to memorize what happened each at-bat. I kept score if I wanted to, but I didn't need the medication to enjoy the game.

As a doctor, I often offer a "use it when you need it" approach to my patients for some medications. If the patient and/or their caregiver are aware and responsible, I feel comfortable telling them that they can try using the medication on an "as needed" basis. This does several things. First, if a medication is not taken for a day or two, it has the potential to produce a greater effect on the days when it is taken. Also, if the person doesn't take it every day, it puts less demand on the person's body. The last, but possibly the most important, thing is that it keeps the patient involved with his own care. It can help a person feel like he is being respected as a *thinking* individual. Note that some situations prohibit using a drug like this. Since every patient and doctor is different, the key lies in the communication.

MS EMOTIONAL LABILITY

For some of us MSers, the loss of the ability to control our emotions is a pain in the jasper.[175] I know I feel slightly foolish when I start crying during a fly-over by the Blue Angels at a football game, but it gets worse when my son asks, "Why are you crying?" I let him know that it's okay to express your emotions, but I don't want him to think that the Super Bowl really means as much to me as the death of a relative. Emotional lability is a major issue for some of us with MS (as well as for people with ALS, traumatic brain injury, Alzheimer's disease, stroke, and other diseases). The system that controls emotions is complex.[176] There is evidence that increasing serotonin levels can be beneficial in improving emotional expression and control of expression, which can then lead to an overall improvement in a person's quality of life.[177, 178] ®In 2010, dextromethorphan and quinidine ([179]Nuedexta® is a registered trademark of Avanir Pharmaceuticals.) came out for the treatment of pseudobulbar affect (another name for emotional lability).

MS TIREDNESS AND SLEEP

Are people with MS also tired? Definitely.[180] There is a greater prevalence of sleep disturbance in people with MS as compared with the general population.[181] Since tiredness can get better with rest, getting proper rest (going through the proper stages of sleep for required amounts of time) can allow a person to not be tired. Unfortunately, when you have a swollen brain, you cannot get into the proper stages of sleep. This is a separate problem from the MS ICE, but some of the causes can be the same (i.e., the swollen MS brain).

There are many players involved in the sleep cycle. Some parts of the brain generate sleepiness while some parts wake us up. Other parts control the timing of sleep. The presence of various neurotransmitters in the blood, from other brain systems, can interfere with these pathways. Of course, the things we decide to put into our bodies (like caffeine, alcohol, and other drugs) can affect the complex systems needed for restful sleep. All of these things can also be affected by the swelling in the MS brain.

There are multiple ways to try to improve sleep. Among the sleep therapies, behavioral changes are a cheap alternative and a good way to avoid medications. If you make the bedroom only for sleeping and other activities that require a bed, your mind can then associate it with rest and sleep. If you work or watch TV in your bedroom, your mind might associate the bedroom with anxiety, producing non-sleep-inducing thoughts. If you keep those activities limited to the rooms outside of the bedroom, then your bed becomes a place of solace.

Of course there is a litany of sleeping medications available, both by prescription and over the counter. As sleep pharmacology continues to evolve, more medications become available. You should work with your doctor and health-care team to find out what is the best thing to do for your sleep.

Personal Sleep Note

I found it interesting that starting three days after my first dose of natalizumab, I stopped waking up with a headache. Every morning for the previous nineteen years, I had woken up with a headache.[182] Additionally, prior to taking natalizumab, I would wake up in the middle of the night drenched in sweat (see the third chapter, "A Day and a Night in an MS Life").

A main point is that tiredness and the MS ICE appear similar but are completely different entities. We, as medical professionals, need to appreciate the difference and treat it accordingly. We, as patients, need to realize that many of our behaviors have been affected by the elevated pressure in our heads, and we need to discuss the MS ICE with the medical professionals in our lives. Hopefully, by making the MS ICE a common phrase, patients and doctors and caregivers and everyone else will be able to get a clearer message about what's causing some of the greatest disabilities in the world of MS.

DEPRESSION AND MS

I'm including depression here because there's an interesting overlap between medications for depression and medications for attention, concentration, and emotional control.

There are definitely people with MS who are depressed.[183] Depression is something that has come to the forefront of medical care over the years. There are many good antidepressant medications available. Many try to increase dopamine, norepinephrine, and/or serotonin levels in the CNS. They increase these neurotransmitters by decreasing their reuptake from the synapse, thus allowing them to continue to stimulate other nerves. Table 11 contains some of the most common antidepressants in use today and how they work.

Table 11. Common medications for depression.

Generic drug	Neurotransmitter(s)	Mechanism of Action
citalopram	Serotonin	Reuptake Inhibitor
escitalopram	Serotonin	Reuptake Inhibitor
paroxetine	Serotonin	Reuptake Inhibitor
fluoxetine	Serotonin	Reuptake Inhibitor
fluvoxamine	Serotonin	Reuptake Inhibitor
sertraline	Serotonin	Reuptake Inhibitor
desvenlafaxine	Serotonin/ Norepinephrine	Reuptake Inhibitor
duloxetine	Serotonin/ Norepinephrine	Reuptake Inhibitor
venlafaxine	Serotonin/ Norepinephrine/ Dopamine	Reuptake Inhibitor
bupropion	Norepinephrine/ Dopamine	Reuptake Inhibitor

Table 12 shows common medications used for ADD. Now, compare the antidepressant mechanism of action with the mechanism of action of the drugs used for ADD. All of the antidepressants listed are reuptake inhibitors. Bupropion, which has indications for treatment of both depression and ADD, is a reuptake inhibitor of dopamine and norepinephrine. The drugs for ADD, however, not only decrease the reuptake of the neurotransmitters dopamine and norepinephrine but also help to push these neurotransmitters out of the nerve terminal where they're made. This action is known as being a *releasing agent*. The difference between a drug that's a reuptake inhibitor and one that's a releasing agent and reuptake inhibitor comes mostly in how quickly it works. If you push the neurotransmitters out of the nerve terminal, there is a quicker increase in the communication between the frontal lobes, basal ganglia, and limbic system. This makes the drug have a quicker onset of action and is more noticeable after taking the medication. The antidepressants do the same thing, but they take longer since they're just decreasing the reuptake of the neurotransmitters.

Table 12. Common medications for attention deficit disorder.

Generic drug	Neurotransmitters	Mechanism of Action
bupropion	Norepinephrine/ Dopamine	Reuptake Inhibitor
dexmethylphenidate	Norepinephrine/ Dopamine	Reuptake Inhibitor/ Releasing agent
methylphenidate	Norepinephrine/ Dopamine	Reuptake Inhibitor/ Releasing agent
amphetamine	Norepinephrine/ Dopamine	Reuptake Inhibitor/ Releasing agent
dextroamphetamine	Norepinephrine/ Dopamine	Reuptake Inhibitor/ Releasing agent
lisdexamphetamine	Norepinephrine/ Dopamine	Reuptake Inhibitor/ Releasing agent

For emotional lability, serotonin is the main neurotransmitter involved. If emotional control is an issue in someone's life, that individual might benefit from using one of the serotonin reuptake inhibitors. If he or she has ADD symptoms and emotional control challenges, venlafaxine might be able to cover both bases in one shot. Then again, since everyone is unique, by using a serotonin reuptake inhibitor and a dopamine/norepinephrine enhancing drug, the doses of each drug can be adjusted independently and achieve the best result for the individual.

WHAT ARE SOME WAYS THAT I, AS A DOCTOR, CAN MELT THE MS ICE?

For us doctors, we can include questions in our intake forms that can help identify areas that we can treat. In addition to my regular intake form, I also give screens for:

1. Attention deficit disorder
2. Hyperactivity disorder
3. Anxiety
4. Depression
5. Addiction

After having the patient answer these questions, and after doing the neurological exam, we as doctors can attend to each issue on the problem list. The following is a simple algorithm that might possibly help make your patient feel better as well as make the time that you spend with your MSers more effective.

(N.B. This algorithm is not peer-reviewed nor is it approved by any medical organization. It is offered as a way to help organize medical thinking.)

Caution should be taken when using dopamine/norepinephrine releasers/reuptake inhibitors in the clinical setting of cardiovascular disease, hyperthyroidism, glaucoma, history of drug dependence, hypertension, the elderly, bipolar disorder, Tourette's syndrome, seizures, breastfeeding, arrhythmias, agitation, atherosclerosis, congenital cardiac disease, cardiomyopathy, and other disorders. Make sure to consult the most recent guidelines as published by the FDA and your area of specialty. If you do not feel comfortable prescribing a medication or a therapy, please educate your patient(s) and caregiver(s) about the neuronal and neurotransmitter systems involved so they can learn and become more empowered in their approach to handling their MS.

AN APPROACH TO WORKING WITH AN MS PATIENT

After complete history, physical and lab work review are completed:

I. Is the patient on a disease-modifying therapy?
   A. If not, start the patient on a disease-modifying therapy.
   B. If on a platform therapy, either continue the therapy if the patient has been stable (both physically and emo-cognitively) or consider discussing the drugs that have a greater efficacy in decreasing the relapse rate (natalizumab, dimethyl fumarate, fingolimod) for reduction in CNS pressure with possible improvement in initiative, concentration, emotional, and behavioral control.
      1. If patient has troubles with coital issues, urinary control, and/ or behavior problems, consider switching patient to a disease modifying therapy that has better effect on reducing the relapse rate and reduces cerebral swelling.
   C. Regardless of current disease-modifying therapy status,
      1. If patient/caregiver reports new onset of deficits in area(s) that can lead to significant physical (vision, walking, or anything important to the patient's daily life) or emo-cognitive (change in relationship with spouse/children/caregiver) disability

               or

      2. Findings on neurological history (patient history of present illness reports onset of new deficits lasting or worsening for longer than twenty-four hours), examination, or neuroimaging studies that lend evidence of increased disease activity, consider:
         a. five-day course of IV steroids if no contraindications (osteoporosis/osteopenia, immunosuppression, allergy, etc.)

               or

         b. adrenocorticotropic hormone therapy if no contraindications (allergy, immunosuppression, etc.)
II. Has the patient had neurocognitive testing (either by a medical professional or computer based)?
   A. If yes, treat the results appropriately.
      1. If there is evidence of attention deficit disorder, start therapy.
         a. Does the patient have any cardiac issues?
            i. If yes, consider bupropion therapy.
            ii. If no, consider dopamine/norepinephrine releasing agent and reuptake inhibitor.
         b. Does the patient have any issues with possible addiction (prior history, family member, social situation)?
            i. If yes, consider bupropion therapy.

   ii. If no, consider dopamine/norepinephrine releasing agent and reuptake inhibitor.

  c. Does the patient have any other psychiatric issues (e.g., bipolar disorder, Tourette's syndrome, etc.)?

   i. If yes, continue, or refer for, management of psychiatric disease.

   ii. If no, consider dopamine/norepinephrine releasing agent and reuptake inhibitor.

 B. If not, get neurocognitive testing done to obtain baseline and treat as indicated.

  1. If depression is present and there are no other contraindications (e.g., bipolar disorder), consider a dopaminergic agent, which could have positive effects on ADD symptoms.

III. Investigate and treat personal issues

 A. If there is evidence of depression, consider starting therapy with an antidepressant that is dopaminergic/noradrenergic (bupropion, citalopram) that could help out with latent ADD if there are no other contraindications (e.g., bipolar disorder, Tourette's syndrome, etc.).

 B. If there are any sexual issues, consider dopaminergic/noradrenergic medications (bupropion, citalopram) before using serotonergic medications (sertraline, paroxetine), which can interfere with the sexual response cycle if there are no other contraindications (e.g., bipolar disorder, Tourette's syndrome, etc.).

  1. Evaluate dynamic between patient and partner/caregiver and direct questions appropriately.

  2. Ask patient if their partner would like to come in to talk about the situation at follow-up.

 C. Inquire about and treat urinary function issues

  1. Urodynamic testing evaluation

  2. Treatment of CNS urinary control issues

   a. Improving cortical control of urination by increasing serotonergic/noradrenergic tone (such as duloxetine) can help.[184]

   b. Consider using or adding muscarinic antagonist (such as tolterodine).

 D. Medications and procedures as appropriate for symptoms affecting the patient's quality of life (painful spasms, paresthesias, hyperacusis,[185, 186] etc.)

    E.   Speech and swallow evaluation as indicated

    F.   Occupational therapy evaluation as indicated

        1.   This is crucial if the patient has any issues with activities of daily living that involve the upper extremities.

    G.   Social work evaluation as indicated

    H.   Nutrition evaluation as indicated

    I.   Physical therapy evaluation as indicated

By bringing up these issues during the interview with the patient, we are letting the MSer and any caregivers in attendance know that feelings of indifference, inconstant thinking, and immature behavior are common symptoms that can be treated.

SO HOW CAN I, AS A PATIENT, HELP MELT THE MS ICE?

For us patients, we can help to make the office visits with our medical professionals go more smoothly by presenting symptoms in a more concise, linear fashion. If it is our first visit, we should make a typed list of the relevant items in the following list. You can ask the receptionist if you should give the list to the receptionist or hold onto it and give it directly to the doctor. If you are told to give it to the doctor, make sure to give it to him or her at the start of your interview.

For those of us who have trouble writing, we should bring along someone with us who can fill out the intake form for us in a legible fashion.

For the following list, we should include only the items that pertain to us.

1.   We need to state the one reason why we came to see the doctor today. It should be something like:

      ➤ Newly diagnosed and are looking for a neurologist

      ➤ Have been diagnosed and am looking for a new neurologist

      ➤ Looking for a second opinion about the diagnosis

      ➤ Looking for another opinion about the therapies that I am currently on

      ➤ Any specific goal that we are trying to attain (starting a more effective therapy, finding someone who has more physical therapy connections, someone who is involved with more clinical trials, etc.)

2. Our doctors, with their contact information
3. The disease-modifying therapies that we have been on, including start and stop dates along with why we stopped each medication (e.g., Copaxone, 12/2002–6/2007, injection site reactions)
4. The steroids or chemotherapies that we have tried to calm down exacerbations (e.g., IV Solumedrol, 1996; cyclophosphamide, 2002)
5. Any experimental or non-FDA approved therapies that we have been on and what effect they had (e.g., bee sting therapy, 1990–1992, helped at first but not so much after three months)
6. All of the medications that we are currently on, including:
   a. the dose of the medication
   b. the frequency with which we take the medication
   c. why we take the medication
   d. who prescribes the medication for us
7. The MS ICE CUBE troubles
   We can list the ones that we have, but we should let the doctor know which one is most important to us!
   a. Initiative
   b. Concentration
   c. Emotional control
   d. Coital issue
   e. Urinary issues
   f. BEhavior issues
8. The physical issues that we currently have.
   We can list the ones that we have, but we should let the doctor know which one is most important to us!
   a. vision
   b. hearing
   c. speech
   d. weakness (include which limb or limbs)
   e. walking problems
   f. balance/fall issues
   g. coordination
   h. sensations

When we go in to see the doctor, we need to remember the golden rule:
Stick to answering the questions asked.
Do not embellish the answers.

If the doctor does not understand something, he or she will ask.

<u>Example of a useful conversation with our doctor:</u>

Doctor:	Hi, Mr. Bond. How are you today?
Mr. Bond:	Crappy.
Doctor:	Why do you feel crappy?
Mr. Bond:	I took my shot today, and it makes me headachy.
Doctor:	Okay. Let's talk about that.

<u>Example of a less useful conversation with our doctor:</u>

Doctor:	Hi, Mr. Bond. How are you today?
Mr. Bond:	Crappy.
Doctor:	Why do you feel crappy?
Mr. Bond:	Well, it all started when my dog, Sir Edmund Hillary, vomited on the policeman who knocked on my door even though I put a sign on the door that says "Please sing the opening lines to 'Modern Major General' from *The Pirates of Penzance* if you would like to come in because knocking scares Sir Edmund, and I wrote it in big, blue letters, because I can't see red because I had optic neuritis three times in 1978 and again in 1979 … or was it 1980 and 1981? … Carol? When did I have the optic neuritises? Was it in 1979 and 1980? No, wait! I know, I know, I know … it was in 1969 because that was the year your father had the heart attack after the Jets won the Super Bowl. Anyway … wait—what did you ask again?

If we are returning for a follow-up visit, we should take a similar, focused approach to our time with our doctor. Instead of taking out a notebook at the end of the visit and reading a list of assorted symptoms that we have assiduously chronicled over the past three months, we need to do our homework. We need to take our list and review it the night before. As we review it, we should note that we marked down on seven different occasions that the tingling in our left foot prevented us from getting a good night's sleep! We then start to realize that that was our biggest problem and it should be brought to the doctor's attention for possible treatment at the start of the visit! Meanwhile, the strange pain that went from our left ankle to our right earlobe, lasting upward of two and a half seconds, which occurred as we left the office after the last visit but has not come back since, doesn't really need to be attended to right now but can be followed, and if it happens seven more times before the next office visit, then we might want to bring it to the doctor's attention straightaway.

Summary

The main thing that makes a good patient/doctor relationship is quite often the same thing that goes into any good relationship—communication. When we as patients can present ourselves with clearly stated issues and well-thought-out questions in a concise fashion, then we as doctors have a better chance of answering questions more clearly and coming up with concrete ways to solve MSer issues. Hopefully, the MS ICE will help to clear a path to mutual understanding of some of the intangible aspects of the disease we drape with the superficial moniker, multiple sclerosis.

---

[112] S. Schacher, "Determination and Differentiation in the Development of the Nervous System," in *Principles of Neural Science*, ed. E. R. Kandel and J. H. Schwartz, (New York: Elsevier Science Publishing Co., Inc., 1985), 729–742.

[113] F. M. Benes, M. Turtle, Y. Khan, and P. Farol, "Myelination of a key relay zone in the hippocampal formation occurs in the human brain during childhood, adolescence, and adulthood," *Archives of General Psychiatry* 51, no. 6 (June 1994): 477–84.

[114] Louis-Antoine Ranvier (2 October 1835–22 March 1922) discovered his Nodes in 1878. It is believed that a year later, in 1879, he discovered his Eardes.

[115] T. S. Shippenberg, R. Bals-Kubik, and A. Herz, "Examination of the neurochemical substrates mediating the motivational effects of opioids: role of the mesolimbic dopamine system and D-1 vs. D-2 dopamine receptors," *Journal of Pharmacology and Experimental Therapeutics* 265 (April 1993): 53–59.

[116] A. Gobert, J.-M. Rivet, F. Lejeune, A. Newman-Tancredi, A. Adhumeau-Auclair, J.-P. Nicolas, L. Cistarelli et al., "Serotonin2C receptors tonically suppress the activity of mesocortical dopaminergic and adrenergic, but not serotonergic, pathways: A combined dialysis and electrophysiological analysis in the rat," Article first published online: 27 APR 2000, doi: 10.1002/(SICI)1098-2396(20000601)36:3<205::AID-SYN5>3.0.CO;2-D; Synapse Volume 36, Issue 3, pages 205–221, 1 June 2000.

[117] Alas, the days of college when the youth are introduced to an elixir that lubricates socially and anesthetizes cortically. The effects on cognition are best seen by those who do not partake and best understood by those found by the commode the next morning. To learn more, you can look up this article: M. Parada, M. Corral, N. Mota, A. Crego, S. Rodríguez Holguín, and F. Cadaveira, "Executive functioning and alcohol binge

drinking in university students," *Addictive Behaviors* 37, no. 2 (February 2012): 167–72. Epub 2011 Sep 25.

[118] "Hope for all aspects of MS—A report from the European Committee for Treatment and Research in Multiple Sclerosis (ECTRIMS)," *Open Door* (November 2009): 6–7; http://www.mstrust.org.uk/information/opendoor/articles/0911_06_07.jsp.

[119] N. M. Stecker and K. Baylor, Department of Neurology and Weis Center for Research, Geisinger Medical Center, Danville, PA, USA, mmstecker@gmail.com, "Peripheral nerve at extreme low temperatures 1: effects of temperature on the action potential," *Cryobiology* 59, no. 1 (August 2009): 1–11. Epub 2009 Jan 31.

[120] W. C. Wetsel, Department of Psychiatry and Behavioral Sciences, Duke University Medical Center, Durham, NC 27710, USA, wetse001@mc.duke.edu, "Hyperthermic effects on behavior," *International Journal of Hyperthermia* 27, no. 4 (2011): 353–73.

[121] A. M. Humm, S. Beer, L. Kool, M. R. Magistris, J. Kesselring, and K. M. Rösler, Department of Neurology, University of Berne, Inselspital, Freiburgstrasse, CH-3010 Bern, Switzerland, "Quantification of Uhthoff's phenomenon in multiple sclerosis: a magnetic stimulation study," *Clinical Neurophysiology* 115, no. 11 (November 2004): 2493–501.

[122] S. Wada, E. Urasaki, C. Kadoya, S. Matsuoka, and M. Mohri, Department of Neurosurgery, School of Medicine, University of Occupational and Environmental Health, Kitakyushu, Japan, "Effects of hyperbaric environment on the P300 component of event-related potentials," *Journal of UOEH* 13, no. 2 (June 1, 1991): 143–8.

[123] D. Shprecher, J. Schwalb, and R. Kurlan, University of Rochester School of Medicine, 1351 Mt. Hope Avenue, Suite 100, Rochester, NY 14620, USA, David_Shprecher@urmc.rochester.edu, "Normal pressure hydrocephalus: diagnosis and treatment," *Current Neurology and Neuroscience Reports* 8, no. 5 (September 2008): 371–6.

[124] Hmmm … sounds like another disease I've heard of.

[125] An army travels on its stomach, and the immune system is no different.

[126] Please note that inflammation is a complex process of getting many other cells to come together. Things like complement, interferons, and interleukins are all players in the inflammatory cascade. It is being appreciated that these molecules also have direct effects on nerve functioning and play a very important role in nerve dysfunction in autoimmune disease. H. Zhang, J. L. Bennett, and A. S. Verkman, Departments of Physiology, University of California at San Francisco, San Francisco, CA; Departments of Medicine, University of California at San Francisco, San Francisco, CA, "Ex vivo spinal cord slice model of neuromyelitis optica reveals novel immunopathogenic mechanisms," *Annals of Neurology* 70, no. 6 (December 2011): 943–54, doi: 10.1002/ana.22551. Epub 2011 Nov 8.

[127] The interstitial space in the CNS is the space between nerve cells. It is not the intracellular space (inside the cell), intraventricular space (inside the ventricles), or the intravascular space (inside the blood vessel).

[128] M. L. Goodwin, M.A., J. E. Harris, M.Ed., A. Hernández, M.A., and L. Bruce Gladden, Ph.D., "Blood Lactate Measurements and Analysis during Exercise: A Guide

for Clinicians," *Journal of Diabetes Science and Technology* 1, no. 4 (July 2007): 558–569. Published online Jul 2007. MCID: PMC2769631.

[129] Thanks to Ted Tierney for his bon mot.

[130] C. Veauthier, H. Radbruch, G. Gaede, C. Pfueller, J. Dörr, J. Bellmann-Strobl, K. D. Wernecke et al., Department of Neurology, Stralsund, Germany, "Fatigue in multiple sclerosis is closely related to sleep disorders: a polysomnographic cross-sectional study," *Multiple Sclerosis* (January 28, 2011). [Epub ahead of print].

[131] T. J. Braley and R. D. Chervin, Multiple Sclerosis Center, Department of Neurology, University of Michigan, Ann Arbor, MI, USA, tbraley@med.umich.edu, "Fatigue in multiple sclerosis: mechanisms, evaluation, and treatment," *Sleep* 33, no. 8 (August 2010): 1061–7.

[132] The orbitofrontal cortex is the same as the frontal-orbital cortex.

[133] E. Niedermeyer, Department of Neurology and Neurosurgery, Johns Hopkins University School of Medicine and Hospital, Baltimore, Maryland, USA, "Frontal lobe functions and dysfunctions," *Clinical Electroencephalography* 29, no. 2 (April 1998): 79–90.

[134] The pathways going to and from the orbitofrontal cortex traverse the orbital, cingulate, and dorsolateral parts of the frontal lobes. They also carry messages to and from the limbic system and basal ganglia and are modulated by input from the hypothalamus.

[135] D. S. Levine, Department of Psychology, 501 South Nedderman Drive, University of Texas at Arlington, Arlington, TX 76019-0528, United States, levine@uta.edu, "Brain pathways for cognitive-emotional decision making in the human animal," *Neural Networks* 22, no. 3 (April 2009): 286–93, doi: 10.1016/j.neunet.2009.03.003. Epub 2009 Mar 24.

[136] P. Sachdev and P. Hay, School of Psychiatry, University of New South Wales, Sydney, Australia, "Does neurosurgery for obsessive-compulsive disorder produce personality change?" *Journal of Nervous and Mental Disease* 183, no. 6 (June 1995): 408–13.

[137] J. Vilkki, "Amnesic syndromes after surgery of anterior communicating artery aneurysms," *Cortex* 21, no. 3 (September 1985): 431–44.

[138] F. Moutaouakil, H. El Otmani, H. Fadel, and I. Slassi, Service de neurologie, hôpital Al-Kortobi, 90000 Tanger, Maroc. mfettouma@hotmail.com, "Severe apathy following head injury: improvement with Selegiline treatment" [article in French], *Neurochirurgie* 55, no. 6 (December 2009): 551–4. Epub 2008 Dec 11.

[139] R. A. Rudick, D. Miller, S. Hass, M. Hutchinson, P. A. Calabresi, C. Confavreux, S. L. Galetta et al., AFFIRM and SENTINEL Investigators, "Health-related quality of life in multiple sclerosis: effects of natalizumab," *Annals of Neurology* 62, no. 4 (October 2007): 335–46.

[140] The Short Form (36) Health Survey (SF-36) is a patient-reported health scale that measures vitality, physical functioning, bodily pain, general health perceptions, physical role functioning, emotional role functioning, social role functioning, and mental health.

[141] R. Zivadinov, A. T. Reder, M. Filippi, A. Minagar, O. Stüve, H. Lassmann, M. K. Racke, M. G. Dwyer, E. M. Frohman, and O. Khan, Buffalo Neuroimaging Analysis Center, Jacobs Neurological Institute, 100 High Street, Buffalo, NY 14203, USA,

rzivadinov@thejni.org, "Mechanisms of action of disease-modifying agents and brain volume changes in multiple sclerosis," *Neurology* 71, no. 2 (July 8, 2008): 136–44.

[142] S. V. Faraone and J. Biederman, Pediatric Psychopharmacology Unit, Massachusetts General Hospital, Boston 02114, USA, "Neurobiology of attention-deficit hyperactivity disorder," *Biological Psychiatry* 44, no. 10 (November 15, 1998): 951–8.

[143] J. A. Staller and S. V. Faraone, Division of Child & Adolescent Psychiatry, SUNY Upstate Medical University, Syracuse, NY 13210, USA, stallerj@upstate.edu, "Targeting the dopamine system in the treatment of attention-deficit/hyperactivity disorder," *Expert Review of Neurotherapeutics* 7, no. 4 (April 2007): 351–62.

[144] B. Baier, H.O. Karnath, M. Dieterich, F. Birklein, C. Heinze, and N. G. Müller, Department of Neurology, University of Mainz, 55131 Mainz, Germany, baierb@uni-mainz.de, "Keeping memory clear and stable—the contribution of human basal ganglia and prefrontal cortex to working memory," *Journal of Neuroscience* 30, no. 29 (July 21, 2010): 9788–92.

[145] R. Zivadinov and J. Sepci, "Cognitive impairment in multiple sclerosis patients" [article in Croatian], *Lijec Vjesn* 126, no. 7–8 (July–August 2004): 204–10.

[146] L. C. Foland-Ross, L. L. Altshuler, S. Y. Bookheimer, M. D. Lieberman, J. Townsend, C. Penfold, T. Moody, K. Ahlf, J. K. Shen, S. K. Madsen et al., Laboratory of Neuro Imaging, Department of Neurology, Department of Psychiatry and Biobehavioral Sciences, and Department of Psychology, University of California, Los Angeles, California 90095, USA, "Amygdala reactivity in healthy adults is correlated with prefrontal cortical thickness," *Journal of Neuroscience* 30, no. 49 (December 8, 2010): 16673–8.

[147] Even though that sentence sounded like I am against socially appropriate behavior, such is not the case. Actually, I am entirely *for* socially appropriate behavior. Unfortunately, as a student of the neural sciences, learning the neural mechanisms for human urinary control was a major pain in the astrocyte.

[148] While the lifespan of Habenular Nuclei was short, their songs were even shorter. They never reached the top four hundred, but their fan will never forget their most powerful song, "Reward Negative," and the follow-up to that, "Avoidance Response." Their one love ballad, "Sleep-Wake-Stress-Repeat," will forever remain in our hearts. And like lead singer Fimbria Septus always said at the end of their one concert just before he passed on, "GABA! GABA! Yeah! It's a neurotransmitter, and it's spelled with only one B, dammit!"

[149] J. K. Rilling and A. G. Sanfey, Department of Anthropology, Emory University, Atlanta, Georgia 30322, USA, jrillin@emory.edu, "The neuroscience of social decision-making," *Annual Review of Psychology* 62 (2011): 23–48.

[150] D. M. Herz, M. S. Christensen, N. Bruggemann, O. J. Hulme, K. R. Ridderinkhof, K. H. Madsen, and H. R. Siebner, "Motivational tuning of fronto-subthalamic connectivity facilitates control of action impulses," *Journal of Neuroscience* 34, no. 9 (February 26, 2014): 3210–7, doi: 10.1523/JNEUROSCI.4081-13.2014.

[151] Please, in the name of all that is good in this wonderful world, I beseech thee, stop using the term "MS fatigue."

[152] X. Montalban, G. Comi, P. O'Connor, S. Gold, A. de Vera, B. Eckert, and L. Kappos, "Oral fingolimod (FTY720) in relapsing multiple sclerosis: impact on health-related quality of life in a phase II study," *Multiple Sclerosis* 17, no. 11 (November 2011): 1341–50, doi: 10.1177/1352458511411061. Epub 2011 Jul 4.

[153] L. Kappos, R. Gold, D. L. Arnold, A. Bar-Or, G. Giovannoni, K. Selmaj, S. P. Sarda et al., "Quality of life outcomes with BG-12 (dimethyl fumarate) in patients with relapsing-remitting multiple sclerosis: the DEFINE study," *Multiple Sclerosis* 20, no. 2 (February 2014): 243–52, doi: 10.1177/1352458513507817. Epub 2013 Oct 22.

[154] A. Svenningsson, E. Falk, E. G. Celius, S. Fuchs, K. Schreiber, S. Berkö, J. Sun, I. K. Penner, Tynergy Trial Investigators, "Natalizumab treatment reduces fatigue in multiple sclerosis. Results from the TYNERGY trial; a study in the real life setting," *PLoS One* 8, no. 3 (2013): e58643, doi: 10.1371/journal.pone.0058643. Epub 2013 Mar 21.

[155] This sentiment is reflected in a phrase, made famous by the incomparable Mr. David Letterman, that many of my MS patients and I use to describe the way we feel when not on natalizumab: "I feel likes my head want to bust open."

[156] G. Michałowska-Wender, J. Losy, J. Biernacka-Łukanty, and M. Wender, Neuroimmunological Unit, Medical Research Center, Polish Academy of Sciences, Przybyszewskiego 49, PL 60-355 Poznań, Poland, grazynawender@wp.pl, "Impact of methylprednisolone treatment on the expression of macrophage inflammatory protein 3alpha and B lymphocyte chemoattractant in serum of multiple sclerosis patients," *Pharmacological Reports* 60, no. 4 (July–August 2008): 549–54.

[157] G. Frisullo, V. Nociti, R. Iorio, A. Katia Patanella, A. Bianco, M. Caggiula, C. Sancricca, P. A. Tonali, M. Mirabella, and A. P. Batocchi, Institute of Neurology, Department of Neurosciences, Catholic University, Largo Agostino Gemelli, 8, 00168 Rome, Italy, "Glucocorticoid treatment reduces T-bet and pSTAT1 expression in mononuclear cells from relapsing remitting multiple sclerosis patients," *Clinical Immunology* 124, no. 3 (September 2007): 284–93. Epub 2007 Jul 12.

[158] L. Xu, Z. Xu, M. Xu, Department of Neurosurgery, Daping Hospital, Third Military Medical University, PLA, Chongqing, China, "Glucocorticoid treatment restores the impaired suppressive function of regulatory T cells in patients with relapsing-remitting multiple sclerosis," *Clinical & Experimental Immunology* 158, no. 1 (October 2009): 26–30.

[159] Eating candy bars is not a currently approved therapy for MS exacerbations and is in no way recommended!

[160] H.P. Acthar® Gel and Questcor® are registered trademarks of Questcor Pharmaceuticals, Inc.

[161] M. Zaidi, L. Sun, L. J. Robinson, I. L. Tourkova, L. Liu, Y. Wang, L. L. Zhu et al., "ACTH protects against glucocorticoid-induced osteonecrosis of bone," *Proceedings of the National Academy of Sciences of the United States of America* 107, no. 19 (May 11, 2010): 8782–7, doi: 10.1073/pnas.0912176107. Epub 2010 Apr 26.

[162] J. F. Evans, A. Fernando, and L. Ragolia, Biomedical Research Core, Winthrop University Hospital, Mineola, NY 11501, United States, jevans@winthrop.org, "Functional melanocortin-2 receptors are expressed by mouse aorta-derived

mesenchymal progenitor cells," *Molecular and Cellular Endocrinology* 355, no. 1 (May 15, 2012): 60–70. Epub 2012 Jan 27.

[163] Granted, there are many other differences in my life during those two time periods. I was a neurology resident while on Avonex and an attending while on Tysabri. The difference in the physical demand placed on a resident and an attending is analogous to the difference in the physical demand placed on a pack-mule and the pack-mule driver. Not many mules have written books.

[164] It was the one where the dog was looking for the bag of dog food, but he couldn't find it because he couldn't read! That really made me tear up.

[165] R. Zivadinov and J. Sepcić, Buffalo Neuroimaging Analysis Center, Department of Neurology, School of Medicine and Biomedical Sciences, Buffalo, NY, USA, "Cognitive impairment in multiple sclerosis patients" [article in Croatian], *Lijec Vjesn* 126, no. 7–8 (July–August 2004): 204–10.

[166] Y. Harel, N. Appleboim, M. Lavie, A. Achiron, Lewenstein Rehabilitation Hospital, Raanana, Israel, yermih@clalit.org.il, "Single dose of methylphenidate improves cognitive performance in multiple sclerosis patients with impaired attention process," *Journal of the Neurological Sciences*, 276, no. 1–2 (January 15, 2009): 38–40. Epub 2008 Sep 24.

[167] I did okay in the other areas, but I really kicked butt in finger tapping. I owe that to the extensive training I did at the Space Invader machines in Penn Station as a young teen.

[168] N. Del Campo, S. R. Chamberlain, B. J. Sahakian, and T. W. Robbins, Department of Psychiatry, University of Cambridge, Cambridge, United Kingdom; Behavioural and Clinical Neuroscience Institute, University of Cambridge, Cambridge, United Kingdom, "The Roles of Dopamine and Noradrenaline in the Pathophysiology and Treatment of Attention-Deficit/Hyperactivity Disorder," *Biological Psychiatry*, 2011 May 5 [Epub ahead of print].

[169] L. J. Bierut, Department of Psychiatry, Washington University School of Medicine, St. Louis, MO 63110, USA, laura@wustl.edu, "Genetic vulnerability and susceptibility to substance dependence," *Neuron* 69, no. 4 (February 24, 2011): 618–27.

[170] N. Aoyama, N. Takahashi, K. Kitaichi, R. Ishihara, S. Saito, N. Maeno, X. Ji et al., Department of Medical Technology, Nagoya University Graduate School of Medicine, Nagoya, Japan, "Association between gene polymorphisms of SLC22A3 and methamphetamine use disorder," *Alcoholism: Clinical and Experimental Research* 30, no. 10 (October 2006): 1644–9.

[171] There are many good resources to learn about addiction. "Addictions and Recovery" is a nonprofit organization that has some good resources. http://www. addictionsandrecovery.org/bibliography.htm. C. A. Prescott and K. S. Kendler, "Genetic and environmental contributions to alcohol abuse and dependence in a population-based sample of male twins," *American Journal of Psychiatry* 156, no. 1 (January 1999): 34–40. M. A. Enoch and D. Goldman, "The genetics of alcoholism and alcohol abuse," *Current Psychiatry Reports* 3, no. 2 (April 2001): 144–51. K. R. Merikangas, M. Stolar, D. E. Stevens, J. Goulet, M. A. Preisig, B. Fenton, H. Zhang, S. S. O'Malley, and B.

J. Rounsaville, "Familial transmission of substance use disorders," *Archives General Psychiatry* 55, no. 11 (November 1998): 973–9.

[172] Note that ADD exists as ADD without hyperactivity (ICD-9 #314.00) and ADD with hyperactivity (ICD-9 #314.01).

[173] It is interesting how some people are fearful of becoming addicted to medication and yet are addicts to many other things that are much worse for them. This list of addictions includes smoking, high-fat foods, high-sugar foods, and doing physical activities that are no more strenuous than changing the channel via infrared transmitters.

[174] In my pharmacology class at Georgetown University School of Medicine, we were always taught that when starting a new medication with a patient we should "start low and go slow." I do this with my patients and with myself. I have also found it to be a wise approach to most things in life.

[175] Jasper is a red-colored type of quartz often used in wood carvings. It also contains a sound that sounds like a bad word when used one way, but that very same word can be found over seventy times in the Bible, including when Yahweh pronounced his Top Ten Commandment List to Moses. Really. It's the one about coveting your neighbor's stuff. Go look it up. It's right there in Exodus, chapter 20, verse 17. I learned a lot about the Bible during my high-school years, which was when I did a lot of biblical exegesis. That was also when I learned that a person truly has to be a cunning linguist when studying the Bible.

[176] It starts with the rostral raphe nuclei in the brainstem, which produce the neurotransmitter serotonin. The raphe nuclei send messages to the mesolimbic system (which is involved with emotions) and then go to both the basal ganglia (which governs motor control) and the prefrontal cortex (which acts as the gatekeeper).

[177] S. Iannaccone and L. Ferini-Strambi, Department of Neurology, State University, Milan, Italy, "Pharmacologic treatment of emotional lability," *Clinical Neuropharmacology* 19, no. 6 (December 1996): 532–5.

[178] Z. Nahas, K. A. Arlinghaus, K. J. Kotrla, R. R. Clearman, and M. S. George, Medical University of South Carolina, Department of Psychiatry, Charleston, SC 29403, USA, "Rapid response of emotional incontinence to selective serotonin reuptake inhibitors," *Journal of Neuropsychiatry and Clinical Neurosciences* 10, no. 4 (Fall 1998): 453–5.

[179] E. P. Pioro, B. R. Brooks, J. Cummings, R. Schiffer, R. A. Thisted, D. Wynn, A. Hepner, and R. Kaye, "Dextromethorphan plus ultra low-dose quinidine reduces pseudobulbar affect"; "Safety, Tolerability, and Efficacy Results Trial of AVP-923 in PBA Investigators," *Annals of Neurology* 68, no. 5 (November 2010): 693–702, doi: 10.1002/ana.22093.

[180] C. Veauthier, H. Radbruch, G. Gaede, C. Pfueller, J. Dörr, J. Bellmann-Strobl, K. D. Wernecke, F. Zipp, F. Paul, and J. Sieb, Hanse-Klinikum, Department of Neurology, Stralsund, Germany, "Fatigue in multiple sclerosis is closely related to sleep disorders: a polysomnographic cross-sectional study," *Multiple Sclerosis* (January 28, 2011) [Epub ahead of print].

[181] A. M. Bamer, K. L. Johnson, D. Amtmann, and G. H. Kraft, Rehabilitation Medicine, University of Washington, Seattle, Washington 98195, USA, adigiaco@u.washington.

edu, "Prevalence of sleep problems in individuals with multiple sclerosis," *Multiple Sclerosis* 14, no. 8 (September 2008): 1127–30. Epub 2008 Jul 16.

[182] Actually, I remember waking up four times during those nineteen years without a headache. Two of those times were after the Yankees had won doubleheaders.

[183] H. A. Demaree, E. Gaudino, and J. DeLuca, "The relationship between depressive symptoms and cognitive dysfunction in multiple sclerosis," *Cognitive Neuropsychiatry* 8, no. 3 (August 2003): 161–71.

[184] K. B. Thor and C. Donatucci, "Central nervous system control of the lower urinary tract: new pharmacological approaches to stress urinary incontinence in women," *Journal of Urology* 172, no. 1 (July 2004): 27–33.

[185] D. Attri and A. N. Nagarkar, Speech and Hearing Unit, Department of Otolaryngology-Head and Neck Surgery, Postgraduate Institute of Medical Education and Research, Chandigarh, India, "Resolution of hyperacusis associated with depression, following lithium administration and directive counselling (sic)," *Journal of Laryngology and Otology* 124, no. 8 (August 2010): 919–21. Epub 2009 Dec 23.

[186] On a personal note, I found that my hyperacusis improved greatly after starting natalizumab, to the point where I no longer needed to wear earplugs when I went to sleep. Additionally, I found that starting amphetamine/dextroamphetamine also greatly reduced my hyperacusis.

Seventeenth

SEX FROM A NEUROLOGICAL POINT OF VIEW

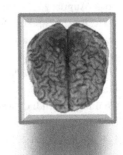

It's a fine line between pleasure and pain.
—The Divinyls, "Pleasure and Pain"

Sex, being the "coital" part of the MS ICE CUBE, is an important issue. It is so important that I have decided to give the topic its own chapter. I remember when I was first diagnosed with MS, one of the things I thought about most often was if I was going to be able to have children. I knew the neurological pathways that were involved with sexual functioning and that a great number of them involved long nerves that were covered in myelin. I knew that if my physical condition prevented my wife and me from having kids the traditional way, I could have my sperm frozen, which could be used for in vitro fertilization. I did not dwell on it for long, though, since no one knew what the future would hold, but it remained a question mark in my mind as a young adult.

My wife, Lauren, was my girlfriend when I was diagnosed with MS. Since we were at different medical schools, we would plan weekend getaways and find a meeting place about halfway between Philadelphia and Washington. While we had our intimate moments, we also enjoyed just being with each other. We would talk about the fact that my MS could affect my sexual functioning. We also discussed parts of her life that would have an effect on me. We discussed these things while we cooked for each other and saw movies and commiserated about whatever rotations we were doing in school at the time. This is when our love was growing. Some might call it "falling in love," but I think that term is too precipitous. We were friends whose love was strong and was, over time, being fortified by the thoughts we shared.

We knew we had the same goals of becoming doctors and having families. However, by getting to know each other, we learned what was different about the other and what was important for the other person to hold on to after becoming one in marriage.

I bring this up because, as you will see, there are physiological and emotional elements of sex that look, smell, and sound like love but are not.

THE SEXUAL RESPONSE CYCLE

The human sexual response cycle is sex from a physiological point of view. The cycle consists of five stages—desire, excitement, plateau, orgasm, and resolution. Each step must follow in sequence in order for the whole cycle to complete. The human sexual cycle is very similar to the sexual cycle of many different animal species.[187] Often, but not always, in the animal kingdom, the female of a species will initiate the sexual response cycle once she is ready to become pregnant. Her desire stage can be brought about by any number of things, including visual, hormonal, and seasonal cues. When interested in having sex, the female might put on a display using parts of her body (neck, feathers, wings, tail, and others) in specific, reflex-mediated movements. She might also perform a well-choreographed, innate "dance" if a male is in the vicinity. She can also make noises or secrete chemical messengers (pheromones) that provoke a physiological response in a male. These maneuvers have the potential to alert one or more males that she is ready for mating.

Depending upon the setting, a male might decide that the sexual notification he gets from the female is a good opportunity to have sex. His desire stage has begun. The male can then make a similar outward gesture to the female, letting her know he is interested. The "courting" can go on for various amounts of time, depending upon the species and the local environment. Once the participants have decided that they have chosen the best candidate with which they can pass on their genes, they commit to continuing the cycle. In many ways, this can be a life-and-death decision in the wild since going through the next stages (excitement, plateau, and orgasm) are among the most vulnerable moments in an animal's life. These three stages commonly happen over the course of seconds to minutes. Vulnerability is at its peak since neither animal can be vigilant for predators while they are engaging their genitals and then trying to elicit the ejaculatory reflex so the male's sperm can be deposited near the egg of the female. If they're lucky and everything works according to plan, the male ejaculates and then disengages from the female. They then ~~spoon snuggle~~ go back to the herd and forage for food.

More often than not, the goal of the male in the wild is passing on his genes as quickly and to as many female partners as is possible. However, the goal of the female is to pick out the male who appears to have the best genes since it will be her that makes the greatest investment in becoming pregnant. She will be vulnerable during gestation. She will carry the fetus, which will increase her need to eat more food. As the fetus grows, their combined weight will cause her to slow down. She will be a target for predators. Getting food will be her primary goal. In some species, the male will stay with the female during gestation. This is called pair-bonding. He will then usually leave after the offspring are born.

Since few of us can speak with animals that are not human, we don't know exactly what role emotions play in the nonhuman animal kingdom. Basic emotions (fear, anger, rage) are rooted in the amygdala, which is found in all animals that live on land (these are the vertebrates). The amygdala is part of the limbic system.[188] The limbic system is one of the main systems that help to keep an organism alive without much thinking being involved. The amygdala gets input from all sensory modalities (but mostly smell— a.k.a. olfaction), the frontal cortex (which manages behavior), and areas in the brain where memories are stored (the temporal lobes).[189] The temporal lobe sends output tracts to the thalamus, which then sends information to the cortex where it is incorporated into thought. It also sends output to the hypothalamus (which regulates heart rate, breathing, and blood pressure) and to the brainstem.[190] When the relatively sophisticated cortex gets involved with the amygdala via the thalamus, we start to have a finer gradation of emotions—apprehension, dislike, appreciation, admiration.[191] While there are degrees of emotions in all vertebrates, the degree of thinking that goes on is most easily seen in us mammals.[192, 193] Exactly how refined the gradation in emotions is across the mammalian class is unknown, as is the expression of those emotions between species. Many of us have creatures in our lives that while the communication is not perfect, an indefinable but certain bond can be sensed. If that bond is secondary to cortical formation and development or due to some unappreciated dimension of our world, no one knows for sure.

THOSE DARN HUMANS

Humans for the most part have working brains that generate useful thoughts that are affected, to varying degrees, by emotions. This allows for another dimension to be added to the sexual equation—sexual satisfaction. This emo-cognitive aspect is separate from the sexual response cycle. It is a layer that can help, and sometimes hurt, the sexual experience.[194, 195] Here is a list of a few things that can affect this very human overlay:

- how you were brought up to view sex
- how your culture views sex
- experiences you have had in prior sexual encounters, if any
- experiences your partner has had in prior sexual encounters, if any
- how you view your inner-self and your body
- how comfortable you are with the person you're with
- how comfortable your partner is with you
- if you know what makes your partner happy
- if your partner knows what makes you happy
- knowing what your partner is comfortable with
- knowing that your partner knows what you're comfortable with
- if you or your partner has any medical and/or physical issues that could be a factor in having a physically or psychologically complete sexual experience
- if your partner knows and understands that a complete sexual experience to you might be different from what he or she thinks a complete sexual experience is
- what current things outside of your relationship are bothering you or your partner (i.e., how each person's life is going at work, school, home, etc.)

These are a few of the issues that everyone has to deal with. If we have MS in our lives, both physical and cognitive issues might or might not add more items to the list.

SEX TALK

When I was in college, I took a course called Sex. It was scheduled right before the course in beer and wine tasting.[196] I still remember one specific line that our professor taught us, which I believe is the most important thing to remember about sex:

> "The most important word, when it comes to sex,
> is a four-letter word and ends with K."

After everybody stopped muttering the obvious answer under their breath,[197] she told us what the word was:

"TALK"

Communication can take a lot of time and understanding to accomplish, but it's worthwhile.[198] Communication between two people in a relationship can be a very difficult thing. Both sides have to understand that while they're speaking the same language, the processing that goes on in the other person's mind can, and most probably will, be completely different from what the speaker intended. This is not just a male-female issue. Each person is different from the next. Remember what was mentioned in the chapter on neurocognitive testing:

"A PERSON'S APPEARANCE DOES NOT INDICATE THE COGNITIVE STATUS OF THAT PERSON!" [199]

Likewise,

"A PERSON'S APPEARANCE DOES NOT INDICATE HOW THAT PERSON IS FEELING!" [200]

The only way to find out what a person is thinking and feeling is to listen to him or her. By trying to understand another person, or at least showing the effort, a deeper bond between individuals can be formed, possibly leading to a more satisfying relationship. And here's the kicker:

Communication is never over.

It's a work in progress that changes every day. We will revisit the importance of talking when we get to the excitement stage.

MS AND SEX

The challenges that people with MS sometimes have to face are as diverse as the disease. I will try to attend to both sides of the sexual coin when addressing the relevant issues, but since I've been a guy for most of my life, I can only write from experience for about half of the stuff. For the purpose of this chapter, it will be assumed that we're talking about people who have a desire for sexual encounters.[201] It should be respected that not everyone feels a need for sexual activity in their lives or that they do not want to participate in a sexual encounter before they've gotten married.

To begin, let's walk through the separate stages of the human sexual response cycle. I will try to identify any potential issues that might interfere with progressing through the cycle, and then come up with ways to get to the end so everyone can have a good time.[202] A crucial element to remember about the human sexual response cycle is that while each of the stages—desire, excitement, plateau, orgasm, and resolution—can take different lengths of time to complete, each one must occur before segueing into the next.

There are two main modalities to start and keep the sexual response cycle going—reflexogenic and psychogenic. Actions that are reflexogenic occur without thought. A common example of reflexes not requiring thinking is when your doctor taps on your knee with a rubber hammer and your leg kicks out. You did not decide to make your leg kick out. It's a reflex arc that starts in the muscle spindle sensory fibers in the quadriceps muscle group. These fibers sense the stretch placed on the quadriceps when the hammer hits the patellar tendon. They send a message to the spinal cord that gets sent directly to the nerve that causes your quadriceps muscle to contract and makes your leg kick out. You and your cortex don't play a role in deciding whether or not to make your leg move. The "decision" was made in your spinal cord, by the reflex arc. The action was produced by a reflex.

Actions that are psychogenic involve you and your mind. Psychogenic actions can elicit or help to elicit a reflex. The description of these modalities is included in the Excitement and Plateau section, but they start in Desire and continue through to Resolution. What roles the reflexogenic and psychogenic arms play are specific to the individual. Therefore, what follows should be adapted accordingly.

DESIRE

Desire for a sexual experience is something that might come up from time to time. Let's say you're watching TV and you saw a provocative program that elicited some thoughts about having sex. A psychogenic desire for sex has been generated in you. Depending on your situation, you start going through a decision tree. You might think that you would like to have sex, but you can't because you have to get ready for your tuba club meeting and you're in charge of bringing the tuning slide grease. So you suppress the desire and decide to sublimate it by really cranking out that riff you came up with for your solo at regionals. If, however, you are still on the disabled list from your last tuba solo (where you slipped on an open tube of tuning slide grease, just before sectionals, that someone left on the floor, which caused you to cut your lip), you might have time for sex.[203] You might start thinking about how to bring up the topic of a sexual encounter with your partner. If you have a partner who shares the same desire at the same time, congratulations! You both can move on to the excitement stage. However, if you're one of the many millions of people who do not have someone on the exact same page as you are, then some more work is needed if you want him or her to be part of the sexual encounter.

Given that hardly any of us live without any responsibilities outside of the bedroom, helping to get to the desire stage set can quite often be a feat. You need to think about multiple things:

- Where is my partner?
- Does my partner want to have sex?
- Where can we have sex?
- Do we have time to have sex before that PBS special about the life cycle of the *Phrynosoma cornutum* comes on?[204]

So you venture to find out what the deal is with your partner. If your partner has stuff going on at that moment that cannot stop, sex will have to wait. If you really wanted to have a sexual encounter, then your desire needs to be fulfilled via another outlet (taking a jog, masturbation, playing hard-rock sousaphone, or whatever floats your boat). If your partner says that he or she is not really in the mood but isn't really doing anything else, this might be a time where you can be proactive in helping him or her get in the mood. This is where some romance might help. Romance will vary for everyone. It can include subtle things like standing near your partner while folding the laundry or bringing home some fragrant flowers for the dinner table or putting on clothes that your partner likes to see you wear. These gestures can open the door to conversations and feelings about sex.

Some of the gestures that we humans can consciously use to open a pathway for psychogenic desire in ourselves and our partners require multiple cognitive processes:

- initiative
- concentration
- attention
- planning
- working memory
- cognitive flexibility
- communication
- self-control

These are many of the functions mediated by our frontal lobes.[205] Coordinating all of these cognitive tasks, in any environment, is difficult for many who are otherwise without disease. In the setting of MS, however, the task of initiating desire by, or for, an MSer can sometimes prove to be an exhausting endeavor.

IMPROVING THE DESIRE STAGE IN THE SETTING OF MS

In the MS ICE chapter, the swelling in the MS brain was described. The swelling can cause an elevated pressure in the brain that causes a global dysfunction of nerves. This dysfunction can impair many functions of the brain. Specifically, it can affect the orbitofrontal cortex, limbic system, basal ganglia, and hypothalamus, all of which play a part in the control of our behavior.[206] Because of this, we MSers sometimes

- demonstrate lack of initiative;
- get distracted easily;
- lose our train of thought;
- act before thinking;
- forget what we wanted to do;

- can't readjust our plan in response to current conditions;
- have trouble communicating what we're thinking; and
- demonstrate poor self-control.

If one of us MSers initiates a sexual encounter, but our partner doesn't want to take part in the encounter, we might start to act immaturely. We might act like a child who wants a piece of candy. If we're told that we have to wait until after dinner until we can have candy, we might say something inappropriate that bothers our partner and "destroys the moment." Those of us with MS do not intend to say something that insults our partner, but it happens more often than it should. This is because our frontal lobe gatekeeper, the orbitofrontal cortex, which is in charge of making us behave in a socially appropriate fashion, is paralyzed by the chronic swelling in our brains. Consequently, we cannot keep our mouths shut![207] When this happens, those of us with MS need to stop talking or defending what we just said and realize what has just happened. Unfortunately, this is incredibly difficult since our frontal lobes, which are not functioning well, are what allow us to understand the consequence of our actions!

After having had this sort of experience enough times, my wife and I made a pact. She promised to look at me in a nonthreatening way that would let me know that I had crossed a line by saying something inappropriate. I would then take a "self-imposed time out." This would give my swollen MS brain a chance to catch up with what had just happened. I would remove myself from the conversation, go to my room, turn on the TV, lie on my bed, and let any emotions that I had accumulated dissipate. After about three to five minutes, I could then look back at what had happened and realize that what I had said or done was wrong. At that point, I would straighten myself up, rejoin the prior situation, and apologize before anything went any further. It usually helps when our partner is an unbelievably caring and patient person who realizes that we didn't really mean to say that she was starting to gain a few pounds and should hit the treadmill more often than the "Cream-o-licious." [208]

Conversely, if the partner of an MSer tries to initiate a sexual encounter, the MSer might have issues with the MS ICE. Commonly, patients report that they don't have the initiative needed for the sexual process. Most research on this point has looked to specific physical disabilities as the nidus for much of the sexual dysfunction in MS.[209, 210, 211] However, many MSers feel like they regain their initiative when they take their medication for ADD.

Others have reported that after they got on natalizumab to slow down their MS, they felt an improvement in their quality of life, including motivation and concentration.[212] Many patients often report a temporary quality of life improvement when they get a five-day course of IV steroids or ACTH injections, which are among the most potent anti-inflammatory medications. Having personally used IV methylprednisolone for exacerbations during the course of my MS, I felt my swollen brain relax and saw my cognition and initiative improve dramatically.

Interestingly, a study was designed in 1995 by Mattson et al.[213] from the University of Rochester, to determine the frequency and nature of sexual dysfunction in MS and its response to medications. The study looked at sixty-five female and thirty-six male MSers. The participants were asked general and specific questions about sexual dysfunction. A person was said to have general sexual dysfunction if he or she responded yes to the question. "Do you have problems with sexual dysfunction?" Specific sexual dysfunction referred to a yes answer to the question, "Have you now or ever had the following?" which was followed by a list of questions. The questions for men included questions about achieving and maintaining erections, ejaculation, and orgasm. Questions for women were about vaginal lubrication, vaginal sensitivity, pain during intercourse, orgasm, and fear of bladder incontinence with sexual activity. They also asked about the correlation of general sexual dysfunction and depression. In reviewing the results, the authors comment on a surprising aspect of their survey.

They noticed that there was a high rate of patients who retrospectively reported an improvement of sexual dysfunction after treatment with corticosteroids.

They postulated that the effect of the corticosteroids could possibly represent the anti-inflammatory effects in spinal cord lesions and edema. They also posit that the patients' "fatigue and depression" improvements were caused by "the increased energy and euphoria caused by corticosteroids." I concur with their medical reasoning.

I would like to put forth another way to interpret some of the results of this study. In table 6 of the paper, retrospective responses of sexual dysfunction to medication were reported. The table compares how patients' sexual dysfunction did after using any one of a list of medications. The medications included corticosteroids, cyclophosphamide, azathioprine, oxybutynin chloride, amitriptyline, fluoxetine hydrochloride, baclofen, and amantadine. As was mentioned, the corticosteroids had the best response. I believe that the anti-inflammatory properties of corticosteroids decreased cerebral inflammation, which causes the MS ICE. Additionally, the steroids possibly decreased the inflammation in spinal cord lesions. By treating the elevated pressure that causes the MS ICE, the MSers regained their initiative to start the human sexual response cycle from the beginning. They could also plan better and be considerate of their partner's feelings.

After desire has been achieved in both individuals, then excitement can begin. It is at this point that the anti-inflammatory effects of the steroids could definitely help to improve sacral spinal cord reflexogenic excitement.[214] Additionally, the improved concentration of the MSer can help to prevent any intrusive thoughts that might disrupt psychogenic excitement, thus allowing vaginal lubrication and erection to start. Taking it one step further, the anti-inflamed brain of the MSer is also better able to deal with change (mental flexibility). If an external event came up that necessitated that the encounter be put on hold, the emotional control of the MSer was better, and the moment was not destroyed by acting childishly.

The other medications that were looked at in the study also yielded interesting results. Ditropan helped a few patients and hurt none. The urinary control provided by ditropan can definitely be a comfort during intimate encounters. It helps to take the concern of incontinence off the table during sex. It should be noted that the frontal lobes and limbic system are crucial for appropriate urinary control.[215] As noted before, improvement in the functioning of these areas has been seen by decreasing pressure in the cortex in the setting of the aforementioned disease, normal pressure hydrocephalus.[216, 217]

Looking at the other medications, amantadine increases dopaminergic tone in the CNS.[218] In the study, four people reported improvement in sexual dysfunction who had taken amantadine, and nobody reported worsening. Amitriptyline improved sexual dysfunction in the study for three patients and worsened it for two. Unlike amantadine, however, amitriptyline is felt to have both dopaminergic and serotonergic actions. While the dopamine-mediated actions of amitriptyline might help improve sexual desire, serotonin is known to decrease it.[219] Fluoxetine is a serotonergic medication. Among the people in the study who were on fluoxetine, one person said that their sexual dysfunction got better while two reported that theirs worsened.

Many of the caregivers who accompany my MS patients to their appointments report the changes that they see after the MSer has been started on medication that improves frontal lobe functioning. They remark on how much more able and reliable the patient has become in doing tasks around the house. They like it when they see their partner doing chores or completing projects. They also like it when they do not have to remind the MSer over and over again about certain things. Helping in household affairs can be very important in initiating psychogenic desire in the partner of a MSer. It helps to shift the MSer caregiver's "I-help-you" role back a little toward the "Let's-help-each-other-which-was-the-way-it-was-when-we-first-got-together" role.

HYPOACTIVE SEXUAL DESIRE DISORDER

There is a syndrome called *hypoactive sexual desire disorder* (HSDD). It is defined by the *Diagnostic and Statistical Manual of Mental Disorders*, Fourth Edition, Text Revision (DSM-IV-TR) as "persistently or recurrently deficient (or absent) sexual fantasies and desire for sexual activity" that cause "marked distress or interpersonal difficulty." In a published study, HSDD occurs in 7–8 percent of adult women, occurring more often in perimenopausal and immediate postmenopausal women.[220] It also affects women much more than men.[221] Several peer-reviewed, randomized, double-blind, placebo-controlled papers have demonstrated the efficacy of using the ADD medication bupropion in the treatment of HSDD.[222, 223]

HSDD is an important player in the MS world for several reasons. First, it affects a large number of women in the general population. In the setting of MS, women outnumber men by about four to one, so the prevalence is even higher. As was discussed in the MS ICE chapter, the pathways that control our initiative use dopamine and norepinephrine as neurotransmitters. If we think of desire as "sexual initiative," the "desire for sexual activity" can possibly be restored by using medications that increase the available dopamine and norepinephrine. These include the ADD drugs. By treating frontal lobe dysfunction in MS patients, the health professional is able to improve another aspect of their patients' lives.

NEURONAL SYSTEMS THAT DECREASE SEXUAL DESIRE

There are neurotransmitters that decrease sexual desire. Along with serotonin, endogenous opioid and cannabinoid receptors become activated when the body wants to inhibit sexual activity.[224, 225] It is well documented that narcotic medication (oxycodone, hydrocodone, etc.), marijuana, and serotonergic medications (like sertraline and paroxetine) can decrease sexual desire.[226]

HORMONES THAT AFFECT DESIRE

Aside from neurotransmitters, hormones can also have a great effect on sexual desire. The hormones that increase sexual desire include estrogen, progesterone, and testosterone. The main hormone that inhibits sexual arousal is prolactin.[227, 228] Prolactin, at baseline, is slightly higher in women than in men.[229, 230] In a woman, prolactin levels are highest during the third trimester of pregnancy.

So to put it all together:

1. The human sexual response cycle is made of desire, excitement, plateau, orgasm, and resolution.
2. Each stage can vary in duration but not in sequence.
3. The therapies that have been found to help improve frontal lobe functioning (reduction in swelling, increasing dopaminergic and noradrenergic tone) can also help to start the desire stage for a person with MS regardless of whether the MSer is male or female.
4. If the MSer is a woman, not only does she have the swollen, paralyzed frontal lobes of the MS brain but she is also much more likely to experience HSDD than a man.
5. Bupropion is a medication indicated for both ADD and HSDD.

PERSONAL MEDICAL/DEPRESSION/SUICIDE SIDEBAR

After I began using more ADD medications with my patients, I noticed that the caregivers of some MS patients began to report that the MSers in their lives were more enjoyable to be around. When the MSer took his or her ADD medication, the caregivers noticed that he or she was able to get things done and not forget so much of what he or she had been asked to do. Additionally, they said that the MSer was behaving slightly better in social situations. Most of the MSers also realized that they behaved better when they took their medication for ADD.

Personally, after starting natalizumab as my MS therapy, I noticed that

I could concentrate better, made fewer immature comments, had better emotional control, and had an improvement in my balance and coordination. When I started amphetamine/methamphetamine, my life improved greatly again. I started listening more and talking less. I noticed that I basically stopped making immature comments. I was more patient with those around me. I was happier. When I did not take my medication, I started to hear myself talking more, being less patient and less polite. I heard the difference in me. I saw the difference in how I affected those around me.

With this newfound knowledge, I tried to approach things differently, especially when talking with others when I had *not* taken my ADD medication. First, I would think at length about what I wanted to say, evaluating whether or not it might possibly be found inappropriate or offensive to anyone who was involved with the conversation. Then I would make my comment. If a person responded by saying something that had the slightest chance of prompting me to make a quick-witted reply, I would then have to summon the good powers of Yahweh, the Pope, Mother Teresa, Gandhi, Allah, Zeus, Apollo, Athena, Superman, Green Lantern, Bono, and my Webelos Pack 406 from 1977 to give me the strength to *keep my mouth shut!* Because of all of the time and energy that it took for me to control my inbred impulse to want to be funny and make people laugh, I would take an uncomfortably long pause before making my reply. People who knew me would then ask, "Are you okay?" I would try to explain myself without letting them know how I had been trying to keep myself from saying exactly what I had been thinking.

What I'm trying to get to is this:

> While I know how to behave better without my medication, it is extremely difficult to consciously do something that had previously been taken care of, automatically, by my frontal lobes.

I often hear people who do not have trouble with their frontal lobes say, "I wouldn't want to put something unnatural like a drug in my body if I can do it myself. I would just work at it. That's all."

Here's an example of where non-MSers have to understand that they cannot understand the mind of an MSer. Once a non-MSer can accept that they cannot understand the mind of another, then they can start to learn why our minds think the way they do.

The following is an analogy describing the nature of frontal lobe dysfunction.

The medulla and pons (located at the top of the spinal cord, just before it transitions into the brain) contain the areas that are in charge of breathing. Suppose these areas got damaged and you had to think about taking a breath every time you needed to.

Sounds like you could do it, right?

Okay, maybe you could, but it would definitely get in the way of things. Actually, aside from just sitting and watching TV, it would be pretty much impossible. Go ahead. Get a timer and set it to go off every ten seconds. Every ten seconds, you would have to think, *Breathe in*, and then think, *Now breathe out*. You might be able to think about something for about seven seconds before your brain would have to start thinking about breathing again.

And that's at rest.

Forget about doing anything more strenuous, like eating a meal. Sure, I guess you could suck on a protein shake while watching C-SPAN, but I think at that point, you've pretty much hit your limit. Any activity that raises your heart rate will require that your respiratory rate go up to keep up with the increased oxygen demand. I guess you could try to lower your metabolic rate using certain yoga techniques to get your heart rate down, but then you would have to concentrate on the yoga when you weren't thinking about breathing.

"But not being able to breathe isn't the same thing as not being able to concentrate or have control over your emotions!" the misbeliever will cry out. "If you stop breathing, you'll die! You're not going to die just because you forget to do some things or you make a stupid comment or people don't want to be around you as much anymore."

The person who says that doesn't get it.

Some of the worst moments of my MS life have been when I felt estranged from family, friends, and other loved ones because of the way I behaved. These feelings produced periods of severe depression. Thankfully, I never had to live alone during those times because someone who's depressed and alone is at the greatest risk for attempting suicide. I bring this up because the suicide rate is higher in MS than in the general population.[231, 232] Suicidal intent, a possible forerunner of suicide, is strongly associated with social isolation, alcohol abuse, and major depression.[233]

If you are depressed (whether you have MS or not), bring your feelings up with your loved ones, doctor, nurse, or other medical professional. If you do not have anyone to speak with when your depression is sucking you down, call 1-800-273-8255, which is the National Suicide Prevention Lifeline.

The take-home message is that some medications can help restore some vital functions that can allow us MSers to lead better lives while also creating better relationships with those around us.

EXCITEMENT AND PLATEAU

The excitement and plateau stages are, physiologically, gradations of each other with a few specific changes that happen toward the end of excitement and signify the start of plateau. Physiologically, during these stages, for both men and women, heart rate, blood pressure, and respiratory rate increase. There is a constriction of the venules (tiny veins) and dilation of the arterioles (tiny arteries) in the penis, testes, clitoris, vulva, and vaginal walls. The vasocongestion in the clitoris causes enlargement and erection while congestion in the walls of the vagina causes a transudate of water and various compounds to be made. This transudate acidifies and lubricates the vagina for intercourse. Bartholin's glands add slightly to the vaginal fluid by secreting a small amount of mucus. In the penis, increased blood flow to the corpora cavernosa fills the spaces that make the penis erect. The seminal fluid is made by Cowper's glands, the seminal vesicles, and the prostate. It contains mucus and other compounds that make it alkaline to offset the acidity of the fluids in the vagina.[234]

It is during these phases that the autonomic nervous system plays a big part. The autonomic nervous system, which starts in certain regions of your spinal cord, is in charge of telling different systems of our bodies to do things automatically (i.e., so we do not have to think about doing them). It controls things like breathing or constricting pupils or making saliva. It has two parts:

1. The sympathetic nervous system, which controls the "fight or flight" response in crisis situations

2. The parasympathetic nervous system, which controls the "rest and digest" activity that goes on when relaxing

REFLEXOGENIC EXCITEMENT

During the excitement stage, the parasympathetic nervous system reflexively causes the erection and lubrication described. The nerves that come out of your spinal cord and subserve these actions are tiny. The blood vessels that feed these nerves are also tiny. Tiny blood vessels are easily blocked by things that travel in the blood like:

> ➤ chemicals from smoking
> ➤ pieces of cholesterol
> ➤ side products of constantly elevated blood-sugar levels

Therefore, if you smoke and/or have high cholesterol and/or have diabetes, you might have some trouble with the excitement stage. There's also a chance that demyelination in the spinal cord could be the cause of the trouble. However, it's far more common for impairment of reflexogenic excitement to come from the causes listed above. Ergo, by not smoking, eating a low-fat diet, and managing your blood-sugar level, chances are that you will be able to enjoy sex more easily for more of your life, whether you have MS or not.

If you're experiencing trouble attaining erection or vaginal lubrication, there are medications available for this phase. For women, vaginal lubrication is available as over-the-counter preparations. For men, drugs like sildenafil, tadalafil, and vardenafil can help to achieve erection. These drugs are by prescription, so you will need to speak with your doctor to find out if they are appropriate for you.

PSYCHOGENIC EXCITEMENT

Psychogenic excitement is sexual stimulation that's generated from levels above the spinal cord. These include the areas that mediate smell, taste, hearing, and vision. These sensory organs send projections (nerves) to the limbic system (involved in emotional control) and the hypothalamus (involved in hormonal/emotional control) that help to modulate behavior during a sexual interaction. These sensory inputs also send messages to the lower thoracic-upper lumbar[235] region of the spinal cord to elicit a parasympathetic response leading to erection.[236] Many of these signals are at work before the thinking part of our brain, the cerebral cortex, gets involved. Once involved, however, the cortex can use imagination to help beget psychogenic excitement and take it to plateau.[237]

Since everyone has a unique brain and mind, the things that go into what is psychogenically exciting are equally diverse. Since we're talking about a sexual interaction between two people, it means that there are two unique minds going through the excitement stage at the same time. In the "Those Darn Humans" section of this chapter, we reviewed one of the most critical aspects of sex—talking. It was mentioned that the better we know our partner, the better we know what things might or might not be exciting to our partner. As things progress through the excitement stage, things that are said will elicit some response in our partner. If you notice that their response or actions do not reflect what you expected they would, it can be beneficial to slow things down and ask why he or she does not appear to be on the same page that you are. It might just be a momentary issue ("When you said, 'Show your world to me,' I thought back to that Dave Matthews concert we were at just before my cat, Snugaginagain, died, but I'm over that now.") or it could be something that brings everything to a halt, and a more lengthy discussion is required.

Changing course in the middle of a mental activity is called cognitive flexibility, which is something that we MSers quite often have trouble with. This is another reason why it's important that we have proper neurocognitive testing done and then be open to starting a treatment for any psychological challenges that have been set before us. Whether it's a medication or talking with a therapist or both or some other therapy, if we rigorously work at improving our cognitive functioning, then there's a better chance that we will have better sex.

Likewise, we physicians have to realize that we can do more than just offer treatments for reflexogenic excitement. Yes, we have limited time because the bean counters say we have to see a patient every fifteen minutes, but that shouldn't prevent us from being able to spend one or two extra minutes to sit down and listen to the patient talk about their most important life stressor that, among other things, is causing trouble in the bedroom. And while most of us are not psychiatrists, we should validate our patients' feelings by saying things like, "It sounds like you're going through some big issues right now, and that's a potential cause of your sexual troubles. I'm sorry that I don't have enough time to listen more, so here's the name of a therapist who's very nice and you might like to share your feelings with."

Going back to us MSers, we need to be able to recognize that we sometimes need to speak with an objective medical professional like a therapist in order to help our mental health. I've had a large number of patients shy away from the idea of going to a therapist. This, I believe, is because the word "therapist" carries a stigma similar to that of using a medication, like amphetamine, or any medication that helps our minds.

While one half of the sex equation is being flexible in how we spend time with our partner, we ourselves have our own baggage that can interfere with the excitement stage. For all of us, we have stressors that come from regular life, but when we add our MS into the mix, it's like putting stress on anabolic steroids. We know we have some cognitive and/or physical disabilities that we're aware of and think other people, like our partner, know about as well. By thinking about what others are thinking about us but not talking about it, we're building a bigger hurdle to get over.

I like to think about it in terms of slumps in baseball. The team is hitting just fine, but then one key batter goes into a slump. The runners are getting on base, but no one scores. Pretty soon, other batters in the lineup get depressed about losing games because no one's driving in any runs. Before you know it, three other players start going one for twenty. Within the next ten days, the team's batting average drops from .305 to .162. They go from being tied for second place in the division to hoping they'll be able to make a wild card spot. The owner starts getting on the manager, and the manager gets on the coaches, and the coaches get on the players. The players start changing their swings or their stances or where they stand in the box. They start trying new diets or supplements or clothes. When they get to the plate, they start intoning Al Pacino quotes from *On Any Given Sunday*. Pretty soon, the entire team, except for the mascot and the heavy hitter who has the $1.6 trillion-dollar contract, is traded for some prospects from the Botswana Bed Bugs Cricket team and the only one who is happy is the team exterminator.

What happened?
The players got trapped in their own minds.
They started thinking about things that got
in the way of their reflex actions.

So how do players get out of their own heads? They have to get back in the moment. They get in the batter's box, and the only thing they should be doing is seeing the ball coming out of the pitcher's hand and taking a swing. For a ball player, this is like breathing. But when you start thinking about breathing, you suddenly feel out of breath. So then you start thinking, "Don't think!" But you can't do that because then you're thinking about thinking, and that makes it worse.

> Think of the instant.
> See the ball.
> Take a swing.
> Repeat.

That's how you get a hit, and that's what leads you out of a slump.

> That's a way to overcome psychogenic sexual
> dysfunction and gets you out of a slump.

> Stay in the instant with your partner. Feel the exciting
> sights, sounds, smells, or touches that are in front of
> you. Take the appropriate action. Repeat.

There is no shame in talking with a professional therapist about the issues floating around in your wonderful, unique mind. Letting out your words to convey your thoughts to another person is a wonderful, healthy way to deal with negative feelings.

And some people find it therapeutic to smash a watermelon with a sledgehammer. That's fine too, as long as no one gets hurt.[238]

PLATEAU

With the arrival of the plateau stage comes the period when the greatest vasogenic pressure develops in the outer one-third of the vagina and in the penis. All of the other physiological changes that started in the excitement phase (heart rate, blood pressure, and respiratory rate) are reaching maximal loads. Plateau is a critical period for most men. A man can get close to the edge and then back away so as to prolong the pleasurable feelings. He can decide to go ahead to orgasm, which is followed by resolution and a refractory period (which is discussed further in the next section). This is different from a woman who can get to plateau, go to orgasm, and go back to plateau and back to orgasm and so on, allowing for multiple orgasms. Again, communication about the approach to orgasm before getting to plateau is crucial so that both partners can have the best time possible.

ORGASM

The definition of orgasm, as defined by Stedman's *Medical Dictionary*, is "The highest point of sexual excitement, marked by strong feelings of pleasure and marked normally by ejaculation of semen by the male and by vaginal contractions within the female. Also called *climax*."[239]

From a neurological point of view, the definition can be more elaborate.

Orgasm starts when the sum of the stimuli, via all senses, leads to a series of reflexes that produce neuroendocrine responses, permitting a loss of cortically-mediated inhibitions, allowing the mind to cease interaction with the external environment and to experience the unmitigated effects of the release of analgesia-inducing neurotransmitters. Orgasm tapers off with a neurotransmitter balance favoring emotions of attraction, more than passion, between partners and a return of normal cerebral blood flow to areas of the brain that are concerned with decision making.[240]

Since MS often causes lesions in the spinal cord, sometimes resulting in loss of function and sensation in the legs and arms, many of the systems that were described above are liable to be affected. Hope is not to be lost, however. In research done by Barry R. Komisaruk, PhD and Beverly Whipple, PhD, RN, FAAN, they have shown that activation of the vagus nerve (see the sixth chapter, table 3, Cranial Nerve X) can bypass a transected spinal cord (at the T10 level and higher) and mediate orgasm. The vagus nerve is one of the cranial nerves and is responsible for sensory input to the brain from the organs of the body (in the gut). Functional MRI (fMRI) studies were done of women who had spinal cord injuries in the lower thoracic cord and higher.[241] The sensory pathways were nonfunctional below the level of the injury in these women. However, by using vaginal-cervical mechanical self-stimulation, the women showed activation of brain areas associated with orgasm. Drs. Komisaruk and Whipple concluded that the vagus nerve must be providing a "bypass" around the damaged spinal cord to transmit sensations from the vagina and cervix to the brain.

SEX AND REPRODUCTION

It should also be recognized that even if an MSer is having trouble with sexual satisfaction from a reproductive point of view, there are ways to get around a dysfunctional spinal cord. For men, the emission and ejaculatory reflexes can be elicited via masturbation, vibratory stimulation, and transrectal electrical stimulation of the prostate and seminal vesicles. If the sperm are motile (if they can swim), they can fertilize the egg in utero or in vitro. If the number of viable and motile sperm is in doubt, the sperm can be injected directly into the egg.[242]

The issues for women are very different from those for men. Ovulation and fertilization can be done separately from the human sexual cycle. There are cases of tetraplegic women with cervical cord lesions who are able to carry pregnancies and have spontaneous vaginal deliveries.[243] The issues that face a woman who has weakness while pregnant include being able to move, toilet, eat, relax, and have the proper emotional support for the nine months of the pregnancy. For women with spinal cord disease, a complete biopsychosocial approach to a pregnancy is needed to ensure that her desires and needs are met.[244]

RESOLUTION

After orgasm, women can return to plateau and then go straight back to orgasm. This is different from men, who have a refractory period after orgasm. During the refractory period, the male is unable to have another orgasm. The refractory period can last anywhere from minutes to days depending upon the individual. There are many things that can affect the length of the refractory period, including age, sexual frequency, and general health. Also, hormones play a big part. At orgasm, certain neurotransmitters are released, including prolactin and oxytocin. Prolactin is known to decrease sexual interest.[245, 246] Prolactin has been found to be elevated in the cerebrospinal fluid in men after orgasm.[247] Oxytocin is slightly more intriguing. It has a pro-erectile effect in the CNS while having an anti-erectile effect in PNS.[248] This might be one of the reasons why men have trouble having multiple orgasms. Like women, some men do have the ability to have multiple orgasms.[249] The main difference between women and men is the glans-vasal reflex. In men, the glans-vasal reflex causes the posterior urethra to fill with seminal fluids from the prostate and the seminal vesicles. The distension caused by this filling helps to enlist both ejaculatory and orgasmic reflexes. It takes time for the seminal fluids to be secreted and build up, which greatly reduces the chance for a man to have another orgasm right after having ejaculated. The glans-vasal reflex does not play a large part in attaining orgasms in women. Additionally during this time, prolactin levels stay elevated.[250] This continues to decrease sexual desire, thus competing with the cerebral, pro-orgasm neurotransmitters and interfering with sensory stimulation.

MEDICATIONS THAT MIGHT CAUSE SEXUAL PROBLEMS

It should be noted that there are a number of medications that people take for medical issues—like hypertension, infections, and psychiatric diseases—that can impair the sexual response cycle. Medications that are commonly used which might impair the sexual response cycle include, but are not limited to, amitriptyline, cimetidine, doxepin, digoxin, finasteride, haloperidol, hydrochlorothiazide, spironolactone, imipramine, ketoconazole, eszopiclone, leuprolide, metoclopramide, nortriptyline, risperidone, and protriptyline. Probably the most common legal drug that impairs nerve functioning is alcohol.

SUMMARY

Talking is the most important part of almost any sexual encounter. There are five stages in the human sexual cycle, and you can't get to the next one until you've gone through the one before it. The first stage is desire, and if overlooked, the human sexual cycle can get bogged down on a road to nowhere.

---

[187] My concentration as an undergraduate at Cornell University was in Neurobiology and Behavior. The paragraph that follows is a severe, anthropocentric oversimplification of the diverse beauty and intricacy of animal behaviors. To learn more about animal behavior, you can visit Cornell's Department of Neurobiology and Behavior website at www.nbb.cornell.edu. Thomas D. Seeley ran the introductory course in neurobiology

and behavior and was one of the most fascinating teachers I had at Cornell. He has studied honeybees for more than thirty years, and his discoveries are amazing.

[188] K. M. Heilman and R. L. Gilmore, Department of Neurology, University of Florida, Gainesville 32610-0236, USA, "Cortical influences in emotion," *Journal of Clinical Neurophysiology* 15, no. 5 (September 1998): 409–23.

[189] The specific areas in the temporal lobe are the entorhinal cortex, parahippocampal cortex, and hippocampus. It is further explained in the paper: P. Sah, E. S. L. Faber, M. Lopez De Armentia, and J. Power, Division of Neuroscience, John Curtin School of Medical Research, Australian National University, Canberra, Australian Capital Territory, Australia, *The Amygdaloid Complex: Anatomy and Physiology*.

[190] I. Kupfermann, "Hypothalamus and Limbic System I: Peptidergic Neurons, Homeostasis, and Emotional Behavior," in *Principles of Neural Science*, ed. E. R. Kandel and J. H. Schwartz, (New York: Elsevier Science Publishing Co., Inc., 1985), 611–625.

[191] R. A. Barton and P. H. Harvey, Evolutionary Anthropology Research Group, Department of Anthropology, University of Durham, Durham DH1 3HN, UK Department of Zoology, University of Oxford, South Parks Road, Oxford OX1 3PS, UK, "Mosaic evolution of brain structure in mammals," *Nature* 405 (June 29, 2000): 1055–1058, doi:10.1038/35016580; Received 1 February 2000; Accepted 4 May 2000.

[192] E. D. Jarvis, O. Gunturkun, L. Bruce, A. Csillag, H. Karten, W. Kuenzel, L. Medina et al., "Avian brains and a new understanding of vertebrate brain evolution," *Nature Reviews Neuroscience* 6, no. 2 (2005): 151–9.

[193] L. J. Wu, S. S. Kim, X. Li, F. Zhang, and M. Zhuo, Department of Physiology, University of Toronto, 1 King's College Circle, Toronto, Ontario M5S 1A8, Canada, longjun.wu@utoronto.ca, "Sexual attraction enhances glutamate transmission in mammalian anterior cingulate cortex," *Molecular Brain* 6, no. 2 (May 2009): 9, doi: 10.1186/1756-6606-2-9.

[194] R. Basson, "Women's sexual desire—disordered or misunderstood?" *Journal of Sex and Marital Therapy* 28, Suppl. 1 (2002): 17–28.

[195] Y. Miyagawa, A. Tsujimura et al., "Differential brain processing of audiovisual sexual stimuli in men: comparative positron emission tomography study of the initiation and maintenance of penile erection during sexual arousal," *Neuroimage* 36, no. 3 (July 1, 2007): 830–42. Epub 2007 Apr 10.

[196] I always thought that the sex class would have been much more interesting if the beer and wine tasting class came first.

[197] Cask. Cornell had a tremendous vat-building department based upon the business they got from Harvard students who, when they came to try and play sport against the Big Red, saw the waterfall that came from Beebe Lake. Having thought that the world of aquatic motion began and ended at the head of the Charles River, they were mesmerized by water existing on a plane orthogonal to their proprietary river. In time, they came to believe that water in a vertical axis would, indeed, allow them to carry on many more effete Crimson activities at altitudes unimaginable. To that end, the eager students would fill cask after cask of the "magic water" and drag it back to Cambridge where, after having several elaborate ceremonies (many of which included spanking and

quoting passages from *Tristram Shandy*), they would release the water with expectations that it would volley skyward and allow for a path more pure to be established between Yahweh and the venerated apostles of John Harvard. While this provided bustling vat, cask, and keg industries in beautiful Ithaca, New York, from 1891 to 1918, it all came to an end when the young "upstart" physicist, Weinegaard Pfloofthroen, after attaining full professorial duties at the "University-Just-Outside-of-Beantown," was able to convince the majority of the Harvard undergraduates, using only a croquet ball and a copy of Newton's *Principia*, that the water was not flowing up into the sky as much as it was flowing down into the creek below it. And while the golden age of cooperage in the Finger Lake region has come and gone, among the Big Red, cask remains the most important four-letter word that ends with K.

[198] Guys, pay attention.

[199] Excuse me for shouting again, but this is the most important idea in the book.

[200] Again, this is the second most important idea in the book.

[201] For purpose of saving space, we will only be dealing with the sexual encounter between two people. While I've heard tale and yarn spun about multiple individuals *in delicto flagrante*, there just isn't enough time or space to go through all of the necessary permutations.

[202] I will be referring to the sexual response cycle from a physiological point of view. There are many different names and stages given to the process, but I will be using desire, excitement, plateau, orgasm, and resolution as the basis of this chapter.

[203] That's right, Newt. I'm looking at you. You're going down. And don't even think for an instant, Karen, that I don't know that you're in on it too.

[204] Also known, inappropriately, as the "horny toad." It's actually a lizard.

[205] R. C. K. Chan, D. Shum, T. Toulopoulou, and E. Y. H. Chen, "Assessment of executive functions: Review of instruments and identification of critical issues," *Archives of Clinical Neuropsychology* 23, no. 2 (2008): 201–216, doi:10.1016/j.acn.2007.08.010. PMID 18096360.

[206] A. Miyake, N. P. Friedman, M. J. Emerson, A. H. Witzki, A. Howerter, and T. D. Wager, Department of Psychology, University of Colorado at Boulder, 80309-0345, USA, "The unity and diversity of executive functions and their contributions to complex 'Frontal Lobe' tasks: a latent variable analysis," *Cognitive Psychology* 41, no. 1 (August 2000): 49–100.

[207] M. Trimble, Institute of Neurology, Queen Square, London, UK, "Psychopathology of frontal lobe syndromes," *Seminars in Neurology* 10, no. 3 (September 1990): 287–94.

[208] This is a purely fictitious example. My wife was an All-Ivy League Field Hockey player. She was raised in a home where a healthy diet, exercise, and hard work were of quintessential importance. She can post up, take a drop step, and shoot a basketball like she's making a loaf of healthy banana bread. She was the one out in the front yard playing with our children almost every day when they were younger. She mowed the lawn with a manual push-mower while she was pregnant. She did this while she ran the newborn nursery at the hospital she worked at after graduating from residency. After I came out of my MS haze by getting on Tysabri and starting Adderall, I picked up some of the slack. My son has become an excellent pitcher, so I went out and bought

a chest protector, mask, shin guards, and a catcher's mitt. I gave them to my wife on our anniversary.

[209] T. M. Kessler, C. J. Fowler, and J. N. Panicker, Department of Uro-Neurology, the National Hospital for Neurology and Neurosurgery, University College London Hospitals, UCL NHS Foundation Trust, UCL Institute of Neurology, London, UK, tkessler@gmx.ch, "Sexual dysfunction in multiple sclerosis," *Expert Review of Neurotherapeutics* 9, no. 3 (March 2009): 341–50.

[210] E. Z. Schmidt, P. Hofmann, G. Niederwieser, H. P. Kapfhammer, R. M. Bonelli, University Clinic of Psychiatry, Medical University of Graz, Graz, Austria, "Sexuality in multiple sclerosis," *Journal of Neural Transmission* 112, no. 9 (September 2005): 1201–11. Epub 2005 Mar 7.

[211] R. DasGupta and C. J. Fowler, Department of Uro-Neurology, National Hospital for Neurology and Neurosurgery, Queen Square, London WC1N 3BG, UK, ranandg@yahoo.co.uk, "Sexual and urological dysfunction in multiple sclerosis: better understanding and improved therapies," *Current Opinion in Neurology* 15, no. 3 (June 2002): 271–8.

[212] R. A. Rudick, D. Miller, S. Hass, M. Hutchinson, P. A. Calabresi, C. Confavreux, S. L. Galetta SL et al., AFFIRM and SENTINEL Investigators, Department of Neurology, Mellen Center for Multiple Sclerosis Treatment and Research, Cleveland Clinic Foundation, Cleveland, OH 44195, USA, "Health-related quality of life in multiple sclerosis: effects of natalizumab," *Annals of Neurology* 62, no. 4 (October 2007): 335–46.

[213] D. Mattson, M. Petrie, D. K. Srivastava, M. McDermott, Department of Neurology, University of Rochester (NY) School of Medicine and Dentistry, USA, "Multiple sclerosis: Sexual dysfunction and its response to medications," *Archives of Neurology* 52, no. 9 (September 1995): 862–8.

[214] To be described in the "Excitement and Plateau" section.

[215] G. Holstege, Center for Uroneurology, University Medical Center Groningen, Groningen, the Netherlands, g.holstege@med.umcg.n, "The emotional motor system and micturition control," *Neurourology and Urodynamics* 29, no. 1 (2010): 42–8.

[216] M. Kiefer and A. Unterberg, Klinik für Neurochirurgie, Universitätsklinikum des Saarlandes, Kirrberger Str., 66421 Homburg, Germany, "The differential diagnosis and treatment of normal-pressure hydrocephalus," *Deutsches Ärzteblatt International* 109, no. 1–2 (January 2012): 15–25; quiz 26. Epub 2012 Jan 9.

[217] D. Tsakanikas and N. Relkin, Department of Neurology and Neuroscience, New York Presbyterian Hospital-Weill Cornell Medical Center, New York, New York 10021, USA, "Normal pressure hydrocephalus," *Seminars in Neurology* 27, no. 1 (February 2007): 58–65.

[218] A. Keller Ashton, R. Hamer, and R. C. Rosen, Buffalo Medical Group, Williamsville, NY 14221, USA, "Serotonin reuptake inhibitor-induced sexual dysfunction and its treatment: a large-scale retrospective study of 596 psychiatric outpatients," *Journal of Sex and Marital Therapy* 23, no. 3 (Fall 1997): 165–75.

[219] H. Sidi, D. Asmidar, R. Hod, N. R. Jaafar, and N. C. Guan, Department of Psychiatry, Universiti Kebangsaan Malaysia Medical Centre, Kuala Lumpur, Malaysia, "Hypoactive

sexual desire among depressed female patients treated with selective serotonin reuptake inhibitors: a comparison between escitalopram and fluoxetine," *International Journal of Psychiatry in Clinical Practice* 16, no. 1 (March 2012): 41–7. Epub 2011 Nov 9.

[220] R. C. Rosen, M. K. Connor, G. Miyasato, C. Link, J. L. Shifren, W. A. Fisher, L. R. Derogatis, and M. J. Schobelock, 1 Department of Epidemiology, New England Research Institutes, Inc., Watertown, Massachusetts, "Sexual Desire Problems in Women Seeking Health care: A Novel Study Design for Ascertaining Prevalence of Hypoactive Sexual Desire Disorder in Clinic-Based Samples of U.S. Women," *Journal of Women's Health* (Larchmt) (2012 Jan 9), [Epub ahead of print].

[221] K. B. Segraves and R. T. Segraves, Department of Psychiatry, Metro Health Medical Center, Cleveland, OH 44109, "Hypoactive sexual desire disorder: prevalence and comorbidity in 906 subjects," *Journal of Sex and Marital Therapy* 17, no. 1 (Spring 1991): 55–8.

[222] R. T. Segraves, A. Clayton, H. Croft, A. Wolf, and J. Warnock, Department of Psychiatry, Case Western Reserve University and Metro-Health Medical System, 2500 MetroHealth Drive, Cleveland, OH 44109-1998, USA, Rsegraves@metrohealth.org, "Bupropion sustained release for the treatment of hypoactive sexual desire disorder in premenopausal women," *Journal of Clinical Psychopharmacology* 24, no. 3 (June 2004): 339–42.

[223] M. R. Safarinejad, S. Y. Hosseini, M. A. Asgari, F. Dadkhah, and A. Taghva, Urology and Nephrology Research Centre, Shahid Modarress Hospital, Shahid Beheshti University, Tehran, Iran, safarinejad@unrc.ir, "A randomized, double-blind, placebo-controlled study of the efficacy and safety of bupropion for treating hypoactive sexual desire disorder in ovulating women," *BJU International* 106, no. 6 (September 2010): 832–9, Epub 2010 Feb 11.

[224] J. G. Pfaus, Center for Studies in Behavioral Neurobiology, Department of Psychology, Concordia University, Montréal, Canada, "Pathways of sexual desire," *Journal of Sexual Medicine* 6, no. 6 (June 2009): 1506–33, Epub 2009 Apr 30.

[225] G. Corona, V. Ricca, E. Bandini, E. Mannucci, F. Lotti, V. Boddi, G. Rastrelli et al., Andrology Unit, Department of Clinical Physiopathology, University of Florence, Florence 50139, Italy, "Selective serotonin reuptake inhibitor-induced sexual dysfunction," *Journal of Sexual Medicine* 6, no. 5 (May 2009): 1259–69.

[226] A. B. Csoka, A. Bahrick, and O. P. Mehtonen, University of Pittsburgh—Medicine, Pittsburgh, PA, USA, csokaA@dom.pitt.edu, "Persistent sexual dysfunction after discontinuation of selective serotonin reuptake inhibitors," *Journal of Sexual Medicine* 5, no. 1 (January 2008): 227–33.

[227] J. A. Simon, Department of Obstetrics and Gynecology, George Washington University, Washington, DC 20036, USA, jsimon@jamesasimonmd.com, "Low sexual desire—is it all in her head? Pathophysiology, diagnosis, and treatment of hypoactive sexual desire disorder," *Postgraduate Medical Journal* 122, no. 6 (November 2010): 128–36.

[228] T. H. Krüger, B. Schiffer, M. Eikermann, P. Haake, E. Gizewski, and M. Schedlowski, Division of Psychology and Behavioral Immunobiology, Swiss Federal Institute of Technology Zürich, Universitätsstrasse 6, 8092 Zürich, Switzerland, krueger@ifv.gess.

ethz.ch, "Serial neurochemical measurement of cerebrospinal fluid during the human sexual response cycle," *European Journal of Neuroscience* 24, no. 12 (December 2006): 3445–52.

[229] T. Mancini, F. F. Casanueva, and A. Giustina, "Hyperprolactinemia and Prolactinomas,"*Endocrinology & Metabolism Clinics of North America* 37 (1) (2008): 67.

[230] Okay, guys, huddle up. In case you didn't get the message, for the majority of women, whether they have MS or not, they're just not in the mood as often as we are to have sex. This is a blanket statement and is not true for all women (likewise, there are some of us guys who are not as much interested in sex as the rest of us are, and that's cool too). But just because your partner isn't interested in sex as much as you are doesn't necessarily make her "frigid." There are ways to help your partner become interested in sex without getting her drunk or showing her what you just bought down at the Vibe-U-Rama. Keep on reading.

[231] A. D. Sadovnik, R. N. Eisen, G. C. Ebers, D. W. Paty, "Cause of death in patients attending multiple sclerosis clinics," *Neurology* 41 (1991): 1193–1196.

[232] E. N. Stenager, E. Stenager, N. Koch-Henrikson, et al., "Suicide and multiple sclerosis: an epidemiological investigation," *Journal of Neurology, Neurosurgery & Psychiatry* 55 (1992): 542–545.

[233] Anthony Feinstein, MD, PhD, From the Department of Psychiatry, University of Toronto and Sunnybrook and Women's College Health Sciences Centre, Toronto, Ontario, Canada, *An Examination of Suicidal Intent in Patients with Multiple Sclerosis.* Address correspondence and reprint requests to Dr. Anthony Feinstein, Department of Psychiatry, University of Toronto and Sunnybrook and Women's College Health Sciences Centre, 2075 Bayview Avenue, Toronto, Ontario, Canada M4N 3M5; e-mail: ant.feinstein@utoronto.ca.

[234] M. Rossato, G. Balercia, G. Lucarelli, C. Foresta, and F. Mantero, Department of Medical and Surgical Sciences, Clinica Medica 3, University of Padova, Italy, marco.rossato@unipd.it, "Role of seminal osmolarity in the reduction of human sperm motility," *International Journal of Andrology* 25, no. 4 (August 2002): 230–5.

[235] T-thoracic spine, L-lumbar spine. The number indicates the vertebral body that the nerve root passes out from. The C (cervical)-spine has seven vertebral bodies, T-spine has twelve, L-spine has five, and S (sacral)-spine has five (which are often fused).

[236] K. Everaert, W. I. de Waard, T. Van Hoof, C. Kiekens, T. Mulliez, and C. D'herde, Department of Urology, Ghent University Hospital, Ghent, Belgium, K.Everaert@ ugent.be, "Neuroanatomy and neurophysiology related to sexual dysfunction in male neurogenic patients with lesions to the spinal cord or peripheral nerves," *Spinal Cord* 48, no. 3 (March 2010): 182–91, Epub 2010 Jan 5.

[237] W. D. Steers, University of Virginia, Health Sciences Center, Department of Urology, Box 800 422, Jefferson Park Avenue, Charlottesville, VA 22908-0422, USA, wds6t@virginia.edu, "Neural pathways and central sites involved in penile erection: neuroanatomy and clinical implications," *Neuroscience & Biobehavioral Reviews* 24, no. 5 (July 2000): 507–16.

238 And while I respect the people in ASPCP (American Society for the Prevention of Cruelty to Plants; http://the antilandscaper.org.) I still contend that if smashing a watermelon can help a person's life, as well as the people around that person, even the watermelon would agree that it is a good idea.

239 "Orgasm." *The American Heritage® Stedman's Medical Dictionary* (Houghton Mifflin Company). 05 Apr. 2012. <Dictionary.com http://dictionary.reference.com/browse/orgasm>.

240 This is a definition that I made up based upon my studies. It is not peer-reviewed and holds no legal value. I think it's a good definition because it helps us realize that orgasm is a complex physiological process. In understanding its complexity, a person who's having some troubles in the bedroom might feel less alone. By splitting up a puzzle into pieces, it can make it easier to figure out where the trouble lies.

241 B. R. Komisaruk and B. Whipple, Department of Psychology, Rutgers, the State University of New Jersey, Newark 07102, USA, brk@psychology.rutgers.edu, "Functional MRI of the brain during orgasm in women," *Annual Review of Sexual Research* 16 (2005): 62–86.

242 M. Fode, S. Krogh-Jespersen, N. L. Brackett, D. A. Ohl, C. M. Lynne, and J. Sønksen, Department of Urology, Herlev Hospital, University of Copenhagen, Denmark, "Male sexual dysfunction and infertility associated with neurological disorders," *Asian Journal of Andrology* 14, no. 1 (January 2012): 61–8, doi: 10.1038/aja.2011.70. Epub 2011 Dec 5.

243 E. Skowronski and K. Hartman, Canberra Hospital, Yamba Drive, Garran, Australian Capital Territory, Australia, emmasko@optusnet.com.au, "Obstetric management following traumatic tetraplegia: case series and literature review," *Aust. N Z Journal of Obstetrical Gynaecology* 48, no. 5 (Oct. 2008): 485–91, doi: 10.1111/j.1479-828X.2008.00909.x.

244 M. Tebbet and P. Kennedy, Oxford Doctoral Course in Clinical Psychology, Isis Education Centre, University of Oxford, Warneford Hospital, United Kingdom, "The experience of childbirth for women with spinal cord injuries: an interpretative phenomenology analysis study," *Disability and Rehabilitation* 34, no. 9 (2012): 762–9, Epub 2011 Oct 19.

245 G. Corona, E. Mannucci, E. A. Jannini, F. Lotti, V. Ricca, M. Monami, V. Boddi et al., Andrology Unit, Department of Clinical Physiopathology, University of Florence, Florence, Italy, "Hypoprolactinemia: a new clinical syndrome in patients with sexual dysfunction," *Journal of Sexual Medicine* 6, no. 5 (May 2009): 1457–66, Epub 2009 Feb 10.

246 T. H. Krüger, P. Haake, D. Chereath, W. Knapp, O. E. Janssen, M. S. Exton, M. Schedlowski, and U. Hartmann, Department of Medical Psychology, University of Essen, Hufelandstr 55, Federal Republic of Germany, tillmann.krueger@web.de, "Specificity of the neuroendocrine response to orgasm during sexual arousal in men," *Journal of Endocrinology* 177, no. 1 (April 2003): 57–64.

247 T. H. Krüger, B. Schiffer, M. Eikermann, P. Haake, E. Gizewski, and M. Schedlowski, Division of Psychology and Behavioral Immunobiology, Swiss Federal Institute of Technology Zürich, Universitätsstrasse 6, 8092 Zürich, Switzerland, krueger@ifv.gess. ethz.ch, "Serial neurochemical measurement of cerebrospinal fluid during the human

sexual response cycle," *European Journal of Neuroscience* 24, no. 12 (December 2006): 3445–52.

[248] R. B. Teng and X. H. Zhang, Institute of Urology and Nephrology, Guangxi Medical University, Nanning, Guangxi 530021, China, "Oxytocin and male sexual function" [article in Chinese], *Zhonghua Nan Ke Xue* 17, no. 6 (June 2011): 558–61.

[249] M. E. Dunn and J. E. Trost, "Male multiple orgasms: a descriptive study," *Archives of Sexual Behavior* 18, no. 5 (October 1989): 377–87.

[250] T. H. Kruger, A. Burri, and M. Schedlowski, "Melatonin plasma levels during sexual arousal and orgasm in males," *Journal of Sexual Medicine* 8, no. 4 (April 2011): 1255–6, doi: 10.1111/j.1743-6109.2010.02048.x. Epub 2010 Oct 4.

Eighteenth

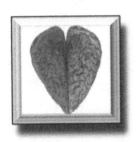

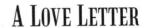

Love
Sex from the other
side of the desk

A LOVE LETTER

I was limited in how I could approach writing this part of the book. If I wrote it from experience, my wife's private life would be compromised, and that would not be respectful of her. If I claimed it was entirely fictional, and writing comes from experience, my wife would want to know where I got the experience.

Ergo …

I offer the following blank page upon which you are invited to begin practice in the art of the handwritten love letter since, in the world of today flooded with lightning fast (and equally ephemeral) e-mail, correspondence that requires the effort of thinking, feeling, and writing, on paper, the emotions we hold for those dear to us, is hovering on the eve of destruction while the mature, penned word is rapidly being sucked out of reality by a fluorescent, unpredictable, cyber-vortex where pixels rise, fall, and dissolve, destined for infinitesimal existence often bearing effect on nothing and no one, yet it is the unassuming paper and crayon that the child takes and thereupon scrawls with fervor and abandon and sees the markings and says it is good and does it again and again until nap time whereupon awakening, he sees the trail of a novice scribe that seemingly had little to offer—aside from being carefree—but soon after, the scratchings began to make sense, for when the girl, who accepted the awkwardly offered but quite formal-appearing letter, looked at him, and then looked at his hand-formed words for what seemed like an eternity, and then back at him with a look that lasted just—a—bit—too—long, causing him to become, for the first time in his life, flustered, since he did not know, but did, for the first time, feel, what purpose she had with her subtle smile and the sweet scent floating from her hair, down her soft face and across the space into his world—a world, which until now, had been tidy and ordered and overflowing with reason, but suddenly had become a domain, while not being broken, was being bent beyond the belief of the former boy, as she became the new, soft, quiet coordinator of his heart and soul and actions and thoughts, as he saw things anew, like the atom's shell being split and light being liberated to cast the world with new shadows and angles, allowing the beauty of the order of the world to finally become realized by appreciating its underlying chaos; where subject and object and verb mean this in this order but that in another and therefore, the instant must be written down, for while the words remain the same, their meaning—at that instant—will never mean the same again, and by having registered them with his hand, a permanent moment was created that incessant Time yielded to them, to become one and create another, and yes, while moments are sometimes copied, they are never to be reduplicated because no one stays there or here, except through the letters they leave, spawned by the heart, interpreted by the mind, and placed by a hand, which, while marking a singular message at that time, begets incalculable life in each mind that sees and reads and feels the palpable words of another.

$\mathcal{N}$ineteenth

HOW STEPHEN COLBERT HAS HELPED ME TO UNDERSTAND MS BETTER

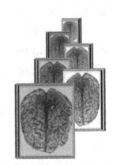

Thou shalt have no other gods before me.
—God, *The Bible*, King James Version

The episode that follows occurred in March 2007. Please note that I no longer watch The Colbert Report *three to four times per day. Ever since I started taking natalizumab and my ADD medication, I have been able to enjoy a show after watching it just once. The rest of my time is now spent writing my own show ...*

I think most people know who Stephen Colbert is and what a quick mind he has. I know he knows how smart he is. However, I am willing to bet that not even he himself knows how much he has added to the world of MS by helping me understand MS better. Much of the MS ICE was developed after I experienced the following event.

It all started with my wife. She's a pediatrician by training, who became a breastfeeding medicine doctor by desire. She helps mommies and babies successfully breastfeed. One of her patients had connections with *The Colbert Report*. When my wife found this out, she said, "That's my husband's favorite show!" Her patient then asked if we would like to see the show. My wife said sure. She asked if we could go on my birthday at the end of the month. She said it was no problem. My wife and I decided we would make a day out of it. We decided that we would close our offices for the day, get some exercise, go into the city to see Dr. Colbert's show, and then go to dinner. We were all set for The Stephen Colbert Experience.

The morning of the show, we decided to go for a jog together. We got our workout clothes on, did our stretching, and then started our jog through town. We usually run next to each other and talk, but at one point we had to run single-file, and so I ran in front.[251] I let my mind drift. I started thinking about how I was looking forward to seeing Stephen Colbert and his perfect hair. I could not wait to see the hallowed pulpit from which he delivered the words from "I am Who am" (which are delivered directly to him, even before they are proofread by the archangel editorial staff). I was thinking about *"Truthiness"* and all things *"Truthy."* I was picturing in my mind's eye how Stephen nonchalantly gives the audience the finger every time he pushes his glasses up on his nose. Nirvana was so close I could ...

Ow!

I had my head so far in the clouds that I didn't see the rock that was in the middle of the sidewalk. When I stepped on the rock, I heard a "pop," and then I started to feel some pain. Within thirty seconds, my ankle was noticeably swollen, and the pain was increasing. I told Lauren I thought I had just royally messed up my ankle and that we had better head home. I had never twisted my ankle so badly. I was weak! I should have seen the rock! I started damning myself for daydreaming about being able to be in the same room as Stephen *and* his mind *and* his hair *and* his product placements.

Oh, the product placements!

I limped home with Lauren acting as my crutch. Lauren asked what I was thinking about when I stepped on the rock. I told her that I wasn't thinking. I was lost in a dreamscape, paralyzed by the great work Stephen was doing for humankind. I tried to numb my pain with positive thoughts of Colbert-almighty's contributions to the Olympics and the United States space program and his ever informative and poignant Word-of-the-Day. I lamented slightly about how Stephen is sometimes not appreciated but garnered courage in knowing that he is always right. *The Colbert Report* was only hours away. I couldn't fall short now after having come so far ...

When we got home, I went to the freezer and got an ice pack. I alternated between icing my ankle and saying novenas. I wrapped my ankle tightly to suppress the swelling. I took some ibuprofen. I got my computer while Lauren brought me my *The Colbert Report* T-shirt. I watched my ankle continue to swell. I sat on the couch with my leg elevated. I knew that if I could just man up, I would still be able to limp into his presence. I went to The Colbert Nation website. I saw Stephen look at me with his left eyebrow arched, daring me to be more than just another medical namby-pamby with a sausage-ankle lying on a couch. It was comforting and inspiring. I knew that even though I would probably not be able to sprint to *The Colbert Report* as I had wanted to, I had to complete my pilgrimage to the place I simply refer to as *"Colberidise."*

As I felt the Power o' Stephen beginning to descend upon my home, the pain in my ankle started to ease. My thoughts became clearer. I started to reflect upon the fortunate life that I had been granted. Sure, I had MS, but I was born in a time when it could be more easily diagnosed. Plus, some treatments had finally been discovered. I was taking natalizumab and reflected on how much better my thinking, memory, and balance had become ever since starting it. I knew the mechanism of action of natalizumab was to prevent the T-cells from getting out of the blood stream and into the brain.

I looked at my swollen ankle again. When I twisted my ankle, my body's immune system called out a whole bunch of inflammatory cells to fix the damage that had been done to my ankle. They all came—white blood cells, extracellular fluid, red blood cells, and other repair cells. They congested the area and made my ankle blow up like a balloon. Now, I could barely use my ankle and the attached foot. It hurt to put weight on it. The range of motion of my ankle was limited by the swelling. I could just barely walk on my twisted ankle, and I sure as heck could not run on it.

It was then that the bulbous being at the end of my leg shouted at me and my bloated brain! Eureka—the connection was finally made! My swollen brain was trapped in the hard shell of my skull. My skull, unlike the skin around my ankle, is unyielding! It cannot expand when the pressure inside of it increases! The WBCs are constantly creeping into my brain. The pressure builds and builds and builds, leading to a global increase of intracerebral pressure. The WBCs cannot be seen on MRI because they're microscopic. They congest and engorge the white matter of my brain. With the inflammation going on everywhere, nerves are going to be affected everywhere, affecting many different tracts of my brain. Initiative, concentration, emotions—they all involve diffuse pathways that cannot be taken down by just one white dot. Or twenty! Or a hundred! Elevated pressure is the silent accomplice of the shiny, deceitful criminal–the enhancing lesion. This menace has caused my cognitive paralysis. Yes, I could still think, but my brain don't be functionin' like it did before it got all swelled up.

Demyelination is bad and has always been the thing doctors mostly focus on when trying to help those of us with MS. But the swelling! The swelling is the thing causing the elevated pressure in our heads that makes nerves not work, and no one can see it. The swelling is the silent marauder in MS!

Then I thought about patients I had taken care of who had encephalitis (an infection of the brain that generates swelling). I thought about how they thought and behaved. Those patients were easily distractible. They could not attend to task. They had disturbed sleep-wake cycles and labile affects (going from laughing to crying easily). Their symptoms got better after their infections were treated with the appropriate medications and the swelling resolved.

Then I thought back on the time I had the opportunity to speak with several groups of doctors and relate my experience taking natalizumab. After explaining to them how distractible and emotionally labile and forgetful I had been before taking a medication that reduced the swelling in my brain, a senior neurologist raised his hand. He said that he had just experienced a similar situation with a syndrome called *normal pressure hydrocephalus*. What happens in this disease is that the fluid that is made in two big holes in our brains (called the *lateral ventricles*) can get backed up because it cannot drain and be reabsorbed properly. This leads to the ventricles swelling and putting pressure on the surrounding brain tissue. The doctor said that he had felt very similar to the situation I was describing. After he had treatment for the NPH (by having a shunt placed, which allows another way for the fluid in the brain to drain) and the pressure returned to normal, he said he was able to think more clearly again.

Once the *pressure-effect idea* crystallized in my mind, I no longer *believed* that I had been touched by a power.

I knew that I had been touched.
All thanks to the One with the Perfect Hair.

Therefore, Dr. Colbert, on behalf of all MS patients who are neurologists who work with their wives and have enough time to watch your show three to four times per day, allow me to give you the credit you deserve in helping to overcome the struggle to better understand the disease known as multiple sclerosis.

SUMMARY

It is important to relax once in a while and let your mind take a vacation.

While on vacation, your brain will have the opportunity to think about whatever it wants to think about.

You might make a discovery.

You might come up with a better way to make chocolate chip cookies.

Or trim your nose hair.

Or cure MS.

A recent study showed that 100 percent of doctors polled believe that watching funny TV, that makes you think, can possibly lead to a cure for MS.[252]

---

[251] To fend off marauders as necessary.

[252] There were flaws in the study design. First of all, the number of responders in the poll was four (me and the three reflections of me in my wife's fancy three-panel bathroom mirror). This number is too small to give the results any power. Second of all, observer bias was rampant because I caught myself laughing in the mirror while I was polling myself. Finally, even though the results of the study overwhelmingly show that funny TV is good for you, the statistical significance of the study is crappy. I calculated the p value, and it showed there was a 99 percent probability that the results were due to pure chance. Based on the full disclosure of these facts, I, as a medical professional, cannot say that it is better for you to watch funny TV than it is for you to get exercise. As a creative medical professional, I can say that it is better for you to take a jog while listening to a standup comedy routine by Jim Gaffigan on a digital music device strapped to your arm. As a comedicaledian, I think it would be *hilarious* to take a jog and listen to Jim Gaffigan while he is strapped to your arm.

Twentieth

FAMILY AND MS FROM A NEUROLOGICAL POINT OF VIEW

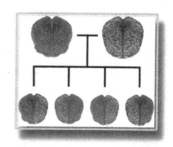

Smile at each other. Smile at your wife, smile at your husband, smile at your children, smile at each other—it doesn't matter who it is— and that will help to grow up in greater love for each other.
—Mother Teresa, Nobel Lecture
December 11, 1979

The family members and dear friends of those of us with MS are quite often our main caregivers.[253] They love us because they know at heart that we're good people, even though some of us might do or say something that's a little left of center. They stand by us and wish that things could return to the way things used to be. They push wheelchairs. They help us get cleaned up. They lay out our meds. Quite often, they put themselves last on the priority list.

After being a doctor for over twenty years,[254] I have had the opportunity to meet and interact with several thousand other MSers. I've heard tremendously inspirational stories about the efforts made by caregivers to help out the MSers in their lives that would soften even the hardest hearts. That's one of the greatest parts about speaking around our beautiful country. Less often, I have heard MSers and others relate accounts of egregious actions by people who found themselves in the role of caregiver before they were ready to become one. These "unexpected" caregivers are regular people who fall in love with another regular person. When the person that they fell in love with goes on to develop MS, the first partner starts to see changes in the other that she cannot understand. She cannot get answers from anyone about what or why this has happened. She starts to think that she made a mistake with whom she chose to spend the rest of her life with. As her partner's MS worsens, she gets scared. She reverts to a childlike state as a defense mechanism. She says something mean ("You're broken. I don't want you anymore."). Then she says that she is taking her toys and going home ("I want a divorce.").

I'd like to think the good stories outweigh the bad. I believe that people are good and that many acts of malfeasance are reactions of fear to the unknown world of MS. Hopefully, by writing this book and explaining the reasons why we MSers can't be judged by the way we appear, others can become empowered to grow and start doing things that they never thought they could do. And while their life might not be what they expected it to be, hopefully caregivers can start to see life for the exciting, relatively unpredictable ride that it is. I know that that's one of the greatest things that MS has taught me.

As a physician, there are certain things I love about having family members actively involved in the care of the MSer (or MSers) in their lives. During an office visit, they can give info about the patient that the patient cannot see themselves:

"I've noticed that Stan forgot to pay the bills
this month, and he never did that before."

Then I'll ask the patient if he noticed that he missed paying the bills and if he had a reason why he didn't pay them:

"Because Jane forgot to leave the checkbook at home after she took
it to buy the tickets for the Bay City Rollers Reunion Tour."[255]

When it comes down to it, as a doctor I get to see my patients for a half hour, plus or minus, every few months. Of course they can always call if something comes up, but if the MSer is not aware of it, he or she cannot call me. Family members might notice something, but they might just sweep it under the rug and say it was a "senior moment" (even though the patient is twenty-nine years old). By me actively bringing it up, I think it helps to let caregivers know that it's good to bring up things that they notice.

I also love it when caregivers step up and become proactive in the care of the MSer in their life. They can become the auxiliary brain for the patient. They remind their partner that they have a doctor's appointment. They might be the same person who helps the MSer get to the appointment. They write things down during the office visit if the list of things that the MSer has to do becomes long (MRI, blood work, physical therapy, etc.). I also like to watch and see how the patient and caregiver regard each other during the interview. If it appears that one is happy and the other is not, I try to help them open a discussion about any unresolved feelings they might have about the other. I know that MS (and just about every other neurological disease) gets worse when a person (or people) have unrequited issues burning inside of them. If the patient and caregiver are married, sometimes more personal issues that are medically relevant might come up, like noticing the start of some skin breakdown because the MSer sits for so long.

Children sometimes come along with the MSer and caregiver. I love meeting them. Some just sit quietly and play on their handheld computer game. Some listen. Some ask questions. I like learning how they view their parent's disease. Usually the tween-aged kids will report all the tasks that they're in charge of to help get Mom or Dad to work on time or what their responsibilities in the house are. It's a positive thing to have children learn about multiple sclerosis, especially if it's affecting one or both of their parents. Children are curious. If they notice something, like Dad walking differently from Mom, they want to know why. If they're told that Dad has a disease called multiple sclerosis that can cause trouble with walking, they then know why Dad walks differently. As they grow, they start to ask more specific questions. It's important to teach them, age appropriately, what's going on. Kids who are in a home with a parent who has a disability have been found to have more positive or neutral feelings about their parents than kids who had "normal" parents. Additionally, kids of parents with disabilities had fewer negative or indifferent feelings about their folks than the kids of "normal" parents.[256] You can see what my kids think about me having MS in the next chapter.

I know some doctors hate it when caregivers are present during an office visit with an MSer. Some doctors get anxious when caregivers ask a lot of questions and write things down. They say the caregivers get in the way of the doctor-patient relationship.

I believe that the caregivers in my MS patients' lives are part of my patient's life and therefore part of my patient's health.

SUMMARY

Caregivers are wonderful people. Some people are thrust into a caregiver's role when they are not ready to handle it. Children are curious. The more they are educated, the stronger people they become. Communication between people is always important. In the world of MS, communication is a crucial part in allowing all of us to take control of the disease.

---

253 I'll use the word "caregiver" to mean "any individual in a person's life who helps out anyone who cannot do a task on their own." I like that definition because everybody needs help at sometime. Please note that help can range from offering maximal physical or psychological support to smiling at someone as you roll down the street in your wheelchair. Yep. It works both ways.

254 I can't believe I just wrote that. That's something an old person says to a little kid. I'm not old. I still listen to rock. I know all the words to "Bonzo Goes to Bitburg" by the Ramones. I jog two miles a few times per week. This past summer, I played goalie in a soccer match and played the best I had ever played in my life (thank you, Mr. Young). I'm still fourteen years old in my head, but a very mature fourteen-year-old. I will agree to the fact that time has passed since yesterday, but until someone can come up with a better way to measure the distance between "now" and "then," I will never accept the concept of old. I will forever be fourteen. Note to my kids: Please remember, when you see in me in the corner of the nursing home that you put me in after you found me walking down the street wearing nothing but a beat-up old Police concert T-shirt, with my ear buds on, plugged into a potato, mumbling something about my light-cone needing to be fixed so I can visit with the other versions of me that exist in the multiverse, that I'm still me. It's just that I found a cooler place to hang out until this damn body is taken away and my mind can roam free.

255 There's not a night that goes by when I don't say a prayer that the legal stuff gets cleared up and we can once again hear that first S roll off the tongues of Les McKeown and the boys as they kick it, Scottish style, on a "S-A-T-U-R-D-A-Y Night!"

256 I. Duvdevany, R. Yahav, and V. Moin, School of Social Work, University of Haifa, Israel, ilana@research.haifa, "Children's feelings toward parents in the context of parental disability," *International Journal of Rehabilitation Research* 28, no. 3 (September 2005): 259–62.

Twenty-first

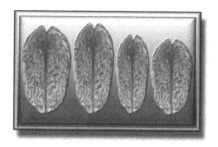

Family and MS from the Other Side of the Desk

This chapter is written by my wife, my daughter, and my son. It's about what it's like to have a person with MS in their lives. Their pieces are unexpurgated.

Several years ago, when I was trying to come up with how to put this chapter together, I was sitting in my living room while my kids were running around.

I asked my son what he thought about me having MS. "Awesome," he answered and then bounced a balloon off my face and ran into the kitchen to get another brownie. He was an eight-year-old boy.

I asked my daughter the same thing. She said she had to think about it. She eventually came back and said, "It's neat." I asked her why, and she said, "Because I get to see what it's like to have MS." She also said that she thinks it's difficult to have MS because even though I look like other people, I sometimes act differently. She had noticed that I get annoyed with people in certain situations when Mommy does not. She was an eleven-year-old girl.

When I asked my wife what she thought about me having MS, she, like my daughter, said she had to think about it. She eventually wrote the two pieces that follow.

I include a piece at the end about the effect that my parents had on me when I was first diagnosed with MS.

WHAT IT'S LIKE LIVING WITH A HUSBAND WITH MS

BY LAUREN G. MACALUSO

PART I

He made me laugh and feel like I was the most wonderful girl on campus within minutes of meeting him. We started walking from ecology to education class together at Cornell. He was funny, handsome, smart, and a gentleman. In a sea of guys drinking and acting like idiots, he was different. He wasn't intimidated that I was premed and focused. He was proud that I was captain of the field hockey team, and he was often the only male, student fan at our weeknight games at Schoelkopf Stadium. It was freezing in Ithaca as the fall athletic season came to an end, yet Vin would be out there with his genetics textbook, cheering me on.

He wrote me a letter when he first got up the nerve to ask me out. He wrote me letters through medical school, as I was in Philadelphia and he in Washington, DC. They were true pieces of art—funny, romantic, occasionally he'd draw a cartoon or picture. I've saved every one of them and recently I read them all again and remembered how wonderful it felt to receive them. I quickly knew at the age of twenty-one what an amazing and special man I was dating. And then he was diagnosed with MS.

I listened intently during the lecture we received on MS during our neurology class in medical school. There weren't many treatments out. We weren't sure exactly what caused it, and we weren't sure how to predict patient outcomes. Yet what I knew was how outstanding my boyfriend was. I knew he was the person I wanted to spend the rest of my life with. We spent most days of our senior year of college together. We studied, laughed, cooked, jogged, and eventually traveled cross-country. I loved every minute of it. I loved him, and I wasn't willing to let MS put an end to that.

There was a moment at our wedding reception when we stopped for a brief moment on the dance floor, and I looked into his eyes and knew this is the path I was meant to take. This is my amazing partner, and I am fortunate to have found him.

Medical school, residency, and our first jobs raced by quickly. We started our family and are fortunate to have our daughter and son. Our children have the same coloring and body build as Vin and I do. When the children were young, we were once stopped by a woman in Manhattan. She said, "Wow, I've never seen people clone themselves the way you have!" Vin quipped that he had been doing a lot of experiments in his lab in the basement, and it seemed to have worked. We both have our own medical practices now, and life is busy, fulfilling, and sometimes overwhelming.

Some days the overwhelming aspect wins. Some days I feel that Vincent is stubborn and set in his ways. Some days I feel that he's being short tempered with the kids. Some days I worry that he's pushing himself too hard and not taking care of himself enough.

Occasionally my thoughts travel to the place of what if his MS worsens. What if his rate of progression speeds up? I remind myself, as Vincent's dad liked to say, I can't worry about the "what-ifs." I have to appreciate every day. I have to be thankful that we are healthy, have two amazing kids, get to help others each day, and have each other.

We share our office space, so I get to see, hear, and feel the care Vin gives his patients. It's wonderful to watch the difference he can make in patients' and their families' lives dealing with MS. I get to hear him speak at conferences and feel proud as he presents MS from a doctor and patient perspective with amazing warmth and humor.

I am blessed. I have learned life has many challenges and sometimes it can feel overwhelming. But I am married to a man who has always been there to face these challenges together. MS is a part of Vincent's life and thus my life, but he has chosen to utilize his talents and help others. And I have chosen to be with a man who I respect and love.

Part II

He sarcastically makes fun of me and others in front of people, which makes me uncomfortable.

He needs to be right. If someone disagrees with him and expresses themselves, he talks over him or her.

He shares personal matters about himself and our family with groups of people in social settings, which makes me uncomfortable.

He needs to go to sleep and separate himself from me and our children very early many nights.

He is frequently at the office on off hours and not with the children and me.

He does not always listen closely to what I ask him to do for the kids and then needs to call me to clarify when I'm working or busy. Then he acts angry when I answer him quickly while I'm in the middle of something.

He can be erratic, funny, and caring one minute and then short and frustrating the next.

HAVING A FATHER WITH MS

BY ABIGAIL MACALUSO, AGE FOURTEEN

Having a father with MS is no different to me than having one without. I treat him the same way I treat my mom, who does not have MS. Sometimes it's difficult to get him to understand what I'm feeling, but then again, he has never been a fourteen-year-old girl. This is when I turn to my mom for help, who has been around him for almost twice as long as I have. She tells me that I have to explain to him what I am feeling, and this helps me to learn how to express myself; I have to learn that he cannot read my mind or infer what's wrong. When I'm lazy and someone is in another room that I have to talk to, I shout to them. This may seem simple, and you probably do it in your own home too, but it hurts my dad. See, I don't know all the scientific stuff of why and how this hurts him, but all I know is that it does and I'm not supposed to do it. Like all other children, my brother and I, we still shout because it doesn't hurt us. My brother hasn't changed this habit as much as me, because it doesn't hurt us. So why would it hurt my dad? Since I'm older than my brother and have developed my frontal lobes more than he has, I don't do it anymore; or at least when I do, it doesn't hurt him, but my brother still does. When the loud noise hurts him, he gets upset—a lot quicker than others. He starts to get angry. He doesn't know how to explain what he's feeling, like I do, except to say that it hurts. He asks my brother, Vincent, to stop shouting, and when he doesn't, he then asks why Vincent still does it even though he knows it hurts him.

My mom, again, tries to help. She does this through talking things out with Vincent and my dad separately and then bringing them together to talk things out. Sometimes this works, and sometimes it doesn't. In the end, the best medicine is laughter. When I say this, I'm talking about my dad and how he's funny. Sometimes, when things are just not working out and we all come together to have dinner, we flip out on each other for no apparent reason. That's when my dad saves the day.

My dad will say something, and it changes the whole mood. My mom and I give each other a look, saying how he could come up with that when a second ago everything was spiraling down the drain and how he's insane. I'm thankful to him for this. That is one of the best things about him.

He also has an extremely good memory, which allows him to do sentimental things. For example, I go to Buckley Country Day School and am in eighth grade. I'm graduating this year. Buckley was where my dad also went for part of elementary and all of middle school. In eighth grade, we make speeches about our time in school. My speech was about the wonderful teachers that we both have had during our times at Buckley. My dad told me about some of the wonderful teachers that he had there. Without those descriptive memories, I could never have had as great of a speech as I did. My dad is speaking at our graduation. That should be filled with memories. And jokes.

> Thank you, Dad, for making life eventful.
> Thank you, Dad, for teaching me.
> Thank you, Dad, for being you.
> I love you.

MY DAD

BY VINCENT P. MACALUSO, AGE ELEVEN

I love it when Dad takes me outside and he catches while I pitch to him. I find it interesting that when my dad throws normally, he throws curve balls even though he doesn't mean to do it. It's just his way of throwing. I think it might have to do with MS.

One time my dad came into my class to read. He read a book that he wrote about me. The story was called *Diary of the Father of a Fourth-Grade Someone*. It was about him waking me up while I was dreaming about striking out Babe Ruth. The Babe was brought back to life with chewing gum and a computer. At the end of the book, my dad leaned down, gave me a big hug, and said, "I love you."

I don't like it when my dad has to leave on a trip to do a talk about MS because I miss him. He has to leave because he has to do his job. His job is when he speaks about MS to patients and their families. I think that it's important to those people so MS doesn't destroy their lives. Knowing this makes me feel less sad.

I really hate it when he doesn't let me pitch to him or play on his computer or iPhone. Sometimes he has to do his work. I like it better when my dad is not writing so I can spend time with him. But I understand that he needs to do his job.

I don't like it when my dad wakes up at three or four in the morning to go to work because he wakes me up. Then I can't go back to sleep. I go and wake up Mom. Then Mom isn't happy because she can't go back to sleep because she has to sleep twelve hours, but she only slept nine hours. I notice that he naps a lot. I'm not sure if that's from MS or not. I get tired sometimes, but I don't have MS.

I think that all of my dad's patients are kind because they're nice to me in the office. They're nice because they think I'm cute.

I like it when he tells jokes. One time, we were eating dinner. My sister, Abby, my mom, my dad, and me were sitting at the table. Abby said something about something she did at school. My dad made a comment that Abby didn't think was funny but I did. I started laughing so hard I fell off my chair onto the floor. I didn't get hurt, but I got angry when my sister and mom started cracking up. My dad didn't laugh at me. He just threw a towel down to me and asked me to start cleaning the floor.

I think my dad is brilliant because he has MS. I think he is brilliant because he takes medicine to help him. When my dad starts the IV for his medication, I think it's a lot bloody. I ask him if it hurts when he puts the needle in. He says it stings like a little pinch, but then it goes away. Then he asks me to put the invisible thing on top of the blood-sucking tube. Sometimes he asks me to get him some water and rarely some potato chips. It's also fun because my mom thinks that I might be a good surgeon if I don't make it to the MLB. But I really want to be a baseball player in the MLB.

At night, I make my dad get in line to put me to bed. He has to go after my mom. He hugs me and says good night. Then I ask him to get water for me. So he gets water for me. Then we say I love you, and I fall asleep.

MY FAMILY AND MS

BY VINCENT F. MACALUSO

My folks were the ones who helped me get through the initial phases of getting used to a diagnosis of MS. My father was my biggest cheerleader. He would call me up whenever he ran across an article in the newspaper (usually the New York Times) about the new advances in MS. There happened to be a lot of stuff going on because I was diagnosed around the same time that the beta-interferons were being approved by the FDA. He was a businessman and always paid attention to the stock market. He would find out the manufacturers of the latest MS drug and do some research into what drugs were making it to the market. This is probably one of the best ways to learn about which drugs are coming out. Usually, on the days after the FDA has approved a drug, the drug company's stock price goes up. Likewise, if a company has to pull a drug, the price goes down. Since the price change occurs right after a drug is approved or taken off the market, the information about the drug is fresh.

My mom was the person who got me interested in medicine. She had been a registered nurse. Her mom had been a registered nurse. My mom stopped practicing as a nurse when she decided to get married and start a family with my dad. She always tried to explain to me, in age-appropriate terms, what was going on in my body. If I scraped my knee, she would explain how the clot would form and why the bruise around it would change color. She made the body logical and predictable to me. This was comforting and was a major reason I went into medicine.

When I was eventually diagnosed with MS, I think they had a tougher time with it than I did. Their perfect son suddenly had a major neurodegenerative disease! But he was supposed to be the first doctor in the family! My mom cried. I remember my dad wore dark glasses to the doctor's office when we went for follow-up. I don't know if he cried, but I knew he cared. I also knew that I needed to help them out. Heck. I was in second year of medical school and was studying about the disease in my neuroanatomy class. I really thought I should be able to figure out the thing about MS that everyone had overlooked.

Hah.

I started having trouble in medical school. My grades were going down. It felt like I couldn't concentrate and memorize like I had always been able to do. About six months after being diagnosed I started worrying about what might happen. I remember sitting with my pathology, pharmacology, and microbiology books lying open at my big, white, Swedish, big-box store desk.[257] I was feeling overwhelmed. Every time I ran my fingers over my head, another ten hairs would leap to their death onto my desk. One time, I called my folks, and they both got on the phone. I started letting them know my concerns about how things were going at school.

"What if I have to go into a wheelchair? How could I be a doctor if I'm in a wheelchair?" As I said it, I remembered that there was a guy in my med school class who was in a wheelchair, and he was doing better than I was. Then I said, "What if I go blind? I can't be a doctor if I'm blind."

That's when my dad interrupted me and said the most important thing I have ever been told in my life.

"Stop," he began. "You can't worry about the what-ifs. You have no control over them. You have control over what's going on right now. You have a pharmacology test tomorrow. Are you ready for it? If not, then study more. You have a pathology test next week? Are you ready for it? If no, then start studying after the pharmacology test. After that, you'll be coming home for Easter break, and you have only two months left before you start your rotations, and then you'll apply for your residency, and once you graduate from that, you'll be a doctor. If anything comes up with your MS, go to see your doctor. Until that time, forget about it."

He made it sound so simple.

According to his thinking, I should be a doctor in a few weeks, and then it would all be wine and roses.

Well, it took a little longer than a few weeks, but what he said still rings true today:

You cannot worry about the what-ifs.
You have no control over them.
You have control over the here and now.

THE "HERE AND NOW"

What we need to concern ourselves with is the "here and now." That's what we have control over. If we have MS and a new symptom comes up, we call our doctors and see if it should be treated. If we need to lose some weight, we need to change our diets and move our bodies more. If we say, "I'll do it tomorrow," we should remember what my daughter, who was nine years old at the time, said to me when I asked her what day is the worst day of her life.

After taking a moment to reflect, she replied.

"Tomorrow," she said.

"Why?" I asked.

"Because it never comes," she answered without a pause.

Wow.

The nine-year-old just hit it out of the park.

Tomorrow never comes.

Today is what has come.

Today is when things happen.

Sure we can plan and have goals, but we need to get things done today. Yes. There are many people and things in our lives and on our MS plates, and while we cannot get everything done today, they will eventually need to be attended to. I like to use a philosophy that Ross Perot uses. When a task needs to be done, he asks himself two questions:

1. If not me, who?
2. If not now, when?

By answering these questions, with specific answers, I then feel obligated to follow what I said. When answering the "who" question, I always make sure I answer with either me or the name of a person I trust. This way, I'm accountable to either myself or someone I can rely on to get the job done. If there's any question as to whether another person can do the job, I put the responsibility on my shoulders. When it comes to the "when" part, "now" is usually (but not always) the best answer. If the answer is not now, then I shoot for the specific time or day when I can do it ("right after church," "after I feed the dogs," "on Monday at three o'clock after flugelhorn practice is over"). I find that by making myself answer these questions in a concrete fashion, I get the task done and can move on with life.

I have been blessed.

My family is the biggest part of my life.

It is important that I respect them.

Knowing that there are people who care about me is comforting.

Knowing that there are people who need me is empowering.

I pray that you have the same.

---

[257] I think it was called the Farfeggnugenbusenhalter, but I could be wrong.

Epilogue

THE BREAKUP

Dear MS –

As I sit here writing, I am overcome with a flood of emotions. When we first met, I was like, "I didn't tell my leg to do that!" and "Is it normal for my back to tingle like that when I look down?" During that first year, people thought I was crazy — and so did I! And yes, after the doctor said I had MS, I was like, "Isn't that like-bad?" But then I thought, "I shouldn't prejudge a disease just because it has a bad reputation." Heck, my cousin had thyroid cancer and everyone was like "OMG! She's so young and she has cancer. I can't believe she is going to die of cancer!" But she had surgery and they got it out, so now she just has to go for check-ups but she's normal and she can dance and everything so I'm all "Don't prejudge a disease."

So when you showed up, you were cute with your tingling and the leg thing (that I was able to cover up by telling my friends it was a new dance move). But then one day, out of nowhere, you spring this "Now you see, now you don't" thing with my left eye. Suddenly, I'm walking into walls.

I looked like a spaz when I tried to pick up a pencil. And yes, while you did eventually give me my vision back, I didn't think of it as a funny little joke like you seemed to think it was. The color vision in my left eye still isn't as good as the right. I knew I should have listened to my mother when she said I should let my neurologist know what you had done to me. But I was just a kid and I thought I knew everything so I just let you be you and I ignored her. But now you have gone too far.

First, you started tingling me in my right toes, then foot and then the calf. Before I knew it, you had gone all the way up my leg and crossed over to the left side. I might have been able to forgive you if you stopped there but you had to push it. I'll never forget when I looked down and saw the pool of water under the dining room table and asked, "Who spilled the lemonade?" If I said I was mortified when my friend laughed as he pointed at my wet pants, I'd be lying.

I could have only wished that death would have been so gracious as to take me then.

You know MS, you're right. You don't kill. You move in, uninvited, and start doing your "thang." You hope that your unsuspecting host will ignore you (like I did). You started chipping away at my life. You took away a little bit here and there from my physical being, which sucked, but then, after awhile, I realized what the worst thing about you was. You're deceitful. While I was thinking about the fact that I couldn't see clearly or walk well, you were, ever so slowly, stealing my initiative and concentration. I didn't realize they were missing until I needed to use them. My family, friends and doctors saw me turn into a scatterbrained layabout but never said anything. My kids kept asking their mother why daddy was crying while watching a T.V. show about the Civil War. She didn't know why so she made something up. Hell, I didn't know why and I felt like a fool so I made something up. You made me lie to my own kids, you bastard!

You really have committed the perfect crime. You distract everyone with a weird assortment of physical troubles with discreet lesions while at the same time maintaining an unrelenting, covert inflammation in my brain and spinal cord – an inflammation that arrested me and stole my life. It made me unable to move even when I had the power to walk. I used to be a nice person but now sometimes I act like a jerk. I feel like an idiot! Meanwhile, the people around me can't see your demonic, noxious swelling.

Well, just because you have fooled others doesn't me you can fool me. While I fell for your game at first, I want you to know something.

It's _over_!

I've made an appointment with my neurologist and we are going to go after you with everything we've got. First, we're going to slap your autoimmune ass with some steroids. Maybe methylprednisolone. Maybe dexamethasone. I don't know. My doc and I will see which one we think will _shut you down_. It'll be our surprise gift to you. I hope you enjoy it because it will be the last gift you ever get from me. And after we knock you down, we're going to put you in a choke hold and keep you down with a platform therapy. And yeah, I know how slimy things like you can sometimes ooze out and get past the platform therapies. That's okay. I'd like you to meet some friends of mine — Nat & Tingo. What's that? They look different. Damn right they're different!

And they're going to be all over
you like a Seal Team on a terrorist
except _not as nice_!

I know you are thinking to yourself that you'll get past them as well. Go ahead. I'm ready to launch the final countdown. I have at least another dozen medical weapons in phase III trials right now. Want more? I've got fifty more in phase II. Nervous yet? No? Okay. There are another _100_ compounds that my scientist buddies are getting ready to roll out of the hangar. And yes, they are all competing to be the one to put the bullet in your _eye_!

Ya hear that, N_S_?

Yeah, it's the sound of your time running out.

I'm getting sick talking about how you're going to be exterminated.

Let's talk about me and how I'm inciting a rally in my body to make my life fantastic!

I've got physical therapy programs for stretching, strengthening, gait and balance. I've got cardiovascular fitness therapy that helps me feel and look great! The heat? Hah. My workouts are in a pool. A clear, cool pool. And to find my center, I've got yoga therapy. Oh, sorry. You're not invited because only positive energy is allowed there. Then after that I move to the mind. I've got cognitive therapies. Some are computer based that I can train on (and have fun with!) Some are with a therapist that I can speak with life about. Some I can do by myself. I can sing or dance or write or talk or shout or just sit quietly and think about how wonderful life tastes as I eat it up.

   By the way, you left some of your crap behind while you took a whirlwind tour of my brain and spinal cord. I know you don't know how to clean up your mess. That's fine. My doctors have provided me with some tools for redecorating — "CNS spackle" if you will. I'm starting some medication to help with my concentration (so I can finish the job of getting you out of my life). Then I've got some dalfampiridine to help out my legs a bit so I can get to the drug store to get my multivitamins, B-complex, zinc, vitamins C & D and fish oil.

Then after that, I'm going to the supermarket and buy my groceries. I'm sorry. I meant to say my healthy groceries. I'm going to feast on the bright colors of vegetables. I'm minimizing fats and maximizing fiber. Since I'm working out and building muscle I need my protein which I am getting from chicken, fish and beans. And yes, I might have a lean, succulent piece of red meat once in awhile to celebrate victory over you. My fallen enemy.

Then again, I could go vegan for awhile
– just to piss you off!

And you know what? Now that we're through, I'm back on the market and I'm looking for someone who makes me tingle and stimulates me in ways you never could. I'm looking for someone who loves me for who I am and who is not going to try and change me (the way you forced me to change). My next relationship is going to be one where we help each other to grow. And we are going to exercise together and eat together and swim and laugh together.

And if the mood is right…

and the relationship is ready…

we're gonna do it.

a lot!

And it's gonna be goooooood....

Then we're gonna have a cool drink of crystal clear water.

And then we're gonna do it *again*.

Because it makes us feel alive!

And that, M.F., is a life you cannot take away from me or any of my friends.

Go ahead.

Try.

I dare you.

You have no idea of the Armageddon you are about to face.

Yours—for never more—

Vince

Conclusion

- MS is demyelination of the axons of nerves in the CNS caused by the immune system, possibly prompted by a combination of certain genes in the person and an environmental factor.
- Nerves work best in a narrow range of both temperature and pressure.
- The influx of immune cells to the CNS in MS causes an elevation in interstitial pressure, akin to a twisted ankle.
- Unlike a swollen ankle, the brain is enclosed in a noncompliant box (the skull).
- The elevated pressure in the CNS in people with MS produces a reversible frontal lobe dysfunction that takes away the MSer's initiative, ability to concentrate, and emotional control.
- The imaging modality that best reflects the diffuse lesion that causes the MS ICE is computer-based neurocognitive testing.
- The inflammatory frontal lobe dysfunction that occurs in MS can be reversed by therapies that prevent inflammatory cells from entering the CNS and by therapies that can reduce inflammation.
- Using a term like the MS ICE (initiative, concentration, emotions) allows patients to better define what they're feeling to a medical professional.
- Using the term MS ICE enables a medical professional to institute therapy(ies) that can greatly improve the life of the MSer and the people around him or her.
- People with MS have better long-term outcomes the sooner they get on a disease-modifying therapy than those who do not.
- MRIs are macroscopic pictures. MS is a microscopic disease. The vast majority of disease activity in MS cannot be seen on an MRI.
- Terms like secondary-progressive or chronic-progressive only create confusion.
- Applying terms like secondary-progressive or chronic-progressive to an individual does nothing more than create excuses for some payers not to pay for medications that actually do help people no matter how long they've had MS or what physical condition they're in.

- Just because a person with MS has to use a wheelchair doesn't mean that he or she still doesn't have relapses.
- Primary progressive MS is a direct attack by immune cells on both myelin and the neuron. This is not MS. The nomenclature should be changed to reflect this.
- Pubmed (http://www.ncbi.nlm.nih.gov/pubmed/) is one of the most reliable places to get valid, peer-reviewed, published, unbiased data when investigating medical topics.
- If you're looking to get involved with a trial for MS therapies, www.clinicaltrials.gov is the place to go. This is the site where FDA-sanctioned drug and therapy trials are listed.
- Relapse = exacerbation = flare up
- MRIs use the 40–50 MHz range of the electromagnetic spectrum. These are radio frequencies that are used in shortwave radio and in police, fire, and highway radio communications. This is different from X-ray frequencies.
- The human sexual response cycle consists of five stages: desire, excitement, plateau, orgasm, and resolution. The stages must occur in sequence.
- The desire stage is facilitated by testosterone, estrogen, progesterone, dopamine, and norepinephrine.
- The desire stage is inhibited by prolactin, serotonin, opioids, and cannabinoids.
- MS caregivers are wonderful people.
- MS caregiving goes both ways.
- Use of ACTH (adrenocorticotropic hormone) or melanocortin receptor agonists might be a useful course for researchers to pursue in helping to improve the quality of life for people who have MS.

About the Author

Vincent F. Macaluso was born to Vincent and Peggy Macaluso in 1968 at North Shore University Hospital in Manhasset, New York. He grew up in Douglaston, New York (where he lives today with his wife and two children). As a child, he played Little League baseball and tennis and did well in school. He watched a lot of PBS television (*Monty Python's Flying Circus*, Carl Sagan's *Cosmos*, David Attenborough's *Life On Earth*, *The Casebook of Sherlock Holmes* on Mystery! with Vincent Price). At his grammar school (Buckley Country Day School), his math teacher, Ms. Salit, started teaching Vincent and some other students about flow charts, probability, and binary numbers. The following year, the school obtained two PET computers. The computers had 1 megahertz MOS processors, 32 K RAM, a monochrome (green) monitor with black background, 80 x 25 text resolution, and an external cassette tape drive on which the students could save their work. The machines each had dual sound systems. This meant that if you made a mistake when typing code, the computer would go "beep." The "dual" part was a switch you could slide to the off position when you got sick of hearing the beep every time your code syntax was wrong. The OS was basic. Vincent thought it was pretty awesome.

One day, Ms. Salit had the students write a program that would add up all the numbers from one to one hundred, inclusive. After typing "Run," the cursor on the screen went away for about two seconds, and then the answer "5050" appeared. When asked why the cursor had disappeared, his teacher said that the computer was "thinking," and it took some time to add up all of the numbers. That summer, Vincent asked a computer-geek friend to add up all the numbers between one and one hundred. After about a second, he answered, "Five thousand fifty." Vincent was stunned. When asked, his friend explained that if you add one to ninety-nine and two to ninety-eight and three to ninety-seven and so on, each answer gives you one hundred. You can do that forty-nine times, all the way up to 49 + 51. The product of those numbers, 100 x 49, equals 4900. Then you can add on the unpaired numbers, fifty and one hundred—5050. That was the last time he would remember seeing a computer work slower than a brain.

At the age of fourteen, he got his first computer—an Apple //e. After spending many hours programming one summer day, his mother shouted down to him in the basement, "Get out of the house and move around and get some exercise! I don't want you to be one of those kids who sit inside all day and don't play and have fun like everyone else!" Ironically, he was writing a program to keep the stats for the kids in town with whom he played softball. Regardless, he listened to his mother and realized that there should be balance in his life.

For secondary school, he attended Regis High School in Manhattan. He continued to learn Latin and French and science as he had in grammar school, but things were different. He had several major awakenings. His classes were challenging, and his teachers made him take advantage of the incredibly stimulating environment around the school and throughout the city. He had an intense American history course, driven by a passionate teacher (Mr. Sabatelli) who wanted to know what his students were thinking. He challenged them to find the primary resources for their papers (usually at the NYC Public Library in midtown) and then use their own minds to figure out what the author was saying. In his English class with Mr. DiMichele, he kept several journals. It was then that he discovered the wonderful world of writing satire. He had also decided to start taking Greek because he thought it sounded interesting. It was not until years later, however, when he was in college, and subsequently medical school, that he understood the importance of having learned Latin and Greek. He found that by knowing where a word came from, he could more specifically express his thoughts. Additionally, he learned these languages from teachers who showed their students the mentality of the people who developed the language. Fr. Kelly's voice rings in his mind, extolling the dualism of ancient Greeks—"The grammatical use of μεν (men) and δε (de) means 'On the one hand and on the other hand.' Gentlemen, there is a balance in the world. ξένος (xenos) means both 'stranger' and 'friend.' Shouldn't we regard all the strangers in our lives as potential friends?"

Throughout his time at Regis, Vincent found that the educational environment created by the Jesuits had fostered a desire to learn. They encouraged thinking that allowed his mind to grow, while at the same time framing his development with an empowering theme of being "a man for others." Theology, like the other classes at Regis, was presented in a fashion more Socratic than dogmatic. During one class, after Mr. Hannon told the students to get comfortable and close their eyes, he read a passage from the Bible where Jesus multiplied the loaves and fishes. At the end, when Jesus went off to pray, he asked the students to put themselves into the passage. He then asked them to think about what Jesus prayed about after feeding the masses. Vincent was initially overcome by the concept of being asked not to think like a messiah but to be and think as the messiah. The nicest part of the exercise was that nobody was right or wrong. The students were allowed to let their thoughts and feelings flow in the light of doing good for others.

While he would eventually go to college at Cornell University (where he met his bride-to-be, Lauren) followed by medical school and neurology residency at Georgetown, he would look back on his times at Buckley and Regis as the moments that gave him a solid foundation for the rest of his life.

It was near the end of his first year in medical school, when he was studying for his neuroanatomy final, that he had the onset of double vision. After school got out, he went to see his ophthalmologist, who, after evaluating him, sent him to a neuro-ophthalmologist, who in turn sent him for an MRI of the brain. The MRI showed lesions. He was told that he should go on with medical school but he probably should go into a medical, rather than surgical, area of medicine. That summer, he just took it easy since he had been granted the job of being editor of the medical school newspaper, *The Scope*. He spent more of his time working on the newspaper than he did studying. He found that he was having more trouble reading and remembering material than he had during college—although he had been having some trouble with his grades toward the end of college as well. He started a humor column (following the style of his favorite author at the time, Dave Barry) called *From Under the Editor's Desk*. Early in the year, he went and spoke with one of the three medical school deans, Jon J. O'Brien, SJ, DO. They spoke and eventually became good friends. Vincent often remarks that Fr. O'Brien was the kindest, most altruistic and intelligent person that he has ever had the pleasure of knowing.

At the start of his second semester of third year in medical school, he decided to propose marriage to his girlfriend, Lauren. He decided to write a book to ask her to marry him. At the time, his grandfather, Vincent Macaluso, who immigrated to America from Italy in 1921, was very ill with prostate cancer. Vincent would fly home most weekends to spend time with his grandfather and family. During his free moments, he would return to the basement where his Apple //e was and write. Over the course of the next eight weeks, he would finish his first book, *Diadochokinesia*. It was about a medical student, Frankie, who was trying to figure out how to ask his girlfriend, Laurae, to marry him. The text made up about sixty pages of the book. During his time as editor of *The Scope*, Vincent had gotten to know the people where the paper was printed up. When he gave them the text of the book to be printed out, he asked them to put in two hundred blank pages at the end. The cover had the name of the book and the author's pseudonym, Francis D. Scrittore ("Francis" is Vincent's middle name, and "scrittore" is Italian for "writer").

When he got the finished book, he took it back to his basement apartment in Burleith (just north of the Georgetown campus). Several weeks earlier, he and his aunt, Ann Macaluso, had gone to the jewelry store of the father of one of his friends from high school, Fred Erker. There, they had bought the engagement ring. The ring was to be mailed down to Vincent in DC. Each day that week, he would race home from his classes to see if the ring had arrived. Each day, Vincent would ask the pleasant, slightly rotund letter carrier if she had a package for him. After several days, the letter carrier asked what the package was so she could make sure it had not been misplaced at the post office. He told her that it was an engagement ring. She said she would keep an eye out for it.

The next day, while waiting on the front stoop, he saw the letter carrier moving as quickly as she could up the street while waving something in her hand, over her head. She handed him the small box, and he saw the return address was the jewelry store. He gave her a hug, thanked her profusely, and took it back into his apartment. There he sat for hours and tried to figure out how exactly he was going to get the ring and the book into her hands. After ordering and eating some Chinese food while watching a few Thursday-night funny shows on TV, he went to work on the book. For the next five hours, using a sharp utility knife, several pieces of ribbon, some heavy-gauge paper, and rubber cement, he began to set the stage for the final scene in the life of Vincent Macaluso, Single Guy. Working from the back page of the book, he carefully carved a one-inch square box through the two hundred blank, white pages, stopping before getting to the last page of text in the book. After making sure the ring fit, he glued a piece of thin ribbon to the inside of the white paper box. He then lined the four sides and the back of the box with pieces of heavy-gauge paper. The ribbon stuck out through a slit cut in the piece of heavy-gauge paper attached to the back of the box. He tied the ring on the ribbon. Using a larger piece of heavy paper, he covered the box and glued it down with rubber cement, leaving a tab of red ribbon hanging out the top so that it could be pulled down to open the box and reveal the ring. Around the box, he wrote, "Lauren, will you marry me? I love you now, forever, and a day ..."

By that time, it was about three in the morning. Now Vincent had to figure out how to get the book with the ring in it into Lauren's hands. He realized that he had to make it such that a person could not open the book if they picked it up before Lauren got to it. He figured he could get it shrink-wrapped somewhere, but it was the middle of the night and most normal people were asleep. Then he remembered that he had some indoor window film insulation that he had used on the basement window-well windows of his walk-down apartment. He wrapped the book with the film and used a hot blow dryer to shrink the film and make the book secure. It looked good. It was now 4:30 a.m. Vincent had to be at the hospital for rounds at seven. He went to bed.

Lauren was to come down later that day to visit for the weekend. After rounds in the hospital, Vincent went to the undergraduate bookstore on campus and arranged a scheme with one of the cashiers. He showed her the book he had written to ask Lauren to marry him. He told her a friend of his would plant it in the store that afternoon. He would bring Lauren to the store and get her to see it, and they would bring it up to be purchased. The cashier was excited to be part of the plot, so she ripped a barcode tag off of a biology textbook and put it on the back of the shrink-wrapped book. He took the book with him back to the hospital and asked a friend of his, John, if he could plant the book in the humor section in the undergrad bookstore at three o'clock and stay with it until Lauren and he got there. He said sure. He was told that the book held an engagement ring. After John congratulated him, Vincent went on to tell him that Lauren knew him by his name but not by face, so he would have to introduce the two of them using a different name. He told John that he would call him Jim Kirk, in honor of the famous Enterprise captain. He said sure and then added that Vincent couldn't be late because he had a softball game to get to at 3:15.

Right, Vincent thought to himself.

At 2:30 p.m., Vincent went to the medical school bookstore to wait for Lauren. He was sweating profusely. He was about to take the greatest leap of his life. If she said yes, then he was about to enter into an entirely new dimension. He would no longer be just "him." It would be "Vincent and Lauren." He knew that he wanted to be with her forever, but he didn't know how much of "him" he would lose in the endeavor. Then he thought about the fact that she was facing the same challenge. *It will all balance out,* he thought. *Men ... and de ...*

At 2:45 p.m., Lauren came walking down the hallway with her book bag slung over her left shoulder. Vincent got up. They exchanged a perfunctory kiss before he explained to her that they had to go over to the undergraduate bookstore because the med school book store didn't have the type of notebook that he liked to use for note taking. She said sure, and they started to walk.

It was then that Lauren asked Vincent if he knew what day it was.

Time slowed down. His heart stopped. The hairs on the back of his head bristled. How could she have found out? No one knew about this except him and the cashier and John. He did the only thing he could think to do. Play dumb. When he told her that he didn't know what day it was, she said it was their anniversary ... which really confused him. When asked which anniversary she was talking about, she reminded him that they had taken the medical college admissions test four years ago that day. Vincent began to breathe again. Then he replied that he knew that it was their anniversary and had already made reservations at a restaurant. He was glad that he had made reservations to celebrate their upcoming engagement, he thought as they continued walking to the bookstore.

Once inside, Vincent made a beeline for the notebook area. Lauren followed. He looked at the assortment and then told Lauren that they didn't have the notebook he needed either. As he led her circuitously out of the bookstore, he saw his accomplice out of the corner of his eye. It was coming together. He told Lauren that he saw a friend of his that he wanted her to meet. They walked over. Vincent put out his hand to shake and said hi to Jim Kirk. He then went on to introduce Lauren. After some small talk, "Jim" mentioned that a girl in their class had just read a book about two medical students who were boyfriend and girlfriend. He started looking back and forth among the books and then pulled out the book Vincent had given to him. Jim handed it to Lauren. She looked at it and flipped it over. Vincent had written $3.29 as the price under the barcode that the cashier had put on the book. Vincent looked at Lauren and said $3.29 was pretty cheap. He wondered if she realized that 3/29 was also his birthday. They decided to buy it.

After saying good-bye to Accomplice #1, they walked toward the checkout area. There were two registers open. The one with the cashier who he had spoken with that morning had a somewhat disheveled, undergraduate student in line, buying a book. The other register was open. Vincent walked directly up behind the student, acting as if he hadn't seen the other register. Immediately, he noticed the student's low-slung jeans and a strong fragrance of last night on the student. He then heard the student start to tell the cashier that he didn't have enough money to pay for the book that he needed. Vincent looked at him and then at Accomplice #2 and then back at the student. Vincent knew that Lauren had seen that the next register was wide open and that she was going to tell Vincent that they should just use the open one. He knew he had come too far and was too close to pulling of the greatest event of his young life to have it blown to bits because a college kid didn't have enough money to buy a copy of Strunk & White.

Vincent asked the student how much money he needed. The kid turned to look at him. It was several seconds later that the question made it to his brain and he was able to formulate an answer. Eventually, he was able to express the concept that the amount was somewhere between two and three dollars, but he wasn't sure. Vincent pulled a five-dollar bill out of his wallet and handed it to the student, emphasizing the concept that the faster that he paid, the better it would be for everybody. The register lady quietly smiled as the college student started proclaiming how such a kind deed was not only noble but had in fact restored his faith in humanity. He started to look for a pencil and some paper to copy Vincent's address down so he could pay him back, but Vincent assured him that the restoration-of-faith-in-humanity-thing was payback enough.

After the transaction was completed, Vincent turned to look at Lauren, who was looking at the checkout display of pencils that had fuzzy hair and googley eyes at the eraser end. Vincent then placed the book on the counter and gave a knowing wink to Accomplice #2. She picked up the book and scanned it; $22.50 showed on the screen above the register. Vincent quickly looked at Lauren. She was spinning one of the fuzzy pencils fast between her hands to make the green hairs splay out sideways. He looked back and saw his accomplice had voided the sale. She told Vincent the price, and he handed her the other five-dollar bill in his wallet. He realized that if Humanity-boy had been a bio major, things might not be going as smoothly as they were. The register lady handed Vincent his change. She then put the book in a bag and handed it to Vincent. He smiled at her and hoped that good things would forever come her way for the crucial role she played in the play he had written. He walked in front of Lauren out of the bookstore. It was a beautiful day, and he recommended they go up to the roof of the student union building. There they could lie in the grass while he did some reading for his medicine rotation and Lauren could whatever reading she wanted to do.

They walked up the stairs to the roof and found a grassy hill under some trees to read. Vincent took out his medical text and went to where he had left off previously. Diabetic ketoacidosis was the topic. He was lying on his stomach with his head facing away from where Lauren had sat down. He could hear her taking the plastic wrap off of the book. He stared at the same line over and over again about ketoacidosis, but his entire focus was on what his ears were picking up. The countdown had begun. Unfortunately, he could not see the clock. He knew she was a fast reader, and the text was widely spaced. Suddenly, he heard her remark that the story sounded a lot like their relationship. He kept looking at his textbook and waved his hand in her direction, letting her know that he eventually wanted to read it and that he didn't want her to give it away.

Vincent went inside of himself transiently and realized that he was in a free fall. He thought about her. He knew he loved Lauren. He had decided to propose marriage after a phone call he had received from a female voice who said that Karen and Dom and Missy and Jim and Paula and Donny were all going to be getting married after med school was over, and they had all put down deposits for their reception halls already, and places were getting booked up quickly, and that her parents were not going to put down a deposit for a reception hall until she had gotten engaged, but that she could not speak for long because she had to go to a pathology review class, and then she hung up. After she had hung up, he sat down on his bed with the phone receiver still in his hand. He was not 100 percent but was really quite, almost positively certain that it had been Lauren who had called and implied that Vincent had to propose to her soon ...

He heard papers rustling as if someone were quietly fighting with a book. When Vincent turned around, he saw Lauren holding the back of the book open. She had a happy but frustrated look on her face as her trembling fingers tried to free the ring from the ribbon. Vincent sat up and moved next to her. After asking if she would like some help, she gave him the book. He took the book and, remembering how he had put it together only hours before, was able to release the gem. He then put the book down, picked up Lauren's hand, and then asked the question that led to his second book.

When Lauren was pregnant with their first child, Vincent had a story channeled to him from his daughter-to-be, Abby, while she was in utero. It was called *A Womb with a View* and described how, at the moment of conception, a life has all the knowledge it needs but loses it as it takes human form so that by the time a person is ready to be born, everything must be learned again. When his daughter was eight, he wrote a children's book, *Daddy, what does my brain do?* In it, he teaches his daughter that everything that she sees, tastes, hears, touches, and smells is eventually sent to her brain to make the person that she is.

Several years later, once his son, Vincent, was in grade school, he wrote another book. This one had his son pitching for the Potatoes, an expansion team from Idaho that had made it to the World Series. The Potatoes were up 4,002–0 over the Yanks. Vincent had a perfect game going. All he had to do was strike out the last batter, Babe Ruth, who had been brought back to life using a computer and some chewing gum. Unfortunately, his father wakes him up to take him to school. At school, Vincent reads a story about his son, who's pitching a shutout and that he just has to strike out Babe Ruth, who was brought back to life using a computer and some chewing gum …

In the course of the completion of this, his first published work, he has discovered much about himself and how much he loves making people feel better—both through medicine and humor. He currently practices adult neurology in New Hyde Park, New York. Over the past sixteen years, he has done shows around the country with patients, doctors, and just about anyone who wants to learn about multiple sclerosis. He gets honoraria for his speaking, which he uses to fund his practice. He calls them shows because he believes people can get more out of a program that deals with an important topic while feeling happy and comfortable. In order to keep people at ease while at a program about multiple sclerosis, he breaks the ice with humor. And after breaking the ice, he puts it in a glass, adds four parts processed knowledge, three parts descriptive movies, two parts family photos, fourteen parts clean humor, an aliquot of refined words, several shots of sarcasm, a scoop of enthusiasm, a heap of caring, and a little pink umbrella. The elixir he makes is educational, good for you, and warms your tummy as it goes down. After performing over five hundred shows, the self dubbed comedicaledian has proven, time and again, that laughter truly is the best medicine.

Unless, of course, you're bleeding internally.

Then you really should go to the emergency room.

Index

R

S

W

Y

Z

Printed in the United States
By Bookmasters